MANUAL of SMALL ANIMAL CARDIOLOGY

MANUAL of SMALL ANIMAL CARDIOLOGY

Larry Patrick Tilley, D.V.M.

Diplomate
American College of Veterinary Internal Medicine
(Internal Medicine)
Staff Consultant, Department of Medicine (Cardiology)
The Animal Medical Center
New York
President, Cardiopet, Inc.
Roslyn, New York

Jerry M. Owens, D.V.M.

Diplomate
American College of Veterinary Radiology
Specialty Referral Practice
Berkeley, California

CHURCHILL LIVINGSTONE
New York, Edinburgh, London, and Melbourne 1985

Acquisitions editor: *Gene C. Kearn*
Copy editor: *Ann Ruzycka*
Production editor: *Michiko Davis*
Production supervisor: *Joe Sita*
Compositor: *Eastern Graphics*
Printer/Binder: *The Maple-Vail Book Manufacturing Group*

Distributed in the United Kingdom by Churchill Livingstone, Robert Stevenson House, 1-3 Baxter's Place, Leith Walk, Edinburgh EH1 3AF and by associated companies, branches and representatives throughout the world.

First published 1985

Printed in U.S.A.

ISBN 0-443-08312-6

9876543

Library of Congress Cataloging in Publication Data
Main entry under title:

Manual of small animal cardiology.

Includes bibliographies and index.
1. Dogs—Diseases. 2. Cats—Diseases. 3. Veterinary cardiology. I. Tilley, Larry Patrick. II. Owens, Jerry M. III. Title: Small animal cardiology.
[DNLM: 1. Cat Diseases. 2. Dog Diseases. 3. Heart Diseases—veterinary. SF 811 M294]
SF992.C37M36 1985 636.7'089612 85-6681
ISBN 0-443-08312-6

Manufactured in the United States of America

To our parents, Dr. and Mrs. Daniel E. Owens and Mrs. Pat Tilley,

and to Geraldine Owens and Jeri Leeds,

without whose inspiration, teaching, and love

our dreams would never have been realized

CONTRIBUTORS

Timothy Bauer, D.V.M.
Lecturer, Department of Medicine, Division of Animal Medicine, University of Washington School of Medicine, Seattle, Washington

Betsy R. Bond, D.V.M.
Diplomate, American College of Veterinary Internal Medicine (Cardiology), Staff Cardiologist, The Animal Medical Center, New York, New York

Clay A. Calvert, D.V.M.
Diplomate, American College of Veterinary Internal Medicine (Internal Medicine), Associate Professor, Department of Small Animal Medicine, University of Georgia, College of Veterinary Medicine, Athens, Georgia

Philip R. Fox, D.V.M., M.S.
Diplomate, American College of Veterinary Internal Medicine (Cardiology), Staff Cardiologist, Director of Clinics, The Animal Medical Center, New York, New York

Rebecca E. Gompf, D.V.M., M.S.
Diplomate, American College of Veterinary Internal Medicine (Cardiology), Associate Professor of Cardiology, Department of Urban Practice, The University of Tennessee, School of Veterinary Medicine, Knoxville, Tennessee

Charla L. Jones, D.V.M., M.S.
Diplomate, American College of Veterinary Internal Medicine (Cardiology), Assistant Professor of Medicine/Cardiology, Department of Companion Animal and Special Species Medicine, North Carolina State University, School of Veterinary Medicine, Raleigh, North Carolina

Mark D. Kittleson, D.V.M., Ph.D.
Diplomate, American College of Veterinary Internal Medicine (Cardiol-

ogy), Assistant Professor, Department of Veterinary Medicine, University of California, Davis, California

Christophe W. Lombard, Dr. Med. Vet.
Diplomate, American College of Veterinary Internal Medicine (Cardiology), Associate Professor of Medicine, Department of Medical Science, College of Veterinary Medicine, University of Florida, Gainesville, Florida

Michael S. Miller, M.S., V.M.D.
Vice President, Clinical Affairs, Cardiopet, Inc., Roslyn; Staff Consultant, Electrocardiography, Staff Clinician, A & A Veterinary Hospital, Franklin Square, New York

Jerry M. Owens, D.V.M.
Diplomate, American College of Veterinary Radiology, Specialty Referral Practice, Berkeley, California

A. Kim Saal, M.D.
Assistant Professor, Department of Medicine, Division of Cardiology, University of Washington; Director, Echocardiography Laboratory, Harborview Medical Center, Seattle, Washington

Glen L. Spaulding, D.V.M.
Diplomate, American College of Veterinary Internal Medicine (Internal Medicine), Director, Laboratory Animal Medicine, Tufts-New England Medical Center; Hospital Veterinarian, Massachusetts General Hospital; Clinical Assistant Professor, Tufts University School of Veterinary Medicine, Boston, Massachusetts

Larry Patrick Tilley, D.V.M.
Diplomate, American College of Veterinary Internal Medicine (Internal Medicine), Staff Consultant, Department of Medicine (Cardiology), The Animal Medical Center, New York; President, Cardiopet, Inc., Roslyn, New York

Wayne E. Wingfield, D.V.M.
Diplomate, American College of Veterinary Surgeons, Professor of Medicine and Chief, Emergency Medicine and Intensive Care, Department of Clinical Sciences, Colorado State University, College of Veterinary Medicine and Biomedical Sciences, Fort Collins, Colorado

PREFACE

In the last decade there have been a number of excellent textbook chapters and journal articles describing new findings in the field of canine and feline cardiology. However, for the practicing veterinarian and veterinary student who are new in the field, the amount of information is overwhelming. The *Manual of Small Animal Cardiology* has been written to meet the need for a textbook that provides useful and practical information on cardiac disease in the dog and cat. This practical approach to the diagnosis and therapy of cardiac disease will be useful to a wide audience, from the veterinary student to the fully trained cardiologist. The approach is largely clinical, and includes the practical as well as the most sophisticated methods for diagnosis and therapy.

Cardiovascular disorders in the dog and cat represent a substantial portion of diseases seen in the average veterinary practice. It is important for veterinary students and practitioners to understand the principles of diagnosis and treatment of the numerous cardiovascular disorders.

The basic examination of a dog or cat with a suspected cardiovascular disorder still consists of obtaining a history and performing a physical examination, routine electrocardiography, and thoracic radiography. More advanced procedures may be indicated in certain situations. For example, in radiography, we can now utilize fluoroscopy, cardiac catheterization, and angiocardiography. In electrocardiography, continuous (Holter) electrocardiographic monitoring and His bundle recordings are now available. Echocardiography is becoming a very important noninvasive diagnostic method in veterinary medicine.

The format of this manual should be beneficial to cardiologists as well as to busy veterinarians who are not specializing in cardiology. The book is in outline form to help the reader review at a glance the facts needed. The manual is not designed as an atlas of cardiology, so only pertinent reproductions, including electrocardiograms, thoracic radiographs, and pressure curves, are used.

The methods of diagnosis of heart disease in the dog and cat are described in Section I. The first four chapters follow the sequence that the veterinarian uses in his approach to the patient. Chapter 1 covers the history and physical examination; Chapter 2, the radiologic examination of the heart; Chapter 3, electrocardiography; and Chapter 4, special diagnostic techniques, including angiocardiography, phonocardiography, and echocardiography.

Section II presents a description of the various cardiac disorders that occur in the dog and cat in a step-by-step fashion, starting with general considerations (e.g., definitions, incidence, pathophysiology, etiology), history, physical examination, electrocardiography, thoracic radiography, special diagnostic techniques, differential diagnosis, and finally, the therapeutic approach.

Section III includes chapters directed toward the treatment of cardiac failure, disturbances of cardiac rhythm, conduction disturbances, and a chapter on cardiopulmonary resuscitation.

Routine dosages of cardiovascular drugs for the dog and cat are listed in the Appendix. Respective chapters should be reviewed for additional details regarding dosages and side-effects.

Although this manual includes discussion of the majority of cardiac disorders, many of these conditions can only be evaluated and treated satisfactorily by a specialist situated in a veterinary school or private practice. Necessary facilities and skills must be available for the evaluation of many cardiac disorders.

Careful attention was given to obtaining as homogeneous a book as possible. When a textbook has many authors, there no doubt will be some duplication and some differences in opinion. As with any specialty, duplication and varied opinions can have an educational value as well as create a stimulus for further studies.

Larry Patrick Tilley, D.V.M.
Jerry M. Owens, D.V.M.

ACKNOWLEDGMENTS

We would like to thank each of the authors for their contributions and for following the format of this type of textbook. The majority of the authors have board certification or are uniquely qualified to give an update and review of their respective disciplines. The authors, including the co-editors, would like to thank the veterinarians who have referred cases. We also express gratitude to each of the veterinary students, interns, and residents who we have had the privilege of teaching.

We gratefully acknowledge the assistance of the numerous secretaries involved in this project. We thank the staff of Churchill Livingstone, particularly Mr. Gene Kearn. We would like to especially thank Nancy Baumoel for her thorough editing. We also acknowledge Desirée Allyn for her illustrations in Chapter 2.

CONTENTS

Section I
DIAGNOSIS OF HEART DISEASE

1

History Taking and Physical Examination of the Cardiovascular System

Rebecca E. Gompf

INTRODUCTION

A patient suspected of having a cardiac problem needs to have a complete history and physical examination; this procedure will establish the correct diagnosis and permit appropriate therapy. The cardiac examination is an extension of the complete physical examination; it includes the signalment (age, breed, sex of the animal), current and previous complaints, clinical history of the complaint, physical examination, radiography, electrocardiography, laboratory examination, and other special procedures (phonocardiography, angiocardiogram, echocardiogram) as indicated. The purposes of performing these examinations are as follows:

1. To determine whether a cardiac problem exists
2. To identify the disease process
3. To determine the severity and prognosis of the disease
4. To determine the best treatment of the disease
5. To determine the expected cost of the therapy

MEDICAL HISTORY

SIGNALMENT

Age

I. Young animals usually have a congenital (e.g., patent ductus arteriosus) or infectious cardiac disease (e.g., parvovirus).

II. Older animals usually have an acquired disease such as degenerative (e.g., mitral and tricuspid insufficiency) or neoplastic disease (e.g., heart base tumor).
III. Exceptions:
  A. Cardiomyopathy can occur in young dogs and cats (e.g., aged 6 months or younger).
  B. Older dogs can have congenital heart defects that were not diagnosed when they were young (e.g., patent ductus arteriosus, atrial septal defect).
IV. The cardiac disease in older animals can be modified or affected by other concurrent disease processes (e.g., collapsing trachea, renal or liver disease).

Breed

I. Certain congenital heart defects are more common in specific breeds of animals:
  A. Patent ductus arteriosus (PDA): Poodles, Collies, Pomeranians, German Shepherds
  B. Aortic stenosis (AS): German Shepherds, Boxers, Newfoundlands
  C. Pulmonic stenosis (PS): English Bulldogs, Fox Terriers, Chihuahuas
  D. Tetralogy of Fallot: Keeshonds
II. Large breeds of dogs (e.g., German Shepherds, Great Danes, Doberman Pinschers) are more susceptible to the development of dilated cardiomyopathy.
III. Boxers are susceptible to neoplasms and myocarditis.
IV. Siamese cats are more susceptible to the development of cardiomyopathy.

Sex of the Animal

Males are more susceptible to cardiac disease (e.g., male Cocker Spaniels to fibrosis of the mitral valve, and large-breed males to dilated cardiomyopathy). Sick sinus syndrome occurs in the female Miniature Schnauzer; PDAs are more common in the female.

Weight

I. The animal's weight influences several aspects of treatment:
   A. Dosing cardiac medication
   B. Evaluating the response to diuretic medication
   C. Monitoring cardiac cachexia
II. A "Pickwickian" syndrome (characterized by severe obesity, somnolence, and hypoventilation) can occur in an animal that is so obese that its ability to breathe is restricted.

Utilization of the Animal

I. A hunting dog with severe heartworm disease may not be able to hunt again after treatment.
II. Some animals with congenital heart defect may have a normal lifespan and make good pets. However, they should not be used for breeding purposes, as the defect could be perpetuated.

History

I. Obtaining a complete history
   A. Establishes the presence of a cardiac problem
   B. Helps differentiate between cardiac and respiratory problems
   C. Determines the course of the disease and the response to therapy
   D. Carefully done to prevent an owner from giving a misleading history
   E. Includes several key questions:
      1. Reason the animal is being presented
      2. Onset and duration of the problem(s)
      3. Progression of the disease
      4. Problems noted by the owner
      5. Any known exposure to infectious diseases, as well as vaccination history
      6. Animal's response to any medications that have been given
      7. Any current medications the animal is receiving
      8. The owner's ability to give the medication

F. Defines the animal's attitude and behavior:
   1. Is the animal listless and depressed or alert and playful?
   2. Does the animal tire easily on exercise?

G. Covers other relevant information to identify the problem:
   1. Appetite (what and how much is being fed)
   2. Water consumption
   3. Urinary habits
   4. Bowel movements
   5. Vomiting or regurgitation
   6. Pruritus, biting, or licking
   7. Seizures or snycopal episodes
   8. Reproductive status
   9. Lameness or paresis
   10. Previous diseases or trauma
   11. Coughing, sneezing, difficult breathing
   12. Environment

H. Includes more specific questions:
   1. Character of the cough
   2. When the cough occurs
   3. Stimuli evoking the cough

II. Symptoms most commonly associated with cardiac disease
   A. Coughing
   B. Swelling (edema or ascites)
   C. Tiring on exercise
   D. Fainting or syncopal episodes
   E. Dyspnea, orthopnea, or difficult breathing
   F. Cyanosis
   G. Poor growth or performance

III. Other symptoms associated with cardiovascular disease
   A. Changes in urinary habits
      1. Polydipsia and polyuria are common in animals on diuretics or having a concurrent disease (e.g., renal disease).
      2. Oliguria occurs with severe left heart failure.
      3. Hemoglobinuria is found with the postcaval syndrome of heartworm disease.
   B. Vomiting and/or diarrhea
      1. Cardiac drugs such as digitalis, quinidine, and procainamide can be responsible.

2. Supplemental drugs such as aminophylline can be causative.
3. Regurgitation occurs with congenital vascular ring anomalies.
4. Right heart failure can cause intestinal edema and a protein-losing enteropathy, which results in diarrhea.
5. Cats with cardiomyopathy can develop a hemorrhagic enteritis secondary to thromboemboli of the gastric or mesenteric arteries.
6. Concurrent diseases can be causative.

C. Sneezing
1. It is a sign of a nasal disease.
2. It is not a cardiac problem.

IV. Specific Symptoms

A. Coughing
1. The most common complaint
2. A sudden, forced expiration; a normal defense mechanism to clear debris from the tracheobronchial tree
3. Can be initiated in the following structures:
   a) Pharynx
   b) Trachea
   c) Bronchi
   d) Bronchioli
   e) Pleura
   f) Pericardium
   g) Diaphragm
4. Causes:
   a) Acute coughs: tonsillitis–pharyngitis, tracheobronchitis, acute bronchitis, pleuritis, or pneumonia
   b) Chronic coughs: right- or left-sided heart disease, heartworm disease, asthma
5. Characteristics that often help determine its cause:
   a) Loud, harsh, dry cough of sudden onset followed by a nonproductive gag: common in tracheobronchitis
   b) Cardiac coughs: usually harsher and lower pitched
   c) Chronic nonproductive cough: may indicate a neoplasm or extrinsic pressure on the trachea, such as that due to an enlarged left atrium with bronchial collapse
   d) Honking, high-pitched cough: often found with a collapsing trachea and/or collapsed bronchi

e) Coughing after drinking: found with cardiac disease, collapsing trachea, chronic tracheitis, tracheobronchitis, laryngeal incompetence, or other other causes of dysphagia
f) Coughing without an inciting factor: may indicate cardiac, pulmonary, or extrapulmonary disease
g) Coughing after eating: found with pharyngeal dysphagia, megaesophagus, vascular ring anomalies, and esophageal diverticula, esophageal foreign bodies and esophageal tumors

6. Harmful effects of chronic coughing:
   a) Dissemination of infection to new areas of the lung
   b) Ruptured lung abscesses
   c) Localized emphysema
   d) Pneumonmediastinum
   e) Pneumothorax
   f) Increased weakness and exhaustion of animal

B. Dyspnea
   1. Difficult, labored, or painful breathing.
   2. Can be accompanied in cardiac patients by the following:
      a) Stridor (harsh, high-pitched respiratory sounds)
      b) Rhonchus (a rattling in the throat)
      c) Wheezing
   3. Characteristics:
      a) Paroxysmal: comes and goes
      b) Exertional: occurs after or during activity
      c) Orthopneic: occurs in recumbency
   4. Occurs whenever anything increases the amount of air that must be breathed.
      a) Decrease in environmental oxygen (high altitudes)
      b) Strenuous exercise
      c) Cardiac disease, primary and secondary
      d) Pulmonary disease, primary and secondary
      e) Central nervous system disorders
   5. Most common cardiac cause of dyspnea: left heart failure causing pulmonary edema
   6. Types of dyspnea:
      a) Inspiratory dyspnea: prolonged and labored on inspiration; due to upper airway obstruction.

b) Expiratory dyspnea: prolonged and labored on expiration; due to lower respiratory obstruction.
c) Mixed dyspnea: due to severe pulmonary edema caused by left heart failure or pneumonia.
d) Simple dyspnea or polypnea: increased rate of respiration due to fever, fear, pain or excitement.

C. Hemoptysis
1. Coughing up of blood
2. Uncommon in animals, as they usually swallow their sputum
3. A sign of very severe pulmonary disease
4. Causes:
a) Trauma causing severe pulmonary contusions
b) Severe heartworm disease
c) Neoplasms
d) Foreign bodies
e) Lung abscesses
f) Fungal infections
g) Lung lobe torsions
h) Acute and chronic bronchitis
i) Severe pneumonia
j) Chronic granulomas
k) Pulmonary embolism (e.g., in heartworm disease)
l) Clotting disorders including disseminated intravascular coagulopathy (DIC)
m) Severe pulmonary edema (e.g., ruptured chordae tendineae)

PHYSICAL EXAMINATION

OBSERVATION

I. Attitude and behavior
A. Depressed or alert?
B. Listless or active?

II. Posture
A. Refusal to lie down may indicate pulmonary edema or pleural effusion.

B. Standing with elbows abducted and head extended as well as open mouth breathing with flared nostrils indicate severe respiratory distress.

III. Rate and rhythm of respiration

A. Tachypnea and panting are usually due to excitement.

B. Expiratory dyspnea usually indicates lower airway disease, while inspiratory dyspnea usually indicates upper airway disease.

C. Coughing

IV. Dependent ventral edema

A. If edema is present in the neck, head, and forelimbs only, it usually indicates an obstruction of the cranial vena cava or a mediastinal mass.

B. If there is edema of the entire body, pleural effusion with or without ascites is usually present. Other causes of edema (e.g. hypoproteinemia) should be considered.

V. Elevated temperature

May be seen with an infectious disease or subacute bacterial endocarditis.

Cardiac Examination

Head

I. Check for any asymmetry and swellings.

II. The eyes should be examined for changes that could indicate systemic diseases.

III. The ears have no significant changes associated with the cardiovascular system. Cyanosis can sometimes be recognized by evaluating the color of the pinna.

IV. Examine the nose for signs of disease and patency.

V. In the mouth, mucous membrane color and perfusion should be noted.

A. A perfusion time of greater than 2 seconds suggests decreased cardiac output.

B. Cyanosis is due to hypoventilation or to poor diffusion across the alveoli produced by:

1. Large airway obstruction (e.g., tracheal collapse)
2. Small airway obstruction (e.g., bronchitis)
3. Fluid-filled small airways (e.g., edema)
4. Right to left vascular shunts (e.g., tetralogy of Fallot)
5. Peripheral extraction of more oxygen from a slow systemic circulation (e.g., severe heart failure)

C. Hyperemic mucous membranes may indicate an increased packed cell volume, which can be secondary to a chronic right-to-left vascular shunt.

D. Pale mucous membrane indicate anemia or poor perfusion.

E. The mucous membranes of the mouth should be compared with the posterior (e.g., vagina, prepuce), as differential cyanosis can occur in a right-to-left shunting PDA.

F. Also check the oral cavity for severe dental tartar, gingivitis, or pyorrhea, which can serve as a source of sepsis leading to bacteremia and possibly endocarditis.

Neck

I. The jugular pulse should be evaluated while the animal is standing, with its head in a normal position. Any pulse going over one-third of the way up to the neck is abnormal and can be due to any of several factors:

A. Right heart failure with tricuspid insufficiency
B. Heart block or premature beat
C. Pulmonic stenosis
D. Pulmonary hypertension
E. Heartworm disease
F. Right heart failure with cardiomyopathy

II. The entire jugular vein can be distended due to congestive heart failure, pericardial disease, or obstruction of cranial vena cava (e.g., heart base tumor)

III. Arterial pulses can mimic a jugular pulse. When light pressure is applied to the area of the jugular pulse, the arterial pulse will continue, while the jugular pulse will stop.

Palpation

Trachea

I. The trachea should be palpated for abnormalities such as collapsing, masses, or increased sensitivity.
II. This step should probably be postponed until after auscultation of the thorax, as a cough may be elicited which makes auscultation difficult.

Thorax

I. The point of maximum intensity (PMI) should be on the left side between the fourth to sixth intercostal spaces. Shifting of the PMI is due to:
  A. Cardiac enlargement
  B. Masses displacing the heart
  C. Collapsed lung lobes allowing the heart to shift
  D. Lying down in right lateral recumbency such that the heart falls to the right
II. A decreased intensity of heartbeat may be due to:
  A. Obesity
  B. Pleural effusion
  C. Pericardial effusion
  D. Thoracic masses
  E. Pneumothorax
III. Loud cardiac murmurs can be palpated as "thrills," which are due to vibrations caused by blood flow.

Abdomen

I. Check for ascites.
II. Check for signs of heptomegaly and splenomegaly due to right-sided heart failure.
III. Palpate for other concurrent related or unrelated masses.

Skin

Palpate for evidence of edema due to right heart failure or venous obstruction.

Femoral Pulse

I. Both pulses should be compared, as one could be obstructed.
II. It is difficult to palpate the femoral pulse in a normal cat; therefore, the absence of palpable femoral pulses in a cat should not be interpreted as definite arterial obstruction.
III. The rate should be taken.
  A. Normal rates in dogs are 70 to 180 beats/min (bpm), with smaller dogs having faster rates. Puppies can have a normal rate of 220 bpm.
  B. Normal rate in cats is 160 to 240 bpm.
IV. The rhythm of the pulses should be noted.
  A. There should be a pulse for every heartbeat.
  B. Pulse deficits usually indicate incomplete ventricular filling, as seen in arrhythmias.
V. The intensity of the pulse should be palpated.
  A. Normal pulses are strong and have a rapid rate of rise and fall.
  B. Hypokinetic (weak) pulses are due to decreased cardiac output or slower rate of rise due to delayed emptying of the left ventricle.
  C. Hyperkinetic (strong) pulses rise and fall quickly and are due to large left ventricular stroke volumes with rapid diastolic runoffs (e.g., PDA and aortic insufficiency). They are called "B-B shot" or "water-hammer" pulses. Fear and fevers can also produce this type of pulse.
  D. Pulsus alternans occurs when the pulse is alternately weak and then strong. It is frequently associated with myocardial failure.
  E. Pulsus paradoxus is an alteration of the pulse strength during respiration due to changes in ventricular filling. This is sometimes a sign of cardiac tamponade.

PERCUSSION

I. Determines the presence of masses or fluid lines, especially in the thorax

II. Elicits a hollow sound over the lungs
III. Elicits a dull sound over solid structures

Auscultation

I. This is the most helpful part of the cardiac examination; it should be done carefully and systematically. The animal should be standing, so that the heart is in its normal position.

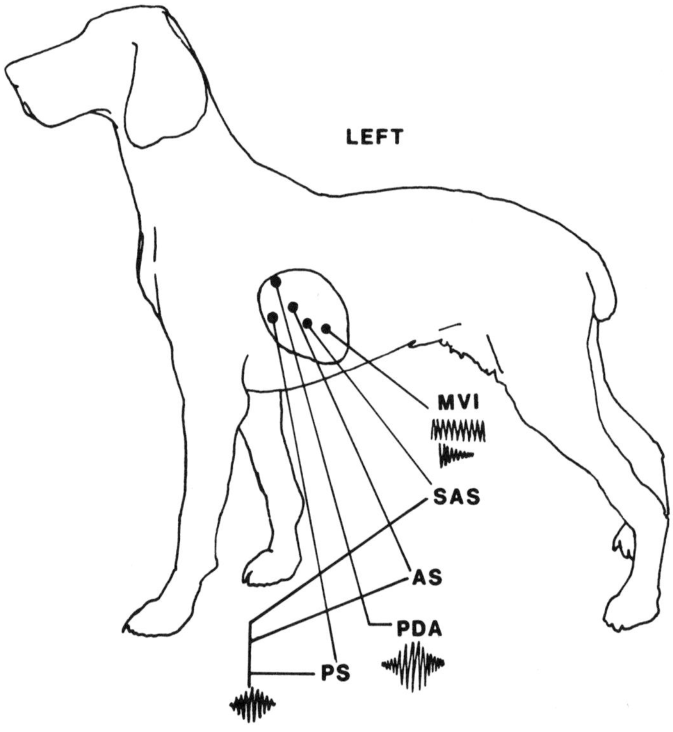

Fig. 1-1. Phonocardiographic configurations of various cardiac murmurs as recorded at the usual points of maximal murmur intensity. View of left hemithorax of the dog. MVI, mitral valve insufficiency; SAS, subaortic stenosis; AS, valvular aortic stenosis; PDA, patent ductus arteriosus; PS, pulmonic stenosis. (From Bonagura JD, Berkwith L: Cardiovascular and pulmonary disorders. p. 119. In Quick Reference to Veterinary Medicine. JB Lippincott, Philadelphia, 1982.)

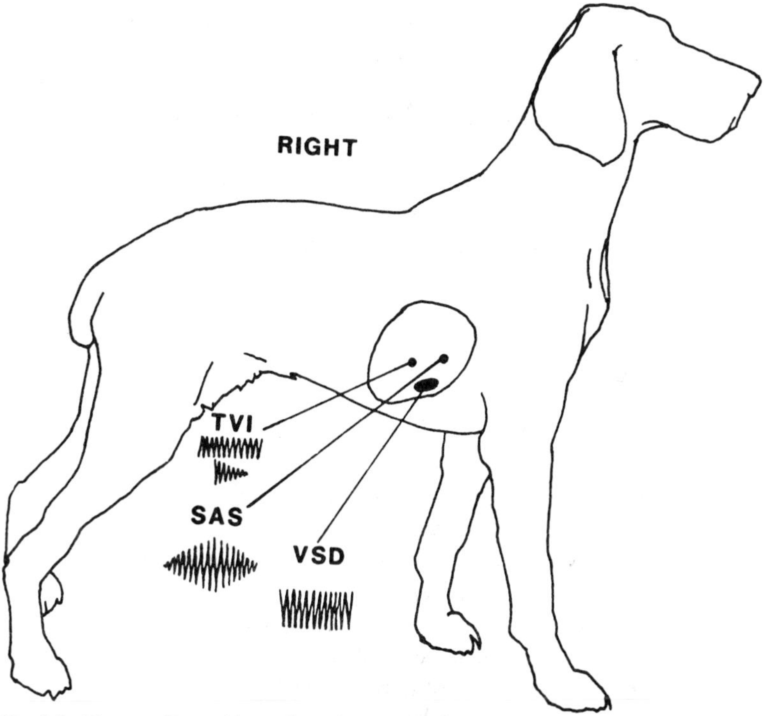

Fig. 1-2. Phonocardiographic configurations of various cardiac murmurs as recorded at the usual points of maximal intensity. View of the right hemithorax of the dog. TVI, tricuspid valve insufficiency; VSD, ventricular septal defect; SAS, subaortic stenosis. (From Bonagura JD, Berkwith L: Cardiovascular and pulmonary disorders. p. 119. In Quick Reference to Veterinary Medicine. JB Lippincott, Philadelphia, 1982.)

A. Common artifacts heard:
   1. Respiratory clicks and murmurs
   2. Rumbles due to shivering and twitching
   3. Movement sounds
   4. Crackling sounds due to the rubbing of hair
   5. Extraneous sounds if auscultation is not performed in a quiet area

B. Auscultate the heart and lungs separately.

II. The areas of auscultation (Figs. 1-1 and 1-2) are as follows:

A. Pulmonic area—left side

1. In the dog, it is between the second and fourth intercostal spaces just above the sternum.
2. In the cat, it is located at the second to third intercostal space one-third to one-half of the way up the thorax from the sternum.

B. Aortic area—left side

1. In the dog, it is at the fourth intercostal space just above the costrochondral junction.
2. In the cat, it is at the second to third intercostal space just dorsal to the pulmonic area.

C. Mitral area—left side

1. In the dog, it is at the fifth intercostal space at the costochondral junction.
2. In the cat, it is at the fifth to sixth intercostal space one-fourth of the way up the thorax from the sternum.

D. Tricuspid area—right side

1. In the dog, it is at the third to fifth intercostal space near the costochrondral junction.
2. In the cat, it is at the fourth or fifth intercostal space, at a level opposite the mitral area.

III. The area in which murmurs are loudest and in which they radiate should be noted. This can help identify the heart problem.

IV. Heart rate and rhythm should be identified.

A. The effects of inspiration and expiration on heart rate, rhythm, and heart sounds should be noted.

B. The presence or absence of heart sounds should be noted.

Normal Heart Sounds

Heart sounds are due to the abrupt acceleration or deceleration of blood and the vibrations of the heart and vessels.

I. The first heart sound (S_1) (Fig. 1-3) is due to passive closure of the mitral and tricuspid valves.

A. S_1 is longer, louder, duller, and lower pitched than the second heart sound.

B. It is loudest over the mitral area.

C. Its intensity increases due to fever, fear, or tachycardia.

D. Its intensity decreases due to obesity, pleural or pericardial effu-

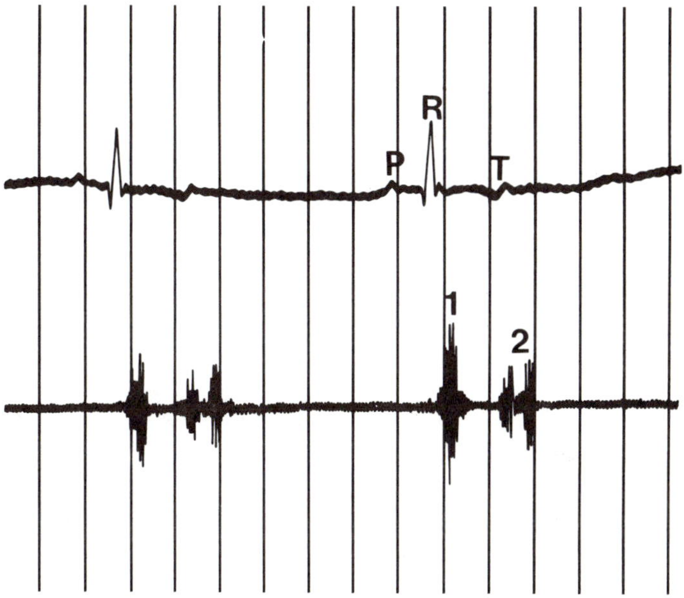

Fig. 1-3. Lead II electrocardiogram recorded simultaneously with medium-frequency band phonocardiogram from a dog. The second heart sound (S_2) is split. First heart sound (S_1). Paper speed, 100 mm/sec. (From Gompf RE: Physical examination of the cardiopulmonary system. Vet Clin North Am 131:210, 1983.)

sion, thoracic masses, diaphragmatic hernias, bradycardias, and insufficient filling of the ventricles.

E. It varies in intensity with arrhythmias.

F. It has four parts which can be seen on a phonocardiogram.

G. It can be split in large breeds of dogs, right bundle branch block, or ventricular premature beats.

II. The second heart sound (S_2) is produced by passive closure of the aortic and pulmonic valves.

A. It is short, high pitched, and sharp.

B. It is loudest over the aortic area.

C. A split S_2 (Figure 1-3) is due to closure of the pulmonic valve after the aortic valve, which occurs in:

1. Pulmonary hypertension (e.g., heartworm disease)
2. Right bundle branch block
3. Ventricular premature beats originating in the left ventricle

4. Atrial septal defect
5. Pulmonic stenosis

D. Paradoxical splitting is due to delayed closure of the aortic valve resulting from:
1. Left bundle branch block
2. Premature beats originating from the right ventricle
3. Subaortic stenosis
4. Severe systemic hypertension
5. Left ventricular failure

E. S_2 may be absent in arrhythmias where there is incomplete filling of the ventricles and insufficient pressure to open the semilunar valves.

Abnormal Heart Sounds

I. The third heart sound (S_3) is due to rapid ventricular filling.
A. It is lower pitched than the second heart sound.
B. It is heard best in the mitral area.
C. In dogs and cats, its presence indicates dilated ventricles, which most commonly occur with dilated cardiomyopathy or decompensated mitral or tricuspid insufficiency.

II. The fourth heart sound (S_4) is due to atrial contraction.
A. It is heard best over the aortic or pulmonic areas but sometimes can be heard over the mitral area as well.
B. It is present in dogs or cats when the atria dilate in response to ventricular diastolic dysfunction such as hypertrophic cardiomyopathy.

III. A gallop rhythm is a S_3, S_4, (Fig. 1-4) or combination of the two.
A. Gallops are of a low frequency and can be difficult to hear.
B. A gallop can be a very early sign of heart failure preceding clinical signs.

IV. Systolic clicks are clicking noises that occur in systole between S_1 and S_2.
A. It may come and go and may change its position in systole (gets closer or further away from S_2).
B. The precise cause of the click is unknown, but many animals develop a mitral insufficiency murmur later in life.

C. This is a benign finding and not usually associated with heart failure.

Arrhythmias Heard on Auscultation

I. Arrhythmias that increase the heart rate

A. Atrial fibrillation, which has a rapid, irregular rhythm with heart sounds varying in intensity.

1. Pulse deficits are present.
2. It has been described as being irregularly irregular and rarely is mistaken for other tachycardias.

B. Ventricular tachycardias are usually intermittent and tend to be more regular than atrial fibrillation. Pulse deficits are frequently present.

C. Sinus and atrial tachycardias are rapid and regular. All the heart

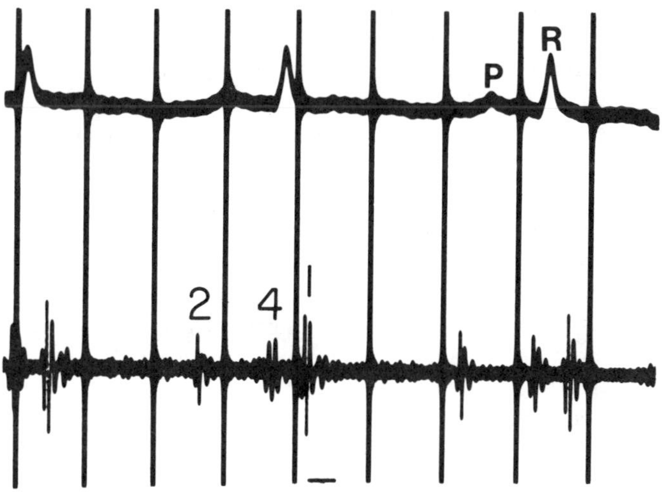

Fig. 1-4. Lead II electrocardiogram recorded simultaneously with a low-frequency band phonocardiogram from a cat with hypertrophic cardiomyopathy. A gallop rhythm or fourth heart sound (S_4) is present. First heart sound (S_1); second heart sound (S_2). Paper speed, 100 mm/sec. (From Gompf RE: Physical examination of the cardiopulmonary system. Vet Clin North Am 131:211, 1983.)

sounds are of a uniform intensity, but an atrial tachycardia tends to be intermittent.

D. An electrocardiogram is necessary to distinguish among sinus, atrial, and ventricular tachycardia.

II. Arrhythmias that decrease the heart rate

A. Sinus arrhythmia has a cyclic pattern.

1. The heart rate will increase during inspiration and decrease during expiration due to changes in vagal tone.
2. The intensity of the pulse and heart sounds may vary.

B. Sinus bradycardia has a very slow rhythm.

1. The heart sounds may vary.
2. The heart rate is 50 to 100 beats/min, depending on the size of the dog.

C. Second- and third-degree heart blocks have slow heart rates.

1. The heart sounds will vary in intensity.
2. A fourth heart sound may be present in third degree block.
3. The pulses will be slow and hyperkinetic, but there are no pulse deficits.
4. A jugular pulse is usually present.
5. Extra sounds may be generated by escape beats.

III. Atrial and ventricular premature beats: Generation of extra sounds that mimic S_3 and S_4

A. It is hard to differentiate between the two types of premature beats as well as S_3 and S_4 on physical examination. An electrocardiogram (ECG) and phonocardiogram may be necessary.

B. Both premature beats interrupt the normal rhythm and are usually followed by a pause.

C. Usually only a S_1 is heard with a premature beat, although sometimes S_1-S_2 is heard very close together. S_2 is usually absent.

D. Ventricular premature beats can also cause a split S_1 or S_2.

IV. Unexpected pauses

A. Sinoatrial (SA) arrest occurs when an impulse does not leave the SA node. The pause continues until the next normal beat or an escape beat occurs.

B. The heart sound following a pause may be louder than usual as the ventricles have had longer to fill and eject a larger amount of blood.

MURMURS

Murmurs are due to turbulent blood flow through the heart and vessels.

I. Classification
   A. Functional murmurs are divided into:
      1. Physiologic murmurs have a known cause such as anemia, hypoproteinemia, hyperkinetic circulation (e.g., fever), and an athletic heart.
      2. Innocent murmurs have no known cause and are not associated with any cardiac problem.
   B. Pathologic murmurs are caused by underlying heart or vessel disease:
      1. Stenosis of valves, outflow tract, or great vessels
      2. Valvular insufficiency
      3. Abnormal intra- or extracardiac shunts

II. Description
   A. Site at which the murmur is loudest (e.g., valve area)
   B. Timing in the cardiac style (e.g., systole or diastole)
   C. Duration of the murmur (e.g., early systolic, holosystolic, pansystolic, continuous)
   D. Intensity of the murmur
      1. Grade 1/6 can only be heard after listening for several minutes and sounds like a prolonged first heart sound.
      2. Grade 2/6 is very soft and can be heard immediately.
      3. Grade 3/6 is low to moderate in intensity.
      4. Grade 4/6 is very loud but a "thrill" cannot be palpated on the thorax.
      5. Grade 5/6 is very loud and a "thrill" can be palpated on the thorax.
      6. Grade 6/6 can be heard without the use of a stethoscope or with the stethoscope slightly off the thoracic wall.
   E. Quality of the murmur: subjective, but can be evaluated according to graphic appearance on phonocardiogram (Figs. 1-1 and 1-2):
      1. Regurgitant murmurs: plateau shaped
      2. Ejection murmurs: decrescendo, crescendo, or diamond shaped
      3. Machinery murmur: diamond shaped and peaking at S_2, continuing through all of systole and most of diastole

4. Blowing murmur: decrescendo murmur

F. Radiation of the murmur: can help identify the problem, as many cardiac problems have murmurs that are loud over one valve area and that radiate to another

Other Sounds Auscultated in the Thorax

I. Normal respiratory sounds
  A. Referred sounds from the trachea are commonly heard over the lungs and bronchi.
  B. Vesicular sounds are due to air moving though the small bronchi and are louder on inspiration.
  C. Bronchial sounds are due to air moving through the large bronchi and trachea and are best heard on expiration.
  D. The combination of the above two are are called bronchovesicular sounds and are heard best over the hilar area.

II. Abnormal respiratory sounds
  A. Attenuated bronchovesicular sounds are due to:
    1. Thoracic masses
    2. Pleural effusion
    3. Pneumothorax
    4. Obesity
    5. Pneumonia
    6. Shallow breathing
    7. Early consolidation of the pulmonary parenchyma
  B. Rhonchi are due to air passing through partially obstructed airways in the bronchial tubes or smallest airways.
    1. Rhonchi from the large bronchi are low pitched, sonorous, and almost continuous. They are heard best on inspiration.
    2. Rhonchi from the small bronchi are high pitched, sibilant, or squeaky and are heard best on expiration.
  C. Rales are interrupted, crepitant, inspiratory sounds heard in many disease conditions and are not pathognomonic for pulmonary edema.
    1. Opening of alveoli or airways that are collapsed or partially filled with fluid
    2. Bubbles bursting in the airways

III. Other sounds auscultated
   A. Pleural friction rubs: grading, rubbing sounds heard during inspiration and expiration due to the moving of two relatively, dry, roughened pleural surfaces over each other
   B. Pericardial friction rubs: short, scratchy noises produced by pericarditis and heart movement
   C. Pericardial knocks: diastolic sounds that occur in animals with constrictive pericarditis

SUGGESTED READINGS

Bonagura JD.: Clinical Cardiology Notes. The Ohio State University, Columbus, Ohio, 1979

Bonagura JD, and Berkwitt L: Cardiovascular and pulmonary disorders. p. 3. In Quick Reference to Veterinary Medicine. JB Lippincott, Philadelphia, 1982

Ettinger SJ: Valvular heart disease. p. 895. In Textbook of Veterinary Internal Medicine. WB Saunders, Philadelphia, 1975

Ettinger SJ, Suter PF: Canine Cardiology. WB Saunders, Philadelphia, 1970

Ettinger SJ, Suter PF: Congenital heart disease. p. 865. In Textbook of Veterinary Internal Medicine. WB Saunders, Philadelphia, 1975

Gompf RE: Physical examination of the cardiopulmonary system. Vet Clin North Am [Small Anim Pract] 13:201, 1983

Harpster NK: Clinical examination of the feline cardiovascular system. Vet Clin North Am [Small Anim Pract] 7:241, 1977

Roudebush P: Lung sounds. J Am Vet Med Assoc 181:122, 1982

Tilley LP: Essentials of Canine & Feline Electrocardiography, Interpretation and Treatment. 2nd Ed. Lea & Febiger, Philadelphia, 1985

2

Radiology of the Heart

Jerry M. Owens

INTRODUCTION

Thoracic radiography is an integral part of the cardiovascular examination. The clinician needs to know both normal radiographic anatomy, including the variables of age, breed conformation, and phases of the respiratory and cardiac cycles, as well as abnormal radiographic anatomy of the heart in disease. In the abnormal state, it is essential to be able to correlate the compensatory and pathophysiologic mechanisms of heart disease and heart failure.

RADIOGRAPHIC TECHNIQUE

Exposure Technique and Film Quality

I. Short exposure time (1/60 or 1/120 second)
II. High-kilovoltage (kV) technique (80 to 120 kVP)
III. High-latitude film–screen combination (e.g., rare earth system or high-speed screens with medium-speed film)
IV. Use of grid to improve image quality when chest is greater than 12 to 15 cm in thickness

Radiographic Projections

Standard Projections

I. Lateral projection (right or left) is exposed at full inspiration.
   A. The same lateral projection should be used on all serial thoracic examinations.

B. In some situations, both right and left lateral projections are helpful.

II. Dorsoventral (DV) or ventrodorsal (VD) projection exposed at full inspiration
   A. The DV projection is usually preferable to the VD projection because the heart shape and position are less variable in this view.
   B. Some radiologists prefer a VD projection over the DV projection.
   C. The same projection (DV or VD) should be used on all serial thoracic examinations.

Supplemental Projections

I. Right and left DV or VD oblique projections are useful in evaluating pleural and mediastinal masses.

II. Horizontal beam projections:
   A. Standing lateral projection: used in evaluating pleural fluid and fluid levels within cavitated masses
   B. Erect ventrodorsal projection: used in evaluating pleural fluid and masses within the cranial mediastinum
   C. Recumbent lateral projection: used in evaluating fluid distribution, in assessing small amounts of pneumothorax, and in evaluating chest wall masses
   D. Recumbent ventrodorsal projection (supine): used in evaluating pleural fluid and diseases of the ventral mediastinum

III. Expiratory radiographs
   A. May aid in detecting small amounts of pleural fluid or pneumothorax
   B. May aid in diagnosing tracheal and/or bronchial collapse

SPECIAL PROCEDURES

Esophagram

I. Indications
   A. Useful in evaluating mediastinal and heart-based masses

B. To localize the esophagus before transthoracic biopsy of mediastinal, pulmonary, or heart-based masses

II. Technique

A. Administer barium paste (e.g., Esophatrast) at a dose of 10 to 30 ml; allowing the patient to swallow adequately a few times to ensure complete esophageal coating.

B. Obtain lateral, ventrodorsal, and right ventrodorsal oblique projections.

Nonselective Angiogram

I. Indications

A. Useful in evaluating the cranial vena cava and heart base

B. Shows the anatomy of the right heart and is useful in determining the presence or absence of pericardial effusion and cardiac wall masses

C. Aids in diagnosing and differentiating cardiomyopathy in the cat

D. Permits diagnosis of some congenital heart defects

II. Technique

A. An indwelling catheter is placed into the cephalic or jugular vein. The size of the needle should be large enough to ensure a bolus injection (e.g., 18 to 20 gauge in the cat, 14 to 18 gauge in the dog)

B. Iodinated contrast media (e.g., Renografin 76) at a dose of 0.3 to 0.5 ml/lb body weight is injected as a bolus.

C. Either a single film or a series of films are then made after injection. The film sequence needed depends on the type of suspected lesion present and on which part of the cardiac anatomy requires observation.

III. Examples

A. In evaluating the cranial vena cava and the right heart, usually only a single lateral projection is needed at the end of contrast injection.

B. In evaluating feline cardiomyopathy, a series of films should be taken 2 to 3 seconds apart using either a rapid film changer or a cassette tunnel system. In the normal cat, the circulation time is approximately 5 to 6 seconds. In hypertrophic cardiomyopathy, the circulation time may be normal or slightly prolonged. In dilated cardiomyopathy, the circulation time is usually moderately prolonged (10 to 20 seconds).

C. In evaluating congenital heart defects, the earliest films (2 to 5 seconds) are best for pulmonic stenosis and right-to-left shunts, while other defects (e.g., aortic stenosis) may not be visualized until 5 to 8 seconds.

Selective Angiocardiography (See also Chapter 4)

I. Indications
  A. Aids in accurate assessment of congenital or acquired heart disease
  B. Permits pressures to be measured and a catheter to be directed toward a specific chamber or vessel

II. Technique
  A. Usually a surgical cutdown is necessary for placement of an angiographic catheter. The most commonly used vessels are the jugular vein, the carotid and femoral arteries.
  B. Iodinated contrast media (e.g., Renografin 76) is injected via a pressure injector.
  C. A series of films are then taken using a rapid film changer, videotape, or cine film to permit adequate demonstration of the circulatory flow of contrast medium from the chamber of injection.

Pneumopericardiography

I. Indications
  A. Permits delineation of the pericardial sac and the epicardial surface of the heart
  B. Useful in the diagnosis of pericardial effusion and other diseases of the pericardium, heart wall, and heart base

II. Technique
  A. The site for pericardiocentesis is in part determined from the survey radiographs. Usually the right fourth to sixth intercostal space near the junction of the lower and middle thirds of the thorax provides the most convenient and safest location for entry.
  B. An indwelling catheter (e.g., Intrafusor, Angiocath), 14 to 16 gauge, is passed through the intercostal space at a 45-degree angle

to the intercostal space in a mediodorsal direction. Electrocardiographic (ECG) monitoring should accompany this procedure in an effort to minimize needle irritation of the epicardium and the production of premature ventricular beats.

C. After safe entrance into the pericardial sac, the pericardial fluid is removed. Pericardial fluid should not clot and its appearance will vary from serous to bloody.

D. After removal of all pericardial fluid, air is slowly infused into the pericardial sac at a dose of approximately two-thirds that of the volume of the fluid that was removed.

E. Ventrodorsal, dorsoventral, right lateral, and left lateral projections are then made.

Radiographic Anatomy

Lateral Thoracic Radiograph

I. The canine heart appears somewhat oval in shape, and its axis is approximately 45 degrees to the sternum.

II. The heart usually extends from the third to the eighth thoracic vertebrae, with the ventricular area occupying approximately three intercostal spaces in a dog with mesomorphic conformation.

III. The caudal heart border touches or overlaps the cranioventral aspect of the diaphragm near its sternal attachment, with the degree of overlap being determined by the phase of respiration (inspiration versus expiration).

IV. The cardiac silhouette occupies approximately 70 percent of the distance from the sternum to the thoracic spine at the point of its greatest dorsal extension.

V. The heart has three borders (see Fig. 2-1):

A. Dorsal border: Includes both atria, the pulmonary arteries and veins, the cranial and caudal vena cavae, and the aortic arch.

B. Cranial border: Formed by the right ventricle and the right atrial appendage, resulting in the "cranial waist."

C. Caudal border: Formed by the left atrium and the left ventricle;

the "caudal waist" corresponds to the atrioventricular groove at the junction of the left atrium and the left ventricle.

VI. The cardiac anatomy of the feline heart is essentially the same as that of the dog, with the following exceptions:

A. The heart is more elongated and elliptical in shape than that of the dog.

B. The ventricular area occupies approximately 2 to 2½ intercostal spaces (compared with approximately 3 intercostal spaces in the dog).

C. Some cats have a more supine cardiac orientation. This is especially common in aged cats and has been called a "lazy" heart.

VII. The main pulmonary artery (pulmonary trunk) cannot be seen on the lateral projection due to a positive silhouette with the craniodorsal base of the heart.

A. The left pulmonary artery can sometimes be seen extending dorsal and caudal to the tracheal bifurcation.

B. The right pulmonary artery is frequently seen on end as it leaves the main pulmonary artery immediately ventral to the carina. This end-on appearance may be confused with a mass lesion.

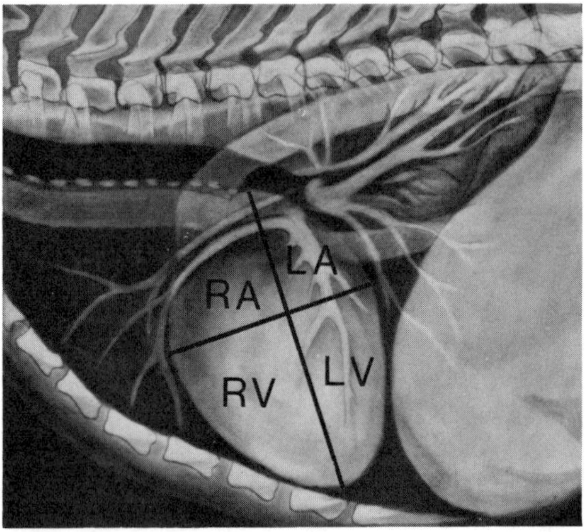

Fig. 2-1. Normal canine heart. Approximate locations of the four heart chambers are depicted. (From Owens JM: Radiographic Interpretation for the Small Animal Clinician. Ralston Purina Co, St Louis, 1982.)

C. The pulmonary veins are best identified as they enter the left atrium caudal to the heart base.

VIII. The pulmonary arteries are located dorsal to their respective bronchi and veins.

A. The vessels to the cranial lungs lobes are usually seen as two pairs of vessels.

B. The more cranial pair of vessels generally corresponds to the side on which the lateral projection was made. For example, in right lateral position, the right cranial lobar vessels are more cranial than are those vessels of the left cranial lung lobe.

IX. The pulmonary arteries and veins are normally the same size. A rule of thumb is that the diameter of the cranial lobar vessels should be approximately 75 percent the width of the narrowest portion of the fourth rib, as seen on the lateral projection.

Dorsoventral and Ventrodorsal Projections

I. The canine heart is somewhat elliptical in shape with its axis oriented approximately 30 degrees to the spine with the cardiac apex slightly to the left of the midline.

II. The heart normally extends from the third to the eighth thoracic vertebrae with the caudal border of the heart usually abutting the diaphragm.

III. The width of the heart across its widest point is usually 60 to 65 percent of the thoracic width in a dog of mesomorphic conformation.

IV. In the cat, the heart is more oval and thinner. The cardiac apex may be located on or to the left of the midline. The ratio of the longitudinal axis to the transverse axis of the heart is approximately 1.4:1. Usually the heart is separated from the diaphragm by one or two intercostal spaces.

V. The atria and ventricles are superimposed; however, the right and left sides of the heart can be estimated by drawing an oblique line from the cranial vena cava to the cardiac apex (see Fig. 2-1).

VI. The margins of the cardiac silhouette are formed by the right at-

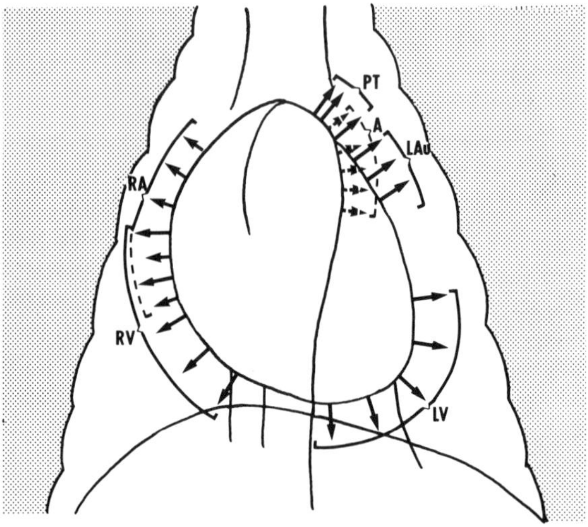

Fig. 2-2. Clock analogy showing the location and direction of enlargement of the cardiac chambers and great vessels. Pulmonary trunk (PT), descending aorta (A), left auricle (LAu), left ventricle (LV), right ventricle (RV), right atrium (RA). (Adapted from Meyer CW, Bonagura JD: Survey radiology of the heart. Vet Clin North Am 12: 217, 1982.)

rium and the right ventricle on the right side, by the left ventricle on the left side, and by the great vessels on its cranial border.

VII. The clock analogy can be used to simplify the anatomy of the cardiac silhouette (see Fig. 2-2).
  A. The aortic arch extends from the 11 to 1 o'clock position.
  B. The main pulmonary artery is located from the 1 to 2 o'clock position.
  C. In the dog, the left atrium is not identified on this projection; in the cat, the left atrium forms the portion of the cardiac border from the 2 to 3 o'clock position.
  D. The left ventricle forms the left heart border from the 2 to 6 o'clock position in the dog and from the 3 to 6 o'clock position in the cat.
  E. The right ventricle is located from the 6 to 11 o'clock position.
  F. The right atrium is located at the 9 to 11 o'clock position.
  G. The pulmonary arteries are sometimes seen superimposed over the heart shadow originating in the main pulmonary artery.

   1. The left pulmonary artery extends beyond the left heart border at approximately the 4 o'clock position.
   2. The right pulmonary artery extends beyond the right heart border at approximately the 8 o'clock position.
  H. The pulmonary veins can usually be seen as they enter the left atrium.
   1. The left caudal lobe pulmonary vein is located at approximately the 5 o'clock position.
   2. The right caudal lobe pulmonary vein is located at approximately the 7 o'clock position.

VIII. Within the lung fields, pulmonary arteries can usually be differentiated from the pulmonary veins.
  A. The cranial and caudal lobar arteries extend into their respective lung lobes lateral to their respective bronchi and veins.
  B. The pulmonary arteries are slightly more radiopaque, taper evenly, are curved, and are equally branched.
  C. The pulmonary veins are usually less well visualized, are straighter, and blunter than arteries, and usually have branches of unequal size.

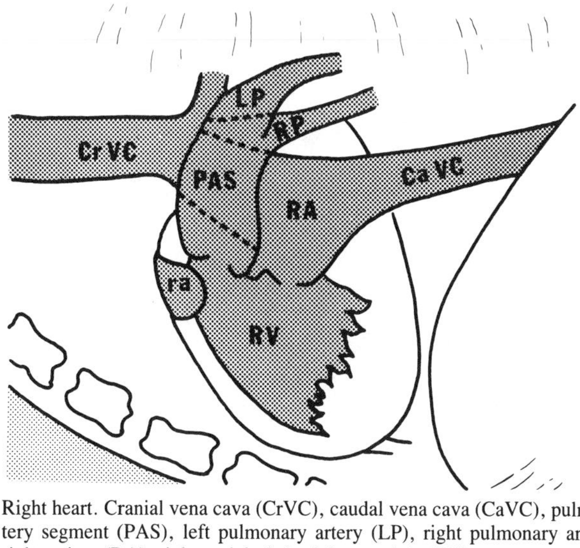

Fig. 2-3. Right heart. Cranial vena cava (CrVC), caudal vena cava (CaVC), pulmonary artery segment (PAS), left pulmonary artery (LP), right pulmonary artery (RP), right atrium (RA), right auricle (ra), right ventricle (RV).

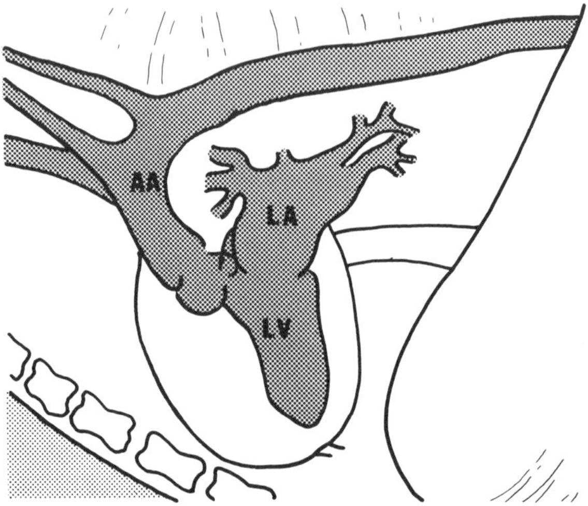

Fig. 2-4. Left heart. Aortic arch (AA), left atrium (LA), left ventricle (LV).

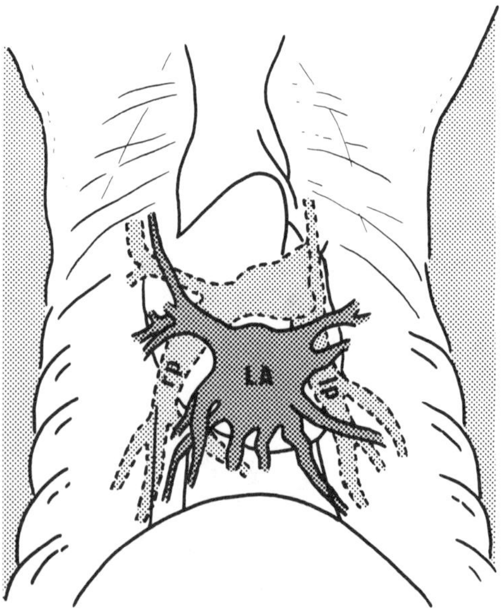

Fig. 2-5. Pulmonary arteries and veins. Left atrium (LA), right pulmonary artery (rp), left pulmonary artery (lp).

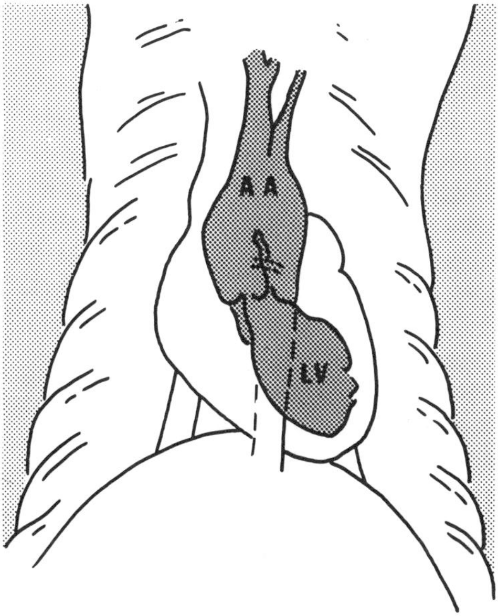

Fig. 2-6. Left ventricle (LV) and aortic arch (AA).

IX. The aortic arch is within the cranial mediastinum at the cranial heart border and is normally not visualized. The descending aorta is seen as a superimposed density over the heart extending caudally, dorsally, and medially. The left lateral border of the aorta can be seen to the left of the vertebral column on the dorsoventral and ventrodorsal projections.

X. The internal anatomy of the heart is depicted in Figures 2-3 through 2-6. The location and appearance of the cardiac chambers and the great vessels, are shown, which form the borders of the cardiac silhouette.

Radiographic Interpretation

Interpretation of the Thoracic Radiographs

A systematic evaluation of the entire chest involves the following steps:

I. Evaluate the radiographs for technical quality, positioning, and proper exposure factors.
II. Determine whether the radiographs were made at inspiration or expiration by observing the position of the diaphragm relative to the heart and the degree of lung inflation.
III. Analyze the extracirculatory strutures, including the spine, sternum, diaphragm, thoracic wall, ribs, thoracic inlet, and cranial abdomen.
IV. Evaluate the position and diameter of the trachea and the tracheal bifurcation.
V. Evaluate the cranial mediastinum for widening, abnormal density, or the presence of an abnormal mass.
VI. Evaluate the aorta and aortic arch, relative to position, size, and degree of radiopacity.
VII. Evaluate the position of the cardiac apex and of the caudal mediastinum.
VIII. Evaluate the size and shape of the main pulmonary artery and of the peripheral pulmonary arteries and veins.
IX. Evaluate the lung for areas of increased or decreased radiopacity.
X. Evaluate the cardiac borders (cranial, caudal, right, and left) for enlargement or abnormal position.

Normal Heart Size in the Dog

Cardiac Mensuration

This system consists of making measurements of the width of the heart shadow relative to the distances between the heart border and the right and left sides of the thoracic wall as seen on the dorsoventral projection.

I. It is based on the assumption that positioning is standardized and that dogs from different breeds have similar heart sizes and shapes.
II. Its disadvantage: Time consuming and frequently inaccurate in the assessment of individual heart chamber enlargement.

Empirical Measurement

I. It uses both the lateral and dorsoventral projections in the assessment of heart size.
  A. Lateral projection: the normal canine heart is approximately three intercostal spaces in width.
  B. Dorsoventral projection: the normal canine heart at its widest point is approximately two-thirds the width of the thoracic cavity.
II. The range of normal in the different breeds is largely determined by individual experience.
III. Individual chamber enlargement or overall heart enlargement is usually more significant if the abnormal changes are seen on both lateral and dorsoventral projections.

Normal Variables for Heart Size and Shape

I. Differences in thoracic conformation
  A. Deep narrow-chested breeds (e.g., Setters, Afghans, Collies)
    1. On the lateral projection, the heart appears more vertical and narrower (approximately 2½ intercostal spaces in width).
    2. On the dorsoventral projection, the heart appears smaller and more rounded.
  B. Shallow wide-chested breeds (e.g., Dachshunds, Bulldogs)
    1. On the lateral projection, the right heart appears more rounded with increased sternal contact and a more dorsal position of the trachea. The heart also appears larger usually measuring 3 to 3 1/2 intercostal spaces in width.
    2. On the dorsoventral projection, the right heart appears enlarged and more rounded.
II. Age difference
  A. Younger animals appear to have larger hearts relative to their thoracic size than they do at maturity.
III. Systole versus diastole
  A. During systole, the heart is slightly smaller than during diastole.

B. However, this difference is usually not well perceived on a radiograph.

IV. Phase of respiration at time of radiographic exposure

A. The heart appears smaller on inspiration than it does on expiration.

B. During expiration, there is increased sternal contact of the right heart and dorsal elevation of the trachea, falsely suggesting right heart enlargement.

Positional Abnormalities of the Heart Size and Shape

Malposition of the cardiac shadow will alter the radiographic interpretation of the heart size and shape.

I. Lateral projection

A. The heart is sometimes positioned away from the sternum. This can be caused by the following conditions:

1. Pneumothorax: The heart is actually dependently moved away from the sternum due to gravitational pull of the heart downward and more pleural air in the upward side of the chest. This condition has been falsely referred to as "elevation" of the heart from the sternum.
2. Mediastinal shift: Occurs in pathological conditions such as lung consolidation, atelectasis, or pleural disease causing shifting of the mediastinum.
3. Marked right heart enlargement. In severe right heart enlargement, such as pulmonic stenosis, tetralogy of Fallot, and heartworm disease, the cardiac apex may move away from the sternum.

II. Dorsoventral or ventrodorsal projection

A. In the dog, there is minimal variation in the cardiac position, while in the cat the cardiac position is more variable.

B. Malposition of the heart to the right (dextroposition, secondary dextrocardia) is the most commonly observed positional abnormality:

1. A normal variant in the cat
2. Frequently due to uneven lung inflation (e.g., as in mediastinal shift)

3. Commonly seen in wide-chested-breed dogs (e.g., Bulldogs, Bassett Hounds)

C. Primary dextrocardia or intrinsic malposition of the heart is a congenital variant and may be seen in the following conditions:
   1. Situs inversus
   2. Kartagener's syndrome (triad of situs inversus, chronic bronchitis, and sinusitis)
   3. Severe cardiac malformations (complex congenital defects)
   4. Pectus excavatum or "funnel chest"—a congenital sternal deformity

D. A shift of the cardiac apex to the left is common in generalized cardiomegaly and in marked right heart enlargement.

E. A shift of the cardiac apex to the right of the midline is common in both normal cats and in cats with left heart enlargement.

Radiographic Assessment of the Heart in Disease (Table 2-1)

The heart has only a limited means of responding to the stress of disease, so that several disease conditions can cause similar morphologic and/or functional cardiac abnormalities.

The abnormalities of cardiac shape and size observed on cardiac radiographs represent variable combinations of functional disorders:

I. Changes of blood volume in the cardiac chambers (e.g., systole versus diastole)
II. Cardiac dilation
III. Changes in muscle mass of the cardiac chambers (e.g., hypertrophy)
IV. Changes in epicardial and pericardial fat
V. Changes in pericardial fluid content

Pertinent Questions

In a patient with heart disease or suspected heart disease, the radiographic assessment should answer the following questions:

I. Is the heart larger or smaller than normal?

TABLE 2-1. TYPICAL RADIOGRAPHIC FINDINGS IN HEART DISEASE

Lesion	RA	RV	LA	LV	Aorta	MPA	Circ	PV	VC	Other Features
Congenial Defects										
Patent ductus arteriosus	N	↑	↑	↑	↑	↑	↑	↑	N↑	Pulmonary edema common
Pulmonic stenosis	↑	↑	N↓	N↓	N	↑	N↓	N↓	↑	Apex displacement mimics left ventricular hypertrophy
Aortic stenosis	N	N↑	N↑	↑	↑	N	N	N↑	N	Widened cranial mediastinum is common
Ventricular septal defect	N	↑	↑	↑	N	N↑	↑	N↑	N↑	Findings vary; may be part of endocardial cushion in cats
Tetralogy of Fallot	N↑	↑	N↓	N↓	N	N↑	↓	↓	N	Aortic position is cranial and may widen cranial mediastinum; apex shift is common
Atrial septal defect	↑	↑	N↑	N	N	N↑	N↑	N	N↑	Generalized cardiomegaly if VSD is also present
Acquired Heart Disease										
Mitral insufficiency	N	N↑	↑	↑	N	N	N	↑	N	Can be secondary to cardiomyopathy, endocarditis or left-to-right shunt
Tricuspid insufficiency	↑	↑	N	N	N	N	N	N	↑	Can be secondary to cardiomyopathy, dirofilariasis or pulmonic stenosis
Aortic insufficiency	N	N↑	↑	↑	N↑	N	N	N↑	N	Caused by endocarditis or as congenital heart defect
Hypertrophic cardiomyopathy	↑	↑	↑	N↑	N	N	N	↑	N↑	"Valentine" shaped heart, apex shift, frequently with pulmonary edema; pleural effusion less common
Congestive (dilated) cardiomyopathy	↑	↑	↑	↑	N↓	N	N↓	↑	↑	Frequently associated with pleural effusion; pulmonary edema less common
Dirofilariasis	↑	↑	N	N	N	↑	↑	N	↑	Enlarged pulmonary arteries, pulmonary infiltrates common
Pericardial effusion	↑	↑	↑	↑	N↓	N	N↓	↑	↑	Globoid cardiac silhouette

RA = right atrium; RV = right ventricle; LA = Left atrium; LV = left ventricle; MPA = main pulmonary artery; PV = pulmonary veins; VC = caudal vena cava; N = normal, ↑ = enlarged or increased, ↓ = smaller or decreased.

Adapted from Meyer CW & Bonagura JD: Survey radiography of the heart. Vet Clin N Am 12, No.2: 223, 1982

II. Is the cardiac apex displaced to the left or the right?
III. Is the cardiac shape normal or abnormal? If abnormal, which cardiac chambers are most severely altered in size and/or configuration?
IV. Are the pulmonary vessels and great vessels normal in size, shape, and position?
V. Is there pleural fluid visible on the radiograph?
VI. Is there evidence of abnormal pulmonary infiltrates? (e.g., as with pulmonary edema)
VII. Can the abnormalities be explained by heart disease alone, or is there concurrent related or unrelated disease present?

Diagnosis

By answering these questions, one or more of the following conclusions can be reached:

I. The radiographs are compatible with heart disease.
II. The radiographs indicate heart failure.
III. It is unlikely that the clinical abnormalities or radiographic impressions are due to heart disease.
IV. Concurrent heart disease with another disease process is likely.
V. The findings are equivocal and additional diagnostic tests and/or special radiographic procedures are needed to arrive at a diagnosis (e.g., diagnostic tests such as biochemical profile, bronchoscopy, fluid analysis, biopsy, or special studies such as esophagram, angiogram)

Cardiac Silhouette

The cardiac silhouette refers to the shadow seen on a radiographic image of the heart, including a summation density of the heart muscle, intracardiac blood, the pericardium, the pericardial content, and the origins of the major vessels, such as the aorta, the pulmonary artery, and the vena cavae. It sometimes includes adjacent extracardiac structures, such as fat in the sternopericardiac ligament, or fluid layered or loculated around the cardiac apex. The cardiac silhouette should be determined as normal in size, enlarged in size (cardiomegaly), or decreased in size (microcardia).

I. Normal heart size with underlying disease: Includes the following possible causes:
   A. Rapidly developing myocardial failure
   B. Endocarditis
   C. Myocarditis
   D. Toxic cardiomyopathy
   E. Conditions in which muscular hypertrophy develops at the expense of ventricular volume (concentric hypertrophy)
   F. Constrictive pericarditis
   G. Cardiac tamponade (e.g., hemopericardium from rupture of the heart due to trauma or neoplasia)
   H. Cardiac contusion
   I. Severe arrhythmias

II. Cardiomegaly: a subjective description of increased heart size; usually but not invariably present in heart failure; can be due to dilation and/or hypertrophy:
   A. Dilation
      1. This is a normal adaptive mechanism that enables the heart to accept an increased venous return or to cope with an insufficient (leaky) valve.
      2. Dilation also occurs as the result of reduced myocardial contractility (e.g., dilated cardiomyopathy).
   B. Hypertrophy
      1. It is a compensatory mechanism that enables the heart to respond to increased wall stress and prevent its increase.
      2. Hypertrophy can be pressure induced (as in pulmonic or aortic stenosis) or can be induced by an increased volume load and ejection tension (e.g., insufficient valve). In the latter example, hypertrophy permits an increase in cardiac output into the aorta or pulmonary artery, despite backflow into the left atrium or right atrium, respectively.

III. Microcardia: The term used to describe a decrease in heart size; it is most commonly associated with the following noncardiac conditions:
   A. Hypovolemic shock
   B. Dehydration

C. Hypocorticism (Addison's disease)
D. Pneumothorax and hyperinflation of the lungs (the heart usually appears smaller due to the relative size of the heart compared with the size of the lungs)

Evaluation of Heart Chamber Enlargement

Right Atrial Enlargement

I. Radiographic signs
  A. Lateral projection
    1. Elevation of the trachea as it courses dorsally over the right atrium
    2. Loss of the cranial waist
  B. Dorsoventral projection
    1. Enlargement of the cardiac border at the 9 to 11 o'clock position tion
II. Causes of right atrial enlargement
  A. Right heart failure
  B. Tricuspid insufficiency
  C. Cardiomyopathy
  D. Right atrial tumor
III. Differential diagnosis
  A. Cranial mediastinal tumor
  B. Heart-based tumor (e.g., chemodectoma)
  C. Hilar lymphadenopathy
  D. Superimposed enlargement of the main pulmonary artery or aortic arch

Right Ventricular Enlargement

I. Radiographic signs
  A. Lateral projection
    1. Increased sternal contact of the right heart

2. Dorsal elevation of the trachea relative to the thoracic spine
3. Rounding of the right heart border
4. Elevation of the caudal vena cava

B Dorsoventral projection

1. An abnormally rounded right heart border
2. In marked enlargement, the right ventricle sometimes assumes an inverted D sign
3. Shift of the cardiac apex to the left

II. Causes of right ventricular enlargement

A. Secondary to left heart failure, frequently caused by decompensated mitral insufficiency
B. Tricuspid insufficiency
C. Cardiomyopathy
D. Cor pulmonale
E. Dirofilariasis (heartworm disease)
F. Congenital heart disease
   1. Pulmonic stenosis
   2. Left to right shunts (e.g., patent ductus arteriosus, ventricular septal defects)
   3. Tetralogy of Fallot

Left Atrial Enlargement

I. Radiographic signs

A. Lateral projection
   1. In the dog
      a) Dorsal elevation of the distal portion of the trachea and carina
      b) Dorsal displacement of the mainstream bronchi (the left bronchus will appear more dorsal than the right bronchus)
      c) Visible prominence of the left atrium with straightening of its border and loss of the caudal waist
   2. In the cat
      a) Slight elevation of the distal trachea and carina
      b) Usually does not displace the left bronchus
B. Dorsoventral projection
   1. Enlargement of the left auricular appendage, which extends beyond the heart border between the 2 to 3 o'clock position
   2. A "double density" of the atrial body over the heart base

II. Causes of left atrial enlargement
  A. Mitral insufficiency
  B. Cardiomyopathy
  C. Congenital heart disease
    1. Congenital mitral insufficiency
    2. Patent ductus arteriosus (PDA)
  D. Left ventricular failure due to any cause
III. Differential diagnosis
  A. Hilar lymphadenopathy
  B. Lung mass adjacent to hilus

Left Ventricular Enlargement

I. Radiographic signs
  A. Lateral projection
    1. Loss of caudal waist
    2. Left heart border straighter and more vertical than normal
  B. Dorsoventral projection
    1. Rounding of the left ventricular border
    2. Shift of the cardiac apex to the right

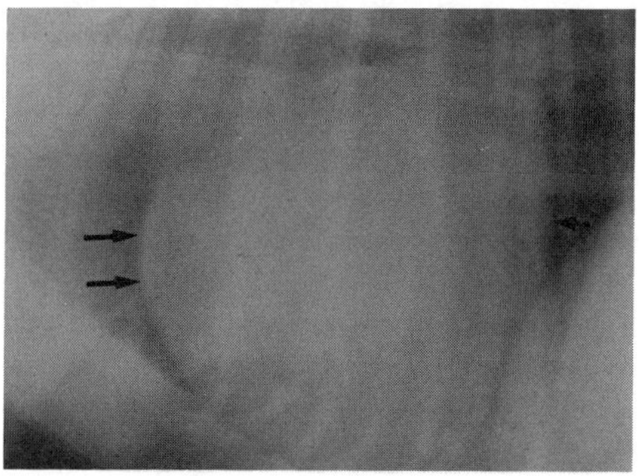

Fig. 2-7. Generalized cardiomegaly. There is increased sternal contact of the right ventricle, bulging of the cranial cardiac border due to right auricular enlargement (arrows), and elevation of the trachea. The caudal cardiac border is straightened due to left ventricular enlargement (arrow), there is loss of the caudal waist due to left atrial enlargement, and elevation of the caudal vena cava. The hilar pulmonary veins and the border of the left atrium are indistinct due to perivascular congestion.

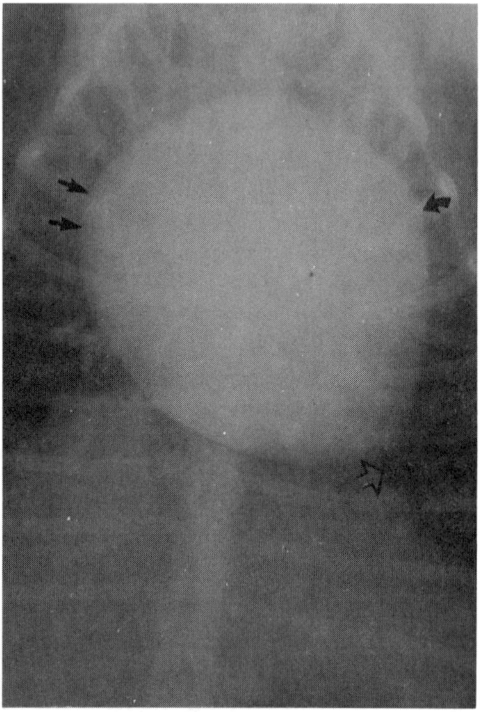

Fig. 2-8. Generalized cardiomegaly. The cardiac silhouette is enlarged and more rounded than normal with bulging of the right atrium (double arrows), left atrium (single arrow), right ventricular enlargement, left ventricular enlargement and displacement of the cardiac apex to the left (open arrow).

II. Causes of left ventricular enlargement
  A. Mitral insufficiency
  B. Cardiomyopathy
  C. Congenital heart disease
    1. Patent ductus arteriosus
    2. Aortic stenosis
    3. Ventricular septal defect (left-to-right shunt)
  D. High-output heart disease
    1. Hypervolemia (e.g., fluid overload)
    2. Chronic anemia
    3. Peripheral arteriovenous fistula

4. Obesity
5. Chronic renal disease

Generalized Heart Enlargement (Figs. 2-7 and 2-8)

I. Radiographic signs
  A. Variable degrees of enlargement of two or more cardiac chambers
  B. Enlargement implies dilation, hypertrophy, or both
II. Causes of generalized heart enlargement
  A. Coexistent right and left heart failure
  B. Chronic mitral and tricuspid insufficiency
  C. Cardiomyopathy
  D. Decompensated congenital heart defects
III. Differential diagnosis
  A. Pericardial effusion
  B. Peritoneal–pericardial diaphragmatic hernia
  C. Obesity

Evaluation of the Major Vessels

Enlargement of the Aortic Arch and Aorta

I. Radiographic signs
  A. Lateral projection
    1. Elongated cardiac silhouette
    2. Protrusion of the craniodorsal heart border
  B. Dorsoventral projection
    1. Widening of the cranial heart border at the 11 to 1 o'clock position
II. Causes of enlarged aortic arch
  A. Patent ductus arteriosus; an aneurysm-like dilation (ductus diver-

ticulum) best seen on the dorsoventral projection to the left of the descending portion of the aortic arch

B. Aortic stenosis with a poststenotic enlargement of the aortic arch

C. Aortic aneurysm (rare)

III. Differential diagnosis

A. Normal variation in some dogs

B. Common in aged cats with a more horizontal heart position and prominence of the aortic knob; particularly prominent on the dorsoventral projection

Enlargement of the Pulmonary Artery Segment

I. Radiographic signs

A. Lateral projection: Protrusion of the craniodorsal heart border

B. Dorsoventral projection: Lateral bulge at the 1 to 2 o'clock position just caudal to the aortic arch

II. Causes of enlarged pulmonary artery segment

A. Pulmonic stenosis (poststenotic dilation)

B. Dirofilariasis

C. Patent ductus arteriosus

D. Septal defects with left-to-right shunting (VSD or ASD)

E. Pulmonary thrombosis

III. Differential diagnosis

A. Positional artifact, usually seen on ventrodorsal projection

Evaluation of the Pulmonary Circulation

Undercirculation

I. Radiographic signs

A. The lung field is more radiolucent than normal.

B. The pulmonary arteries are smaller than normal and may be less than their corresponding veins.

II. Causes of undercirculation
  A. Right-to-left shunting (e.g., tetralogy of Fallot)
  B. Pulmonic stenosis (relative undercirculation)
  C. Hypovolemia (the heart is also smaller than normal)
  D Hypocorticism (Addison's disease); the heart may also be smaller than normal
III. Differential diagnosis
  A. Emphysema
  B. Overinflation
  C. Pneumothorax
  D. Overexposure

Overcirculation

I. Radiographic signs
  A. The pulmonary arteries and veins are enlarged.
  B. The arteries are frequently larger than corresponding veins.
  C. The lung field appears more opaque than normal due to increased pulmonary vasculature.
II. Causes for overcirculation and/or enlarged vessels
  A. Dirofilariasis (arteries are larger than corresponding veins)
  B. Patent ductus arteriosus (PDA)
  C. Left-to-right shunts (VSD, ASD)
  D. Congestive heart failure (veins may be larger than the arteries)
  E. Fluid overload
III. Differential diagnosis
  A. Underexposure
  B. Expiratory radiograph

Radiographic Diagnosis of Heart Failure

The radiographic diagnosis of heart failure is based on the recognition of imbalances in the blood and fluid distribution within the body. This circulatory imbalance is the result of diminished cardiac output into the pulmonary or systemic vascular bed and/or a reduced acceptance of blood by the failing ventricle. Depending on which side of the heart is most severely affected, blood is shifted from the systemic to the pulmonary circulation (left heart failure) or from the pulmonary to the systemic circulation (right heart failure).

Right Heart Failure

I. In right heart failure, an inadequate right ventricular output into the pulmonary arteries exists concurrently with a reduced acceptance of blood from the systemic veins. The blood volume and pressure in the splanchnic and systemic veins are elevated.
   A. The venous congestion causes hepatomegaly.
   B. There is a progressive increase in the amounts of fluid, solutes, and protein that escape from the capillary beds of the liver and bowel.
   C. When this excessive fluid can no longer be disposed of by an increased lymph flow, fluid exudes into the serosal cavities, causing pleural effusion, ascites, and pericardial effusion.

II. Pleural effusion
   A. Radiographic signs
      1. Visualization of interlobar fissures
      2. Separation of visceral pleura away from the chest wall
      3. "Leafing" of the lung lobes
   B. Causes of pleural effusion due to right heart failure
      1. Decompensated mitral and tricuspid insufficiencies
      2. Decompensated pulmonic stenosis
      3. Decompensated tetralogy of Fallot
      4. Dirofilariasis (caval syndrome)
      5. Pericardial effusion (due to any cause)
      6. Restrictive pericarditis
   C. Differential diagnosis
      1. Pleuritis
      2. Chylothorax
      3. Hemothorax
      4. Pyothorax
      5. Hypoproteinemia
      6. Neoplasia (primary or metastatic)

III. Hepatomegaly
  A. Radiographic signs
    1. Rounded liver margin
    2. Liver margin extends caudal to last rib
    3. Displacement of the stomach caudally and to the left
  B. Causes of cardiac-related hepatomegaly
    1. Any cardiac disease that is decompensated to produce right heart failure (congenital or acquired)
    2. Increased venous pressure of the caudal vena cava
  C. Differential diagnosis
    1. Hepatitis
    2. Congestion
    3. Neoplasia (primary or metastatic)
    4. Lipidosis
    5. Steroid-induced hepatopathy

IV. Ascites
  A. Radiographic signs
    1. Loss of abdominal detail
    2. Distended abdomen
    3. Hepatomegaly usually present
  B. Causes of cardiac-related ascites
    1. Any decompensated heart disease producing right heart failure (congenital or acquired)
    2. Increased venous pressure in the caudal vena cava or within the portal system
  C. Differential diagnosis
    1. Hypoproteinemia
    2. Peritonitis
    3. Carcinomatosis
    4. Hemoperitoneum (e.g., trauma, ruptured abdominal tumor)
    5. Ruptured urinary bladder

Left Heart Failure

I. In left heart failure, there is inadequate left ventricular output into the aorta and a diminished acceptance of blood from the pulmonary veins entering the left atrium. This ongoing process ultimately causes pulmonary edema. This edema can be divided into three distinct phases of failure, which can be correlated radiographically and clinically: pulmonary congestion, interstitial lung edema, alveolar edema.

A. Pulmonary congestion
   1. Radiographic signs
      a) Engorgement and distention of the pulmonary veins, especially in the hilar area as they enter the left atrium
      b) The diameter and density of the veins is equal to or slightly greater than that of the corresponding pulmonary arteries.
      c) The radiopacity of the lung fields away from the hilus is unchanged.
B. Interstitial lung edema
   1. Radiographic signs
      a) There is a diffuse increased radiopacity of the lung fields due to a hazy interstitial density.
      b) The borders of the pulmonary veins and arteries are indistinct due to perivascular edema.
      c) In some patients, fluid accumulates around the major bronchi, producing prominent bronchial markings.
C. Alveolar edema
   1. Radiographic signs
      a) Fluid enters the alveolar airspaces and peripheral bronchioles, causing a coalescent fluffy alveolar infiltrate. Air bronchograms and air alveolograms are usually present.
      b) The borders of the pulmonary vessels are usually completely obscured especially in marked alveolar flooding of the airspaces. The alveolar infiltrate is usually of greatest opacity in the perihilar area fading peripherally. In some animals, asymmetric alveolar edema affects one lung more than the other.
      c) Small amounts of pleural fluid can occur as seen by the presence of pleural fissure lines, indicating either pleural edema or small amounts of pleural effusion.

II. Radiographic signs of left heart failure
   A. Venous congestion and perivascular edema
   B. Interstitial edema
   C. Alveolar edema with increased opacity in the hilar area radiating peripherally

   D. Increased bronchial markings in some cases
   E. Small amounts of pleural effusion in some cases

III. Causes of pulmonary edema
   A. Cardiogenic
      1. Decompensated mitral insufficiency
      2. Decompensated cardiomyopathy
      3. Arrhythmias (acute or chronic) with decompensation
   B. Noncardiogenic
      1. Neurogenic
         a) Electrocution
         b) Head trauma
         c) Postictal
         d) Encephalitis, brain tumor
      2. Fluid overload
      3. ANTU poisoning
      4. Drowning

SUGGESTED READINGS

Ettinger SJ, Suter PF: Canine Cardiology.WB Saunders, Philadelphia, 1970

Hamlin RL: Radiographic diagnosis of heart disease in dogs. J Am Vet Med Assoc 137:458, 1963

Lord PF, Zontine WJ: Radiographic examination of the feline cardiovascular system. Vet Clin North Am [Small Anim Pract] 7:291, 1977.

Myer CW, Bonagura JD: Survey radiography of the heart. Vet Clin North Am [Small Anim Pract] 12:213, 1982

Owens JM, Twedt DC: Nonselective angiography in the cat. Vet Clin North Am [Small Anim Pract] 7:309, 1977

Owens JM: Radiographic Interpretation for the Small Animal Clinician. Ralston Purina Co, St Louis, 1982

Rhodes WH, Patterson DF, Detweiler DK: Radiographic anatomy of the canine heart. Part I. J Am Vet Med Assoc 137:283, 1960

Rhodes WH, Patterson DF, Detweiler DK: Radiographic anatomy of the canine heart. Part II. J Am Vet Med Assoc 143:137, 1963

Silverman S, Suter PF: Influence of inspiration and expiration on canine thoracic radiographs. J Am Vet Med Assoc 166:502, 1975

Suter PF: The radiographic diagnosis of canine and feline heart disease. Comp Cont Ed 3:441, 1981

Suter PF, Gomez, JA: Diseases of the Thorax: Radiographic Diagnosis. Venture Press, Davis, Calif, 1981

Suter PF, Lord PF: A critical evaluation of the radiographic findings in canine cardiovascular diseases. J Am Vet Med Assoc 158:358, 1971

Suter PF, Lord PF: Thoracic Radiography: A Text Atlas of Thoracic Disease of the Dog and Cat. Peter F. Suter, Wettswil, Switzerland, 1984

Watters JW: Radiographic signs of cardiovascular disease. Comp Cont Ed 1:766, 1979

3

Electrocardiography

Charla L. Jones

PRINCIPLES OF ELECTROCARDIOGRAPHY

ELECTROPHYSIOLOGY

I. Definition
  A. The electrocardiogram (ECG) is a recording of the voltage and direction of electrical activity during depolarization and repolarization of cardiac muscle cells plotted against time.
  B. Normally, electrical activation of the cells or "depolarization" stimulates myocardial contraction.
  C. "Repolarization," or restoration of the electrical potential of the cells, occurs towards the end of cardiac contraction.

II. Procedure for performing the technique
  A. Electrodes attached to the skin serve as positive and negative terminals of a lead system used for monitoring the electrical activity throughout the electrical cycle.
  B. An electrical wave moving toward the positive electrode registers a positive deflection on the ECG, while an electrical wave moving away from the electrode registers a negative deflection.
  C. When the wave is moving perpendicular to the positive or negative electrode, the deflections are small or absent.

III. Clinical use
  A. Examination of the electrical activity from multiple leads permits evaluation of the site of origination of an electrical stimulus, its anatomic progress as a wave of depolarization, and the repolarization process.

B. Results can be compared with activity considered normal in animals of similar species, conformation, size, and age.

Application of the Technique

I. The ECG serves as a valuable tool:
  A. In diagnosing cardiac arrhythmias
  B. In evaluating response to therapy
  C. In providing information regarding some pathologic or physiologic processes affecting the heart
II. Serial ECG recordings may be particularly useful in monitoring progressive cardiac disease processes or the responses to therapy.
III. The ECG is best used in conjunction with a complete clinical history, physical examination, and other cardiovascular diagnostic procedures:
  A. Significant cardiovascular disease may exist, producing only minor alterations in the ECG or no electrocardiographic abnormalities at all.
  B. The ECG does not directly indicate mechanical function of the heart, and a diagnosis should not rest on the basis of an ECG recording alone.

RECORDING THE ELECTROCARDIOGRAM

Recording techniques vary depending on the status of the patient, the purpose of the desired information, and the equipment available. Ideally, the more versatile the equipment, the more effectively it can be used. However, even relatively simple equipment can be an asset in patient evaluation and monitoring.

Use of Equipment

I. Equipment
  A. Basically, the electrocardiograph is a voltage meter and amplifier that feeds electrical information into a display system such as a strip recorder or an oscilloscope.

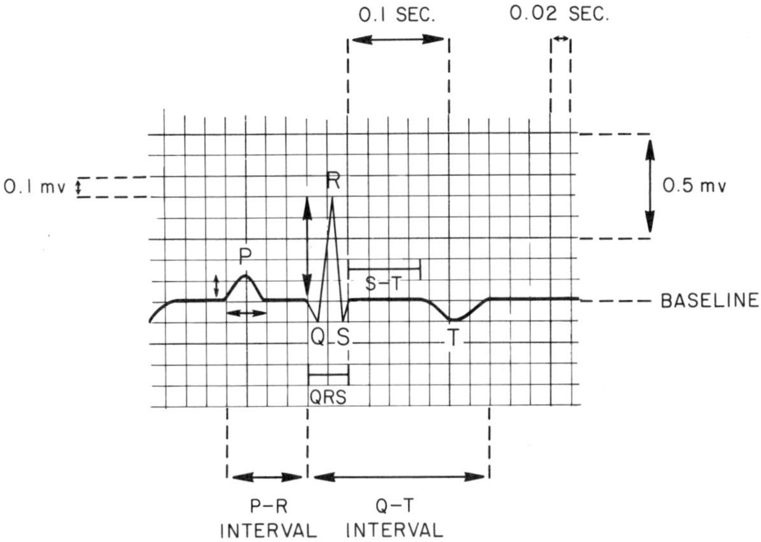

Fig. 3-1. Closeup of a normal feline lead II P-QRS-T complex with labels and intervals. Measurements for amplitude (millivolts) are indicated by positive (+) and negative (−) movement; time intervals (hundredths of a second) are indicated from left to right. Paper speed, 50 mm/sec; sensitivity 1 cm = 1 mV. (From Tilley LP: Essentials of Cainine and Feline Electrocardiography—Interpretation and Treatment. Lea & Febiger, Philadelphia, 1985.)

B. In its simplest form, the ECG may be capable of monitoring only one to three leads.

C. More sophisticated equipment has the capacity to select multiple leads of observation, to adjust the recording sensitivity and paper speed, and to adjust stylus position and stylus heat to improve the clarity of the trace.

II. Settings

A. Sensitivity normally used in recording is 1 cm = 1 mV:

1. If the complexes are too large, the sensitivity may be reduced to 0.5 cm = 1 mV.
2. If the complexes are too small, they can be amplified by increasing the sensitivity to 2 cm = 1 mV.

B. Recording speed may be 25 mm/sec or 50 mm/sec; if the heart rate is very rapid, 50 mm/sec spreads the complexes in order to increase the ease and accuracy of measurements.

C. Stylus position should be centered on the paper such that all portions of complexes remain within the margins of the recording paper.

III. Paper

A. The electrocardiographic paper is marked with a grid of 1-mm horizontal and vertical lines and heavier lines at every fifth millimeter (Fig. 3-1):

1. The vertical lines marking 1 mm would equal 0.04 seconds at a paper speed of 25 mm/sec and 0.02 seconds at 50 mm/sec.
2. Horizontal 1-mm markings would equal 0.1 mV at a sensitivity setting of 1 (1 cm = 1 mV), 0.05 mV at a sensitivity of 2 (2 cm = 1 mV), and 0.2 mV at a sensitivity of ½ (0.5 cm = 1 mV).

B. Time markers are spaced on the paper margin every 75 mm.

Recording Technique

I. Electrodes

A. The standard electrocardiogram uses five electrodes attached to the left (LA) and right (RA) forelegs, in close proximity to and equidistant from the olecranon, left (LL) and right (RL) hindlegs, equidistant from the patella, and an exploring precordial chest electrode (C).

B. To facilitate conduction, a contact medium such as alcohol, commercial electrode gels or paste, or phisohex should be used to moisten the skin at the site of electrode attachment.

II. Body position

A. Right lateral recumbent

1. The animal is positioned with the legs extended perpendicular to the long axis of the body.
2. In this position, all 10 leads used for dogs and cats can be recorded.

B. Sternal recumbent, standing, or sitting position

1. A monitoring ECG, such as a lead II or base–apex lead, may be recorded quickly and easily.
2. This position is particularly useful for monitoring cardiac rhythm when the animal is difficult to restrain, in pain, or exhibiting respiratory distress.

III. Restraint
  A. Manual restraint is usually adequate if care is taken to calm the animal and minimize discomfort.
  B. Chemical restraint can affect cardiac rhythm, rate, and complex intervals and therefore should be used only when necessary.

IV. Recording identification
  A. The identity of the animal, date, time, animal position, recording sensitivity, paper speed, and lead identification should be clearly indicated on the recording.
  B. Any changes in these parameters and special conditions such as anesthesia used during the recording should be noted.

LEADS

Table 3-1 specifies the electrode terminal positions for the standard limb and special chest and base–apex leads.

I. Recording sequence

TABLE 3-1. LEAD SYSTEMS USED IN CANINE AND FELINE ELECTROCARDIOGRAPHY

Standard limb leads
Bipolar limb leads
I right arm (−) compared with left arm (+)
II right arm (−) compared with left leg (+)
III left arm (−) compared with left leg (+)
Augmented unipolar limb leads
aVR right arm (+) compared with average voltage of left arm and left leg (−)
aVL left arm (+) compared with average voltage of right arm and left leg (−)
aVF left leg (+) compared with average voltage of right arm and left arm (−)
Unipolar precordial chest leads
plus exploring electrode located as follows:
CV6LL (V2) sixth left intercostal space near costosternal junction
CV6LU (V4) sixth left intercostal space at costochondral junction
V10 over dorsal spinous process of seventh thoracic vertebra
CV5RL (rV2) fifth right intercostal space near costosternal junction
Base–Apex Bipolar Monitoring Lead
Record on lead I of selector. Position electrodes as follows:
LA electrode over left sixth intercostal space at costosternal junction
RA electrode over spine of right scapula near the vertebra
Complexes resemble lead II.

A. The typical recording sequence is standard limb lead I, II, III, aVR, aVL, aVF.
B. Chest leads are CV6LL, CV6LU, V10, and CV5RL.
C. The RL electrode always serves as an electrical ground in all leads.
D. An electrical abnormality may not be apparent in all leads, so that multiple leads are desirable and advantageous in a detailed electrocardiographic evaluation.

II. Standard limb leads
   A. The standard limb leads examine the electrical activity in the frontal plane of the body.
   B. Leads I, II, and III are bipolar leads that record electrical activity between the two electrodes used in each.
   C. Leads aVR, aVL, and aVF are augmented unipolar limb leads that use three electrodes each, in which the reference limb (+ terminal) is compared with the sum of the electrical activity of the two other limbs (− terminal).

III. Unipolar precordial chest leads
   A. The unipolar precordial chest leads use a positive exploring electrode positioned at indicated locations over the chest.
   B. The RA, LA, and LL electrodes are internally connected by the electrocardiograph to serve as a zero reference equivalent to the center of the heart in the chest leads.
   C. When recorded on the V position of the lead selector switch, the chest leads record the direction and voltage of electrical activity from the heart to the electrode position.
   D. The chest leads are necessary in determining electrical activity in the sagittal and horizontal planes of the body.

ANALYZING THE ELECTROCARDIOGRAM

Analysis should be both thorough and systematic. Interpretation should include determinations of heart rate, cardiac rhythm and rhythm disturbances, measurements of amplitudes and intervals, and determination of the mean electrical axis. (The range of normal values for dogs and cats is listed in Table 3-2.) Measurements should be taken at several locations in

TABLE 3-2. NORMAL ELECTROCARDIOGRAPHIC MEASUREMENTS

Parameter	Canine	Feline
Heart rate (beats/min)	70 to 160 for adults Up to 180 for toy breeds Up to 220 for puppies	160 to 240
Rhythm	Normal sinus rhythm Sinus arrhythmia Wandering atrial pacemaker	Normal sinus rhythm Sinus tachycardia
Intervals (sec)		
P	Maximum 0.04	Maximum 0.04
PR	0.06 to 0.13	0.05 to 0.09
QRS	Maximum 0.06 in large breeds Maximum 0.05 in toy breeds	0.04
QT	0.15 to 0.25	0.12 to 0.18
Amplitudes (mV) in lead II		
P	Maximum 0.4	0.2
R	Maximum 3.0 in large breeds Maximum 2.5 in small breeds	0.9
T	No greater than one-fourth the amplitude of the R wave +, − or biphasic	0.3 +, − or biphasic
in CV6LL		
R	Maximum 2.5	
S	Maximum 0.8	
in CV6LU		
R	Maximum 3.0	Maximum 1.0
S	Maximum 0.7	
Mean electrical axis in frontal plane	+40 to +100 degrees	0 to + 160 degrees

order to adjust for normal variation with respiration or heart rate and because full duration of an electrical event may not be apparent in every lead.

I. Heart rate

A. Heart rate can be determined by counting the number of complexes between two sets of time markers and multiplying by 10 or 20 if the paper speed is 25 or 50 mm/sec, respectively.

B. If the rhythm is very regular or the strip is too short to use this technique, the R-R interval can be counted and the number of millimeters divided into 1,500 mm/min (for a speed of 25 mm/sec) or 3,000 mm/min (for a speed of 50 mm/sec), which would give the number of beats per minute.

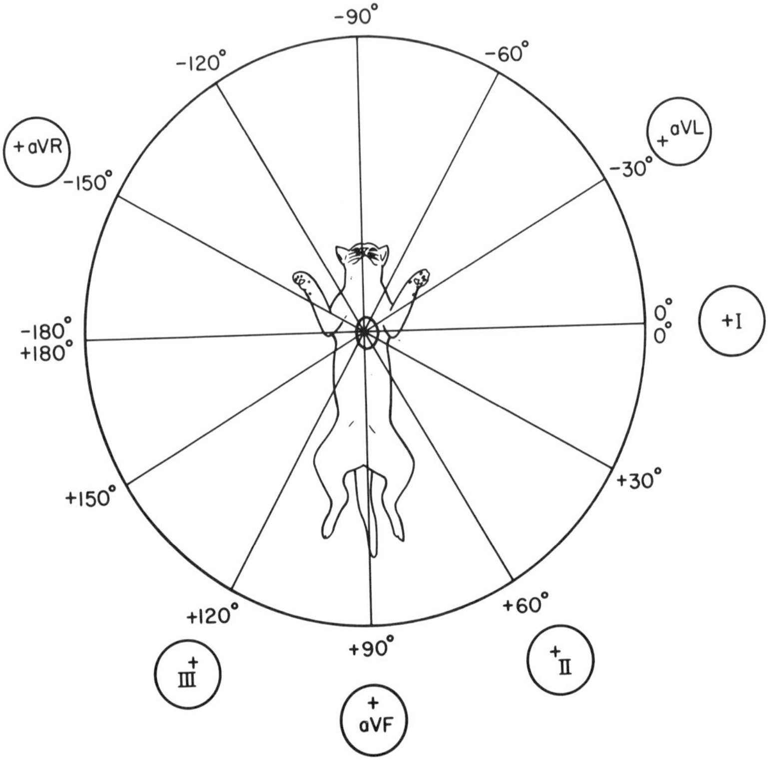

Fig. 3-2. The hexaxial lead system can be enclosed in a circle superimposed on the frontal plane of the animal's body with the heart at the center. The leads are marked with a + sign at the positive electrode. Left ventricular enlargement produces greater amplitude of ventricular electrical forces to the animal's left, while right ventricular enlargement produces a shift in the sum of the forces to the right. Normal mean electrical axis for the feline is 0 to + 160 degrees, and for the dog + 40 to + 100 degrees. (From Tilley LP: Essentials of Canine and Feline Electrocardiography—Interpretation and Treatment, Lea & Febiger, Philadelphia, 1985.).

C. The heart rate varies normally with age, breed size, physical fitness, and degree of excitation.

II. Rhythm

A. Rhythm determination requires recognition of all components of the P–QRS–T complexes, evaluation of their configuration and spatial relationships, and a knowledge of what is normal as opposed to abnormal.

B. An understanding of the propagation sequence of the normal cardiac impulse is essential in order to determine the nature of a disturbance in conduction.

III. Intervals

A. Interval measurements may be performed in any lead in which the complexes are of adequate size to make measurements possible. Figure 3-1 demonstrates where intervals should be measured.

B. The longest measurements found in any one lead are considered correct.

C. Prolongation of an interval indicates a delay in conduction, depolarization, or repolarization.

1. P interval: The time necessary for atrial depolarization
2. P-R or P-Q interval: The time from initiation of the atrial depolarization, conduction through the atrioventricular (AV) node, bundle of His, bundle branches, and Purkinje fibers
3. QRS interval: The time of ventricular cell depolarization
4. Q-T interval: The time in which ventricular depolarization and repolarization occur

IV. Amplitudes

A. Amplitudes are measured in lead II from the baseline to peak of the deflection for each wave.

B. Figure 3-1 demonstrates where measurements of amplitudes are taken. The P, Q, R, S, and T wave measurements are considered important.

V. Mean electrical axis

A. The MEA is a determination of the sum of voltage and direction of the heart's ventricular electrical activity in a 360-degree circle assigned to the frontal plane of the body (Fig. 3-2).

B. A similar axis determination can be calculated for the atrial depolarization, ventricular depolarization, and repolarization in the frontal, sagittal, and horizontal planes of the body.

1. An abnormal rotation or deviation of this axis is most frequently seen in right ventricular enlargement and intraventricular conduction disturbances in cats and dogs.
2. Rapid determination of the frontal MEA can generally be performed:

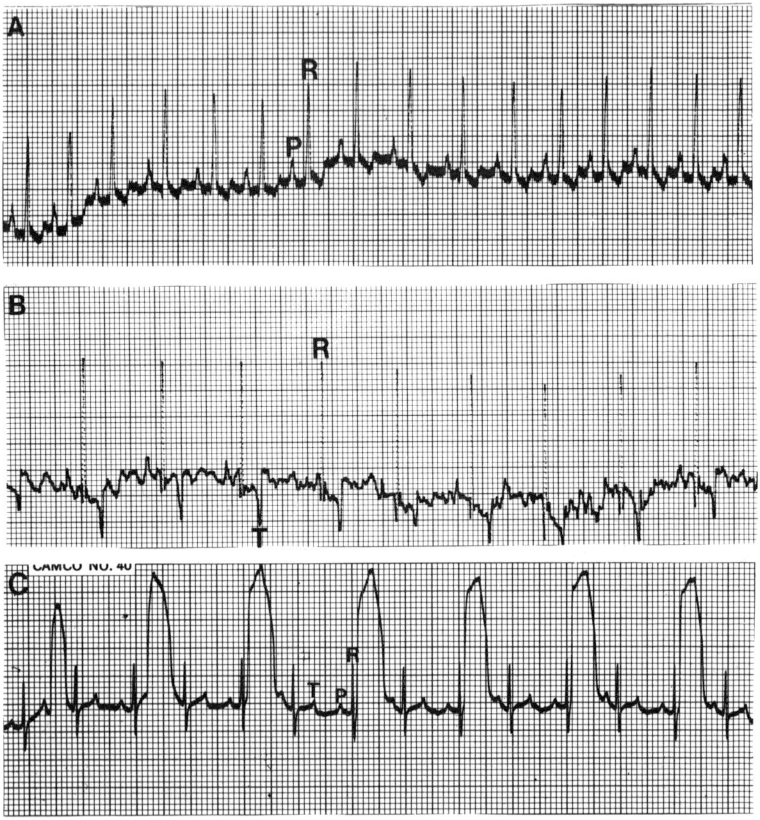

Fig. 3-3. Artifacts may make interpretation of the ECG difficult, as illustrated in these three canine tracings recorded at 1 cm = 1 mV and 25 mm/sec. (A) Sixty-cycle interference produces heavy, regular sawtooth undulations of the baseline interfering with interval measurements in this lead II recording. (B) Shivering in this lead II recording produces irregular, rapid baseline undulations that distort complex shapes and amplitudes. (C) Hiccups at a rate of 80 per minute in this lead aVF recording produce regular baseline motion that has no effect on the cardiac sinus rhythm and heart rate of 140 beats/min.

a) By first identifying the most isoelectric QRS in a standard limb lead (I, II, III, aVR, aVL, aVF).
b) Next determine the sum of the QRS deflections in the lead which is perpendicular to the isoelectric lead in the hexaxial system.

c) The positive or negative sum of the QRS voltages indicate the direction of the axis.

3. In some cases, the MEA cannot be determined by this method due to the existence of multiple isoelectric leads. (For other methods of axis determination refer to the electrocardiology reference texts listed in the Suggested References.)

NORMAL ELECTROCARDIOGRAM

The range of normal parameters for the ECG of the adult dog and cat is listed in Table 3-2.

I. In the young of both cats and dogs, the heart rates may be faster and intervals shorter.

II. In animals conditioned to exercise, heart rates may be slower than the range given and P-R and Q-T intervals longer than the range given.

III. Lean animals may have higher amplitudes, while obesity or heavy muscle mass will result in lower amplitudes due to damping of electric voltages.

IV. Typically, feline heart rates are more rapid, intervals are shorter, and amplitudes are lower than in dogs.

V. Values that appear to be outside the range of normal for that species may still be normal for the individual animal. Age, body size, conditioning, and degree of excitation must be considered when evaluating the ECG. When possible it is best to use the animal as its own control by recording serial ECGs.

ABNORMAL ELECTROCARDIOGRAM

ARTIFACTS

Abnormalities of the ECG that are not caused by cardiac disorders are known as artifacts. These may result from technical or mechanical errors or from malfunctions during recording. Several artifacts are commonly seen and can usually be corrected with patience and perseverance.

I. 60-cycle interference
  A. This regular sawtooth appearance of the baseline results from improper grounding of the patient, electrocardiograph, or electrical source (Fig. 3-3A).
  B. The artifact may obscure small waveforms and make interval determination difficult or impossible.
  C. Several measures can be taken to alleviate the artifact:
    1. Reapply the electrodes and contact medium directly to the skin.
    2. Avoid attendant contact with the electrodes and table during recording.
    3. Prevent hair or skin contact with electrodes on the adjacent limb.
    4. Place a nonconducting surface (i.e., a rubber mat) under all parts of the animal's body and the ECG cable.
    5. Remove collars or halters with metal parts.
    6. Clean electrode clips and attach them securely to the cables and animal.
    7. The auxiliary electrocardiograph ground (if one is necessary) should be attached to a water pipe.
    8. The electrical outlet servicing the ECG equipment should be a three-pronged plug when possible.
    9. It may be necessary to unplug or turn off other electrical equipment in the room.

II. Tremor of the patient
  A. Muscle fasciculation, panting, shivering, or purring produces an irregular, rapid sawtooth vibration of the baseline that is greater in amplitude as the body motion increases in severity (Fig. 3-3B).
  B. Attempts to calm the animal, make it more comfortable, or stop the purring may reduce the artifact.
  C. In some cases, sedation may be necessary.

III. Wandering of the baseline
  A. More severe limb or body movements, heavy breathing, hiccups, or coughing may produce this artifact (Fig. 3-3C).
  B. Proper restraint or holding the animal's mouth closed for a few seconds may permit recording of strips without baseline motion.
  C. Animals in respiratory distress should be restrained in positions that do not produce further respiratory compromise.

IV. Electrode misplacement
  A. Complexes can be reversed in polarity or be mirror images to what they should be, resembling aberrant conduction patterns.

B. Electrode placement should be checked routinely in every recording.

C. Coding of the limb electrodes by color commonly varies between electrocardiograph equipment, so the alphabetic designation of the electrode should be used for checking limb placement.

P-QRS-T Abnormalities

I. P-wave abnormalities associated with chamber enlargement
   A. Left atrial enlargement
      1. P waves are produced that are wider than normal and often notched, particularly in lead II (Fig. 3-4B).
      2. Because of its common association with mitral valve insufficiency, this P-wave configuration is called p mitrale.
      3. Causes of prolonged-duration P waves would include acquired or congenital cardiovascular diseases resulting in disturbances in the atrial conduction pathway from the sinoatrial (SA) to atrioventricular (AV) node or in left atrial volume or pressure overload:
         a) Mitral valve insufficiency
         b) Patent ductus arteriosus
         c) Aortic stenosis
   B. Right atrial enlargement
      1. P waves of increased amplitude are produced (Fig. 3-4B) in leads II, III, and aVF.
      2. This abnormality is termed p pulmonale, as it is often associated with chronic pulmonary disease causing pulmonary hypertension (e.g., collapsing trachea, bronchitis, pneumonia).
      3. Other causes:
         a) Tricuspid insufficiency
         b) Interatrial septal defects
         c) Rapid heart rates
   C. Biatrial enlargement
      1. P waves result which are tall and wide.
      2. The waves may also be notched and slurred (Fig. 3-4B).
II. QRS abnormalities associated with chamber enlargement
   A. Left ventricular enlargement
      1. The QRS complex is altered resulting in high-amplitude R waves

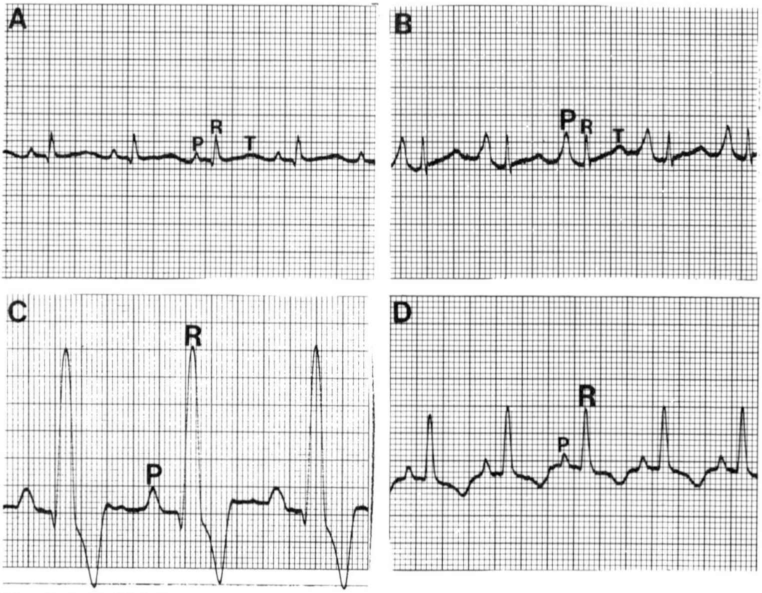

Fig. 3-4. P-QRS-T abnormalities. (A) Normal feline tracing. Note the normal small amplitudes of complexes. (B) Tall (0.5-mV) and wide (0.05-second) P waves in this feline lead II recording indicate right and left atrial enlargement. (C) Left atrial and left ventricular enlargement in a canine. Note the wide P waves (0.06-second) and tall (3.1-mV) and wide (0.07-second) QRS complexes and the S-T segment coving. Left bundle branch block would have to be considered, especially if heart is not enlarged on radiographs. (D) Left ventricular enlargement in a cat. The R waves are high (1.1-mV).

associated with increased ventricular muscle mass (Fig. 3-4C,D).

2. The QRS may be prolonged in duration due to conduction delays associated with severe hypertrophy and/or dilatation.
3. Other features seen in enlargement may include increased T-wave amplitudes, ST-segment depression or coving into the T wave, and MEA deviations to the left.
4. Criteria for LV enlargement in the dog:
   a) R waves 3.0 in lead CV6LU and 2.5 mV in CV6LL
   b) R waves 2.5 in leads II and aVF for dogs older than 2 years of age

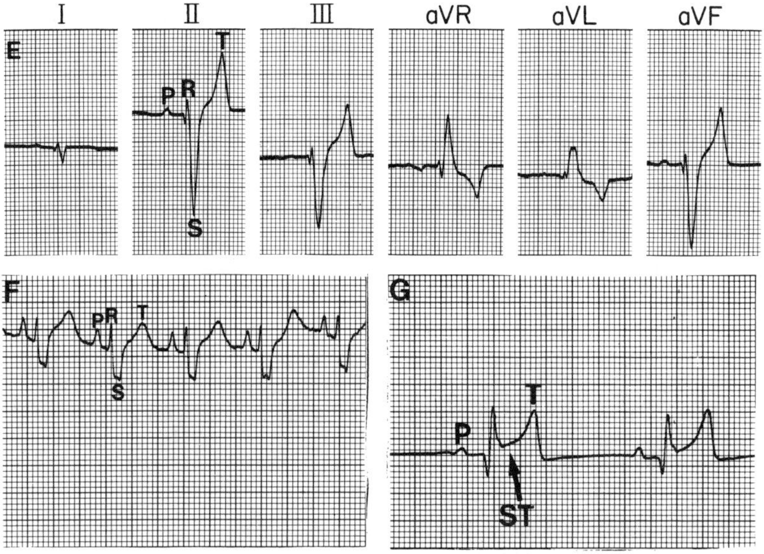

Fig. 3-4(*Cont.*) (E) Right bundle branch block in a dog. The QRS duration is 0.09 seconds, and there are large S waves in I, II, III, and aVF. Right ventricular enlargement should also be considered. (F) Right bundle branch block in a cat. QRS duration is 0.06 second with a large S wave (also present in I, II, III, and aVF). (G) ST segment elevation, large T waves, and small QRS complexes in a dog with pericardial effusion. Paper speed, 50 mm/sec, 1 cm = 1 mV. Single strips are all lead II.

   c) R waves 3.0 mV in II and aVF in dogs less than 2 years of age
5. In the cat, R-wave amplitudes 0.9 mV in lead II and 1.0 mV in CV6LU suggest LV enlargement.
6. Causes of LV enlargement:
   a) Congenital anomalies (e.g., PDA, aortic stenosis)
   b) Acquired diseases (e.g., mitral insufficiency, cardiomyopathy)

B. Right ventricular enlargement
1. This abnormality is detectable with the ECG only in severe cases.
2. It produces a MEA deviation to the right greater than + 103 degrees in the dog and greater than + 160 degrees in the cat.

3. Axis deviation is often more extreme in cases of hypertrophy in congenital right heart disease than in acquired disease.
4. Deep S waves are present in leads I, II, III, aVF, CV6LL, and CV6LU (Fig. 3-4E).
5. Positive T waves in lead V10 also suggest RV enlargement, except in Chihuahuas.
6. Criteria for abnormally deep S waves in the dog:
   a) > 0.05 mV in lead I
   b) > 0.35 mV in lead II
   c) > 0.8 mV in CV6LL
   d) > 0.7 mV in CV6LU
   e) > R:S wave ratio of 0.87 in CV6LU
7. In the cat, normal S waves should not exceed 0.5 mV in leads I, II, III, and aVF, and 0.7 mV in CV6LL and CV6LU.
8. Deep Q waves 0.5 mV in leads I, II, III, and aVF in dogs may be supportive of RV enlargement.
9. Causes of RV enlargement:
   a) Congenital anomalies, (e.g., pulmonic stenosis, tetralogy of Fallot)
   b) Acquired diseases (e.g., tricuspid insufficiency, chronic or acute pulmonary disease, heartworm disease)

C. Biventricular enlargement
1. This abnormality may be present without ECG abnormalities.
2. Some ECG features that may suggest biventricular enlargement include:
   a) Prolongation of the QRS
   b) High-amplitude R waves
   c) Deep amplitude Q waves in I, II, III, and aVF
3. The mean electrical axis may or may not be deviated to the right.

III. QRS abnormalities associated with intraventricular conduction disturbances

These abnormalities result in prolongation of the QRS interval. The disturbance may involve the right bundle branch and/or anterior or posterior fascicle of the left bundle branch and may or may not be associated with chamber enlargement. Thoracic radiographs are helpful in the differentiation of ventricular enlargement and intraventricular conduction defects without chamber enlargement. Intraventricular conduction disturbances may be associated with ischemic cardiac disease, chronic valve disease, cardiomyopathy, congenital heart disease, neoplastic heart disease, trauma or no other evidence of cardiac disease.

A. Right bundle branch block
   1. RBBB results in normal left ventricular activation but in delayed right ventricular activation.
   2. The QRS is wide, and right axis deviation is usually present.
   3. In leads I, II, III, aVF, CV6LL, and CV6LU, the QRS exhibits a small R wave and a large wide S wave (Fig. 3-4E,F).
   4. The QRS is positive in aVR, aVL, and CV5RL.

B. Left bundle branch block
   1. LBBB of the main branch or both fascicles results in delayed activation and depolarization of the left ventricle with normal depolarization of the right ventricle.
   2. On the ECG, the QRS complex appears wide and positive in leads I, II, III, aVF, CV6LL, and CV6LU and negative in aVR, aVL, and CV5RL (Fig. 3-4C).
   3. A small Q wave may precede the R wave in lead I and the left chest leads.

C. Fascicular block
   1. The problem in either the anterior or posterior branch of the left bundle produces a slight prolongation of the QRS.
   2. The direction of the LV depolarization is shifted in the direction of the blocked fascicle and corresponding papillary muscle.
   3. Data on ECG diagnostic features are available only for left anterior fascicular block due to the rarity of fascicular lesions in animals.
   4. Left anterior fascicular block (LAFB) produces:
      a) Normal QRS duration
      b) Left axis deviation
      c) Deep S waves in leads II, III, and aVF
      d) Sometimes a small Q wave and large R wave in I and aVL
   5. RBBB and LAFB produce:
      a) Wide QRS with marked left axis deviation in the frontal plane
      b) Wide deep S waves in I, II, III, aVF, and CV6LU
      c) Tall R waves and small Q waves in leads I and aVL

IV. Low-voltage QRS complexes

A. This abnormality may occur with:
   1. Obesity

2. Heavy muscle mass
3. Pericardial or pleural effusion
4. Pneumothorax
5. Pulmonary consolidation
6. Large thoracic masses

B. When seen, abnormal conditions should be ruled out using thoracic radiographs.

V. Electrical alternans

A. This alteration of the QRS or P, QRS and T complex configuration occurs on every second, third, or fourth beat (See Chapter 9).

B. There is no change in cardiac rhythm or origin of each beat.

C. Electric alternans is most commonly associated with pericardial effusion but may be seen with supraventricular tachycardia or alternating bundle branch block.

D. The configuration changes may be due to actual anatomic motion of the heart or to alteration of myocardial conduction pathway.

VI. Q-T segment abnormalities

A. These are seen as prolongation or shortening of the interval from the onset of the Q wave to the end of the T wave.

B. Because the Q-T prolongs with slow heart rates and shortens with rapid rates, only dramatic changes in interval can be considered significant.

C. In the dog, the Q-T should be approximately less than one-half the preceding R-R interval for normal heart rates.

D. Q-T prolongation is seen with:

1. Hypocalcemia, hypokalemia, or hyperkalemia (Fig. 3-6A)
2. Hypothermia
3. Quinidine administration
4. Ethylene glycol toxicity
5. Strenuous exercise
6. Left ventricular enlargement
7. Intraventricular conduction defects

E. Shortened Q-T intervals are associated with:

1. Hypercalcemia
2. Digitalis administration

VII. ST segment abnormalities

A. The ST segment should arise from the same level as the baseline or T-P segment and may normally be isoelectric or slightly concave or convex.

B. It represents the period of time from the end of ventricular depolarization (QRS interval) to the onset of ventricular repolarization (T wave).
C. Significant deviations or alteration in shape of the ST segment suggest myocardial hypoxia (Fig. 3-4G).
   1. Such changes are most often associated with:
      a) Myocardial ischemia
      b) Congestive heart failure and other causes of respiratory distress
      c) Myocardial trauma or infarction
      d) Hyperkalemia or hypokalemia
      e) Digitalis toxicity
      f) Myocarditis or pericarditis
      g) Accompanying intraventricular conduction disturbances or arrhythmias
   2. Abnormal deviations of the ST segment in the dog would include:
      a) Depression of −0.2 mV or elevation of +0.15 mV in the limb leads
      b) Depression of −0.3 mV in CV6LL or elevation of +0.3 mV in CV6LL and CV6LU
   3. In the cat, any deviation of + or − 0.1 mV or greater in the limb leads is considered significant.

VIII. T-wave abnormalities
A. The T wave is the most labile portion of the ECG, and as such may be altered by virtually any perturbation of the animal's metabolic or neurologic state.
B. The T-wave normally may be positive, negative, biphasic, or notched.
C. Serial ECG recordings from the same animal are most valuable in evaluation of T-wave configuration.
D. A change in T-wave polarity is usually abnormal but nonspecific.
   1. Criteria considered abnormal in the dog (Fig. 3-4G):
      a) T waves greater than 25 percent of the R-wave amplitude, sharply pointed or notched
      b) Positive in polarity in V10 (except in the Chihuahua)
      c) Negative in polarity in CV5RL in dogs over 2 months of age
   2. In the cat, T waves normally should not exceed 0.3 mV.
   3. Abnormal T waves have been associated with electrolyte imbal-

ances, myocardial hypoxia, infarction, intraventricular conduction defects, ventricular enlargement, metabolic or drug toxicities, respiratory abnormalities, and autonomic neural control, as well as normal healthy animals. Spiked, high-amplitude T waves are often suggestive of hyperkalemia as in hypocorticism (Addison's disease) or urinary tract obstruction (Fig. 3-6A).

ARRHYTHMIAS

Arrhythmias are disturbances in cardiac rhythm that result from abnormalities in impulse formation and/or conduction. Systematic evaluation of any rhythm disturbance will simplify diagnosis. Use of multiple leads and longer rhythm strips often aids in evaluation of the waveforms of an arrhythmia. An accurate diagnosis is essential to determining probable cause, severity of the arrhythmia, and the appropriate therapeutic approach. Arrhythmias are also discussed in detail, including treatment in Chapter 13.

Terminology of Classification

I. A general inspection of the ECG strip should be made to determine the predominant rhythm and the type, frequency, and pattern of occurrence of an arrhythmia.
   A. Tachycardia: Persistent arrhythmia that is regular and rapid
   B. Paroxysmal/intermittent: An arrhythmia that occurs intermittently
   C. Premature beat: A beat that occurs earlier than the beats of the predominant rhythm
   D. Escape beat: An abnormal beat that follows an abnormally long period of asystole
   E. Bradycardia: An unusually slow rhythm
   F. Conduction block: A disturbance resulting in delay of transmission of an impulse or prevention of depolarization through normal pathways

II. To differentiate the site of the arrhythmia, determine whether the QRS configuration is normal and preceded by a P wave.

A. Normal QRS: Indicates that ventricular depolarization is normal and therefore that the rhythm disturbance is supraventricular (i.e., originating above the bundle branches in the atria, AV node, or bundle of His)
B. Wide QRS: indicates abnormal ventricular depolarization:
   1. Wide QRS complexes preceded by related P waves: Suggests aberrancy of the ventricular conduction pathway, as in bundle branch block or ventricular enlargement
   2. Wide QRS complexes not associated with P waves: Suggests a ventricular origin of the beat

III. To further differentiate the site of the disturbance, determine whether P waves (atrial activity) are present and related to QRS complexes.
A. Identification of P waves may be particularly difficult in cases of tachyarrhythmias (where they are hidden in preceding T waves) and in cases of low-voltage P waves.
B. Often, differentiation of supraventricular tachycardias is impossible until the rate slows sufficiently to evaluate for the presence of P waves.
   1. P waves that precede and appear related to the QRS: Indicate a disturbance from an atrial focus
   2. P waves unrelated to QRS complexes: Suggests a junctional or ventricular arrhythmia
   3. Absence of P waves: Can occur in atrial, junctional, or ventricular arrhythmias

IV. Once the characteristics of the rhythm disturbance are determined, it can be classified by terminology indicating its site and type of abnormality.

Supraventricular Rhythms and Arrhythmias

I. Sinus rhythms
A. Normal sinus rhythm:
   1. SA node depolarization that stimulates atrial activation, producing a P wave at an inherent pacemaker rate of 70 to 180 beats/min (bpm) in dogs and 160 to 240 bpm in cats (Fig. 3-4A)

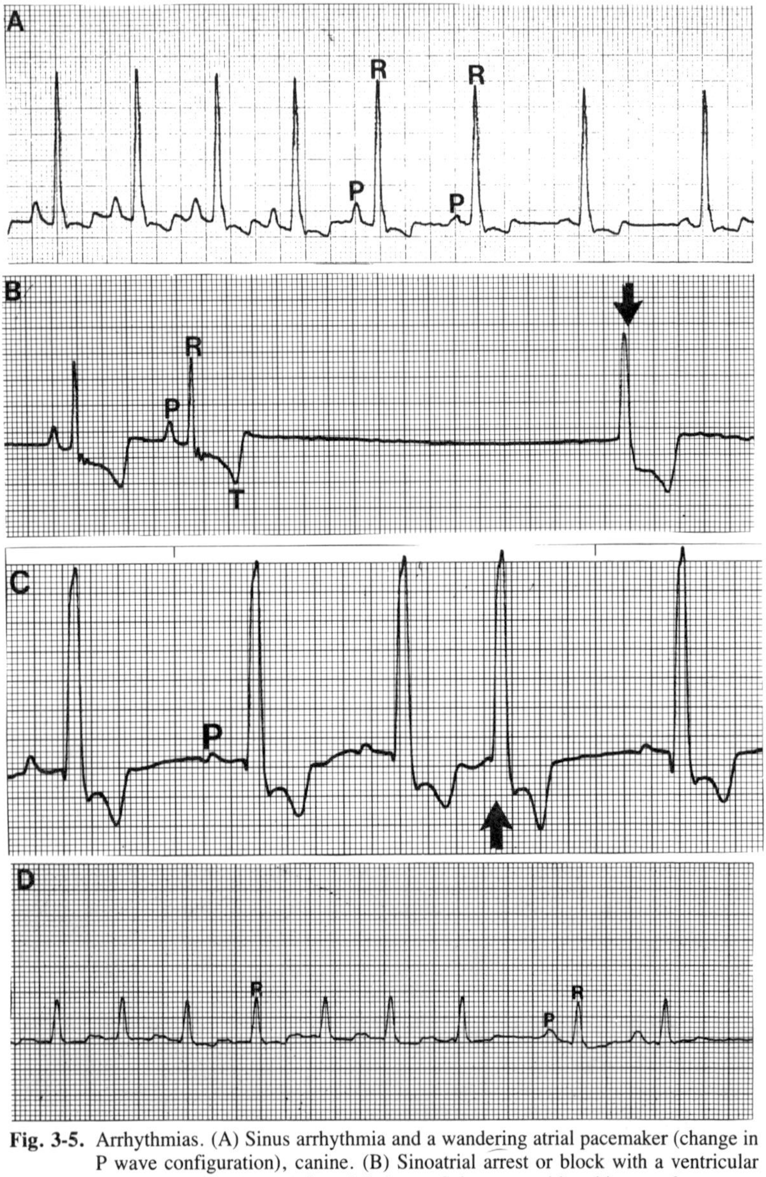

Fig. 3-5. Arrhythmias. (A) Sinus arrhythmia and a wandering atrial pacemaker (change in P wave configuration), canine. (B) Sinoatrial arrest or block with a ventricular escape complex (arrow) in a Miniature Schnauzer with a history of syncope. Large T waves may represent hypoxia. (C) Supraventricular premature complex (arrow) in a dog with heart failure. Tall, wide QRS complexes and ST segment coving are compatible with left heart enlargement. (D) Paroxysmal atrial tachycardia in a cat. The last two complexes are sinus in origin.

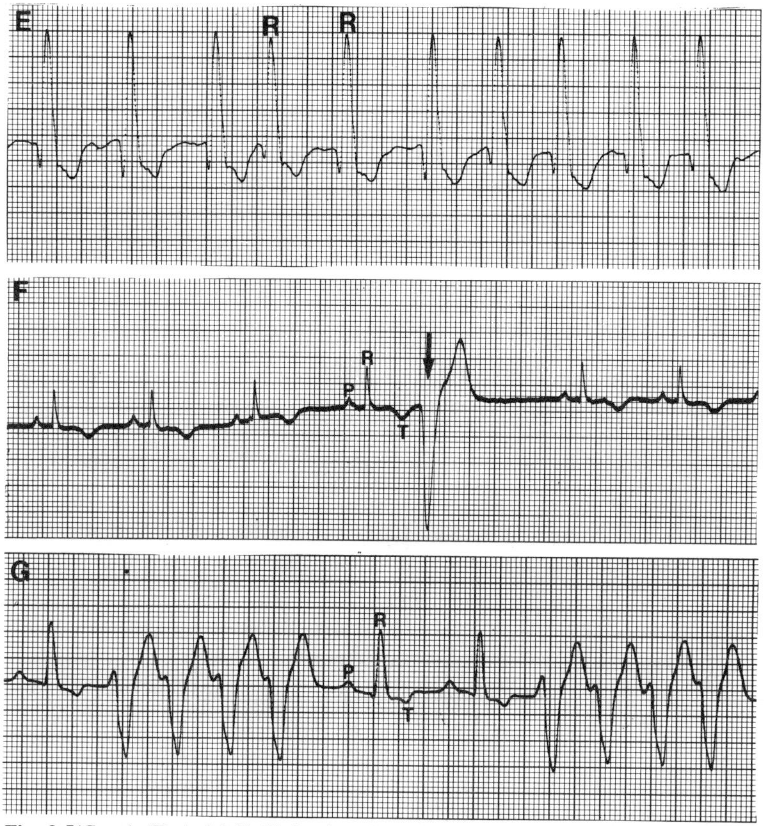

Fig. 3-5(*Cont.*) (E) Atrial fibrillation in a dog with cardiomyopathy. (F) Ventricular premature complex (arrow) in a cat. (G) Intermittent ventricular tachycardia in a dog. The rhythm is interrupted by sinus complexes. Paper speed, 50 mm/sec. 1 cm = 1 mV. Lead II tracings.

2. Slightly irregular rhythms that exhibit a P-P interval variation of < 0.12 second in dogs or 0.10 second in cats

B. Sinus tachycardia: Sinus node depolarization that is more rapid than the normal range for each species

C. Sinus bradycardia: Depolarization rate that is slower than the normal range

D. Sinus arrhythmia:
1. A more irregular sinus rhythm with greater P-P interval variation (Fig. 3-5A)

2. Exhibits a pattern of alternating periods of slower and more rapid heart rates and is often related to respiration

II. Atrial arrhythmias

A. Wandering atrial pacemaker/wandering sinus pacemaker:

1. Frequently observed as a normal form of sinus arrhythmia in dogs
2. Consists of a changing heart rate accompanied by a shifting of the pacemaker site within the SA node and/or atrium
3. P-wave morphology varies with the change in heart rate and may become biphasic or reverse its polarity (Fig. 3-5A)
4. P-R interval may vary from normal to short in duration
5. Must be differentiated from atrial premature beats

B. Atrial premature contractions/beats:

1. Result from an ectopic focus in the atria
2. P wave usually different in configuration from the P wave of sinus beats (Fig. 3-5C)
3. AV node and ventricular tissue repolarized and receptive to an electrical stimulus: premature impulse will follow the normal pathway of conduction, producing normal QRS-T complexes
4. Tissues not yet receptive to a new stimulus: impulse may be blocked and no QRS-T complexes will be formed
5. Partial recovery of the AV node or ventricular tissues: P-R interval of the APC may be prolonged and the QRS morphology altered
6. Premature beat usually resets pacing cycle of the sinus node
7. Sinus node not depolarized by the premature beat: compensatory pause may follow the APC, permitting SA node to resume its previous cycle rhythm
8. Commonly associated with atrial disease or enlargement
9. May be drug induced (e.g., digitalis, anesthetics, diuretics)

C. Atrial tachycardia:

1. An arrhythmia originating from an ectopic atrial focus outside the SA node with a rapid depolarization rate
2. Paroxysmal atrial tachycardia
   a) May be persistent or may occur in an intermittent burst of activity (Fig. 3-5D): called paroxysmal atrial tachycardia
   b) QRS complexes: Usually normal but may be bizarre with intraventricular conduction disturbances
   c) P waves: May be superimposed on preceding T waves

3. Multifocal atrial tachycardia:
   a) Irregular tachycardia rhythm
   b) Configuration of P wave varies
   c) Causes similar to those of atrial premature contractions
   d) Signifies more widespread disease of a serious nature
   e) Can result in syncope, sudden death, congestive heart failure

D. Atrial flutter:
   1. Regular, rapid atrial rhythm with an atrial depolarization rate of 300 to 500 bpm
   2. AV node cannot conduct impulses that rapidly, so most atrial depolarizations are blocked at the AV node
   3. Conduction to the ventricles may vary in a ratio 2:1, 3:1, 4:1, and so on.
      a) With a stethoscope, this arrhythmia sounds irregular, as does atrial fibrillation.
      b) On the ECG, the rapid flutter waves (F waves) have a sawtooth configuration seen between the normal QRS complexes. T waves may be distorted by the superimposed F waves.
      c) Causes are similar to those of APCs.

E. Atrial fibrillation: Occurs when atrial depolarization is so rapid it becomes disorganized. Ventricular rates are irregular and usually rapid as the AV node attempts to conduct the chaotic atrial impulses.
   1. Diagnostic ECG features of atrial fibrillation are the absence of P waves and the irregular ventricular rate with normal QRS configuration (Fig.3-5E). Fibrillation or f waves are oscillations of the baseline that may or may not be apparent.
   2. At rapid ventricular rates, the heart will sound more irregular than the R-R intervals appear.
   3. Atrial fibrillation is usually associated with diseases causing marked atrial enlargement, but may also occur secondary to cardiac trauma, anesthesia, or digitalis toxicity and occasionally in absence of cardiac disease.
   4. High vagal tone or drugs that prolong the refractory period of the AV node will reduce the ventricular response rate.

F. Sinoatrial block (sinoatrial arrest): Results from a failure of the SA node to fire or a block in conduction from the SA node.
   1. The ECG exhibits prolonged pauses in sinus rhythm with the absence of P-QRS-T complexes until the sinus pacemaker or an ec-

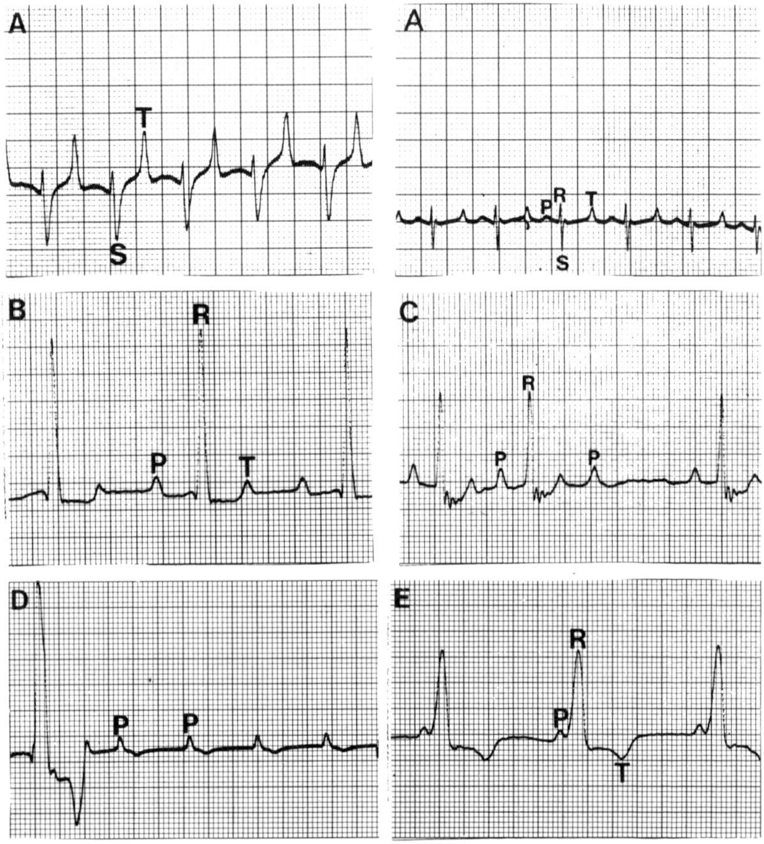

Fig. 3-6. Abnormalities of impulse conduction. (A) Hyperkalemia associated with urethral obstruction in a cat, producing bradycardia, flattening of the P waves, QRS and Q-T prolongation, and tall spiked T waves. The right strip was recorded a few minutes after therapy; the P-QRS-T waves have a more normal appearance. (B) First-degree AV block in a dog, P-R interval is prolonged (0.15-second). (C) Second-degree AV block in a dog; P wave is present without a QRS complex. (D) Third-degree AV block in a dog with an idioventricular escape rhythm. Numerous P waves are present without QRS complexes. (E) Ventricular preexcitation in a cat. P-R interval is short and the QRS complex is wide and tall. Slurring is present in the upstroke of the R wave. Strips A, paper speed, 25 mm/sec, while other strips are 50 mm/sec. 1 cm = 1 mV. Lead II tracings.

topic focus assumes the pacemaking function (Fig. 3-5B). The P-R interval is usually constant. The sinus beat complexes are usually of normal configuration.

2. The SA arrest may accompany an exaggerated sinus arrhythmia or follow a paroxysm of tachycardia.
3. SA block is occasionally seen in brachycephalic breeds due to high vagal tone during inspiration. It is also associated with SA node dysfunction (sick sinus syndrome), atrial disease, vagal nerve irritation, and drug toxicities (e.g., digitalis, propranolol, quinidine, procainamide).

G. Persistent atrial standstill (silent atrium): A rare arrhythmia characterized by complete absence of atrial activity and a slow regular junctional or ventricular escape pacemaker; has been reported in Springer Spaniels and Old English Sheepdogs and may represent a form of neuromuscular disease.

III. Junctional arrhythmias

These arrhythmias arise from the cells in the area of the AV node and bundle of His called the junctional tissue. The cells are capable of spontaneous depolarization which can be conducted along normal ventricular pathways and backward or retrograde to the atria. The QRS of impulses originating at the junction is usually normal in configuration and may be of similar or higher amplitudes than that of sinus beats. The retrograde atrial conduction results in a P′ wave that is usually negative and may precede, be superimposed on or follow the QRS. When the P′ precedes the QRS, the P′-R interval may be normal or short in duration making differentiation from atrial arrhythmias difficult.

A. Junctional premature contractions and junctional tachycardia: More commonly seen junctional arrhythmias associated with conditions similar to those that produce atrial premature contractions and atrial tachycardia.
B. Junctional escape beats: Occur after a period of ventricular asystole, when the atrial pacemaker slows down, stops, or is blocked as seen in sinoatrial block or third-degree AV block.
C. Idiojunctional rhythm: A slow, regular rhythm which occurs when the junctional tissue assumes the role of the dominant cardiac pacemaker.

IV. Atrioventricular node block

Conduction block within the AV node can vary in degree from partial to complete.

A. First degree AV block: Consists of a conduction delay in the AV node that results in a prolongation of the P-R or P-Q interval (Fig. 3-6B). The delay may be due to intrinsic nodal disease, related to electrolyte imbalances, associated with increased vagal stimulation, or induced by drugs (e.g., digitalis, quinidine, procainamide, propranolol).

B. Second-degree AV block: A temporary failure of conduction through the AV node for one or more beats. The nonconducted impulses are often referred to as "dropped beats." There are two types of second-degree block.

   1. Mobitz type I (Wenckebach phenomenon) exhibits a progressive delay in AV conduction. The P-R interval progressively lengthens on each beat until conduction is completely blocked and the P wave is not followed by a QRS complex.
   2. In Mobitz type II there is no P-R interval prolongation leading up to the sudden block (Fig. 3-6C).
   3. Second-degree AV block is sometimes associated with supraventricular tachycardias, disease of the AV node and bundle of His, electrolyte imbalances, increased vagal tone and sinus arrhythmia in normal dogs, or use of drugs (e.g., anesthetics, digitalis, antiarrhythmic agents).

C. Third-degree AV block: Involves a complete blockage of conduction, so that atrial activity has no correlation with ventricular depolarization. A slow, ectopic junctional or ventricular focus below the location of the block becomes the pacemaker for the ventricles.

   1. On the ECG, P waves have a regular rhythm and are normal in configuration but have no constant relationship with the QRS complexes (Fig. 3-6D). The QRS complexes may be normal in configuration with a junctional pacemaker or be bizarre in appearance with a ventricular pacemaker. Idiojunctional rhythm has an inherently faster rate than an idioventricular rhythm, while both are slower than the atrial rate.
   2. Causes of complete blockage include congenital defects, infiltrative lesions, fibrosis, hypoxia or ischemia, inflammation, hypertrophic cardiomyopathy, intracardiac trauma from surgery or catherization, hyperkalemia, and toxicities such as digitalis.

Ventricular Arrhythmias

Ventricular tissue is capable of spontaneous depolarization that can be conducted from the ectopic focus throughout the myocardial cells. The abnormal pathway and slow conduction result in bizarre, wide QRS complexes not preceded by a related P wave.

I. Ventricular premature contraction: Premature ectopic complex (Fig. 3-5F).
   A. VPCs occur frequently in the dog and cat in association with cardiac diseases, drugs, alteration in autonomic nervous tone, electrolyte imbalances, hypoxia, hypothermia, anemia, pyometra, gastrointestinal and renal disease.
   B. VPCs may or may not be followed by a compensatory pause. Failure of repolarization of the myocardium and junctional tissue in time to conduct the next sinoatrial depolarization results in a pause in ventricular activity until the sinus rhythm can be restored.
   C. When all the VPCs are similar in configuration they are assumed to originate from a single focus and are termed *unifocal* (Fig. 3-5G). If the VPCs differ in configuration, they are termed *multifocal*.
   D. *Fusion beats* arise from a sinus beat and ventricular beat occurring synchronously, producing a QRS complex that is intermediate in form and preceded by a P wave.
   E. A regular arrhythmia in which every second beat is a unifocal VPC is called *bigeminy*, while a VPC every third beat is called *trigeminy*.
   F. Frequent VPCs and multifocal VPCs are dangerous arrhythmias that should be treated aggressively.

II. Ventricular tachycardia: Three or more ventricular beats in rapid succession (Fig. 3-5G).
   A. Ventricular tachycardia may be paroxysmal or sustained.
   B. If the R wave of a VPC falls on the preceding T wave, it is called *R-on-T phenomenon*. The peak of the T wave represents a period of increased ventricular vulnerability. A stimulus during this period can induce ventricular tachycardia or fibrillation.
   C. Multiple VPCs in succession and R-on-T phenomenon are considered dangerous arrhythmias requiring prompt, aggressive therapy.
   D. Causes of ventricular tachycardia are similar to those of VPCs.

III. Ventricular fibrillation: Occurs when the ventricular depolarization rate increases and becomes chaotic. Fibrillation is a terminal arrhythmia unless corrected immediately. In fibrillation, the ECG baseline appears to undulate rapidly with no recognizable P-QRS-T complexes. The oscillations may be small or large, characterizing "fine" or "coarse" ventricular fibrillation.

IV. Ventricular asystole: The absence of any ventricular activity and is also a terminal event.

V. Ventricular escape beats: Ventricular depolarizations that occur after a period of ventricular asystole when no faster pacemaker rescues the heart rhythm (Fig. 3-5B).

VI. If a ventricular focus assumes the role of a dominant pacemaker, the slow regular rhythm is termed *idioventricular rhythm* (Fig. 3-6D). Idioventricular rhythms frequently occur associated with third-degree AV block or atrial standstill.

VII. *Atrioventricular* (AV) *dissociation*: A complicated rhythm disturbance that may be intermittent or sustained. The dissociation is characterized by a ventricular pacemaker, which is firing independently and faster than the sinoatrial pacemaker.

A. The intermittent periods of AV dissociation are usually initiated by a premature beat. When the waves of atrial depolarization reach the AV node while it is refractory, conduction is blocked and the two pacemakers continue to fire independently. If, however, the atrial wave reaches the AV node when it is receptive, the impulse may follow the normal intraventricular pathway and "capture" the cardiac rhythm.

B. During the dissociation, the QRS complex will have a configuration suggesting a junctional or ventricular origin, and P waves will be out of synchrony with the ventricular beats. With capture of the AV node, the beats will take on a normal appearance of sinus beats.

C. In the dog, the term AV dissociation is used when the idioventricular rate is faster than the atrial rate but <100 bpm whereas ventricular tachycardia implies a rate >100 bpm. By comparison, third-degree AV block differs in that the atrial rate always exceeds the ventricular rate.

D. Causes of AV dissociation are similar to those of VPCs.

VIII. *Ventricular preexcitation syndrome*: A clinical condition in which an accessory conduction pathway between the atrium and ventricles permits a wave of depolarization to bypass the AV node and activate the ventricular tissue early.

A. One type of preexcitation syndrome that produces paroxysmal supraventricular tachycardia in dogs and cats is *Wolff–Parkinson–White syndrome* (WPW).
B. The classic ECG features of preexcitation include a normal P wave, short P-R intervals and a wide QRS complex with a notch (delta wave) on the upstroke of the R wave (Fig. 3-6E).
C. The major significance of WPW syndrome is the mechanism for producing recurrent tachycardias. An impulse traveling to the ventricles via the normal AV node conduction pathway can reenter the atria by way of the accessory pathway and continue to repeat the conduction circuit, producing very rapid supraventricular tachycardia.
D. Ventricular preexcitation syndrome may occur as a congenital or an acquired abnormality sometimes associated with other cardiac anomalies or disease processes.

Electrolyte and Drug-Induced Arrhythmias

I. *Hyperkalemia* in dogs and cats produces tall, spiked T waves. As the potassium level increases, there is prolongation of the P-R, QRS, and Q-T intervals, decreased amplitude of the R wave. In severe hyperkalemia, the QRS becomes bizarre in configuration, the P waves decrease in amplitude and finally disappear, and the ventricular rate becomes very slow (Fig. 3-6A). Finally, ventricular fibrillation and asystole result.
II. *Hypokalemia* and *hypocalcemia* may cause prolongation of the Q-T interval and inversion of the T wave.
III. *Hypercalcemia* can produce shortening of the Q-T interval and result in ventricular arrhythmias.
IV. *Digitalis* may slow the heart rate and prolong the P-R intervals by slowing AV node conduction. Toxicity can produce S-T segment abnormalities and every type of cardiac arrhythmia.

V. *Quinidine* produces prolongation of the QRS and Q-T interval. Toxicity may result in AV block and atrial and ventricular arrhythmias.

SUGGESTED READINGS

Bolton GR: Handbook of Canine Electrocardiography. WB Saunders, Philadelphia, 1975

Cattcot EJ (Ed): Feline Medicine and Surgery. ed 2. American Veterinary Publication, Santa Barbara, Calif, 1975

Ettinger SJ, Suter PF: Canine Cardiology. WB Saunders, Philadelphia, 1970

Hurst JW, Logue RB, Schlant RC, Wenger NK: The Heart, Arteries and Veins. McGraw-Hill, New York, 1978

Tilley LP, Gompf RE: Feline electrocardiography. Vet Clin North Am 7:257,1977

Tilley LP: Essentials of Canine and Feline Electrocardiography—Managment and Treatment. Lea & Febiger, Philadelphia, 1984

Watanabe Y, Dreifus LS: Cardiac Arrhythmias. Grune & Stratton, New York, 1977

Wellens HJJ, Lie KI, Janse MJ: The Conduction System of the Heart. Lea & Febiger, Philadelphia, 1976

4

Special Diagnostic Techniques for the Evaluation of Cardiac Disease

Timothy Bauer
A. Kim Saal

INTRODUCTION

During the past 10 years, the practice of human and veterinary cardiology has become increasingly dependent on sophisticated noninvasive diagnostic techniques. The purpose of this chapter is to familiarize the clinician with these newer techniques and compare them with the more traditional and invasive means of evaluation, such as cardiac catheterization and ventriculography. The clinical merits and limitations are presented in hopes that it will allow the clinician in the general practice of veterinary medicine to choose the most appropriate and cost-effective means available to solve the clinical problems at hand. Likewise, it is the authors' impression that many of the more invasive diagnostic modalities pose an unnecessary and unacceptable risk to the animal when less invasive means are available that will ultimately allow the delivery of primary care with a more accurate anatomic diagnosis and physiologic assessment.

While the authors recognize that there are areas of the United States and Canada without the availability of a referral veterinary institution, it should be noted that there are numerous hospitals and ambulatory diagnostic services in most communities that are able to obtain the studies described in this chapter. If there are questions regarding the interpretation, the case material may easily be forwarded to a referral center for evaluation.

EXTERNAL PULSE RECORDINGS AND PHONOCARDIOGRAPHY

Phonocardiography and pulse-form recordings provide graphic representation of cardiac sounds and pulsatile events and correlate them to the cardiac cycle.

TECHNIQUE

Recordings are obtained by placing a phonocardiographic transducer on the precordium; different cardiac sounds are best recorded in their respective anatomic areas.

I. The transducer's electrical crystals convert sound waves into an amplified electrical signal, which in turn is recorded concurrently with an electrocardiogram.
II. Similar technique with the use of an inductant displacement transducer will provide graphic representation of arterial or venous waveforms. These are likewise timed by simultaneous electrocardiographic recordings.

CLINICAL APPLICATION

Because of advances in other noninvasive means of cardiac evaluation and imaging, the value of phonocardiography has become somewhat limited. The most important application remains the timing of cardiac events:

I. Identification of cardiac sounds that are difficult to place in relationship to the cardiac cycle (e.g., S_3, S_4, and early ejection sounds (see Chapter 1)
II. Determination of the temporal relationships of sound and pulsatile cardiac events, with systolic time intervals determined by simulta-

neous recording of phonocardiogram, electrocardiogram, and arterial pulse tracings

III. Recognition of heart sounds and waveforms—not pathognomonic for specific disorders, but may provide supportive evidence for the diagnosis of specific valvular, myocardial, or pericardial disorders

IV. As a valuable teaching tool, the graphic representation of cardiac sounds and events aid in teaching physical diagnosis

Limitations

While the studies are noninvasive and can document specific physical findings, they often do not significantly add to the diagnosis, because these studies are unable to assess the significance or magnitude of cardiac events.

AMBULATORY ELECTROCARDIOGRAPHIC MONITORING (HOLTER MONITORING)

The most frequent use of ambulatory electrocardiography is the substantiation of suspected transient rhythm disturbances. It is most frequently employed in the evaluation of the animal with apparent syncope, where the resting electrocardiogram is unremarkable.

Hardware and Acquisition of Holter Recordings

The most commonly used recorders are those that will continuously record the electrocardiogram for a period of 24 hours:

I. Electrodes
   A. The most frequently used electrodes are those of the disposable adhesive variety.
   B. It is important to lightly abrade the skin following the removal of hair.

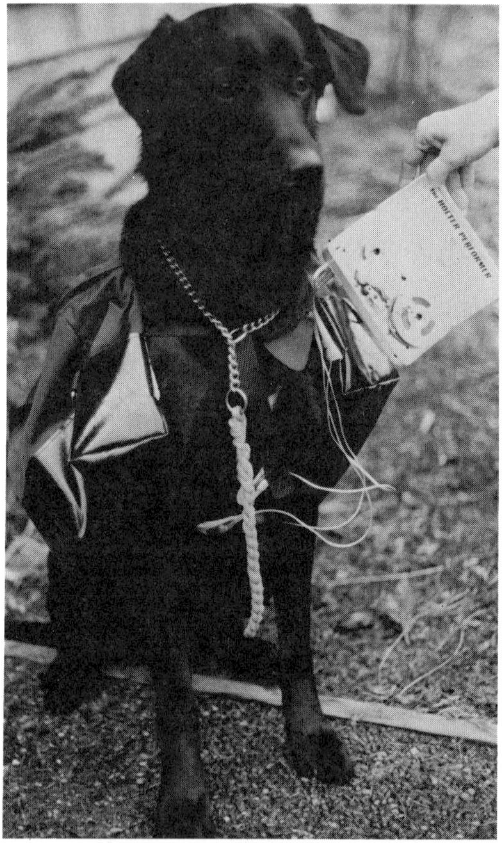

Fig. 4-1. Dog with Holter monitor.

   C. Preparing the surface with a tincture of benzoine solution may aid in the adhesion of the electrode.

II. Recorder
   A. In most instances, the recorder is held in a backpack (Fig. 4-1) or affixed to the patient by elastic bandages.
   B. There are many commercially available backpacks that will accommodate dogs of various sizes.

III. Data retrieval
   A. A growing number of computerized scanning units will analyze the Holter recording.

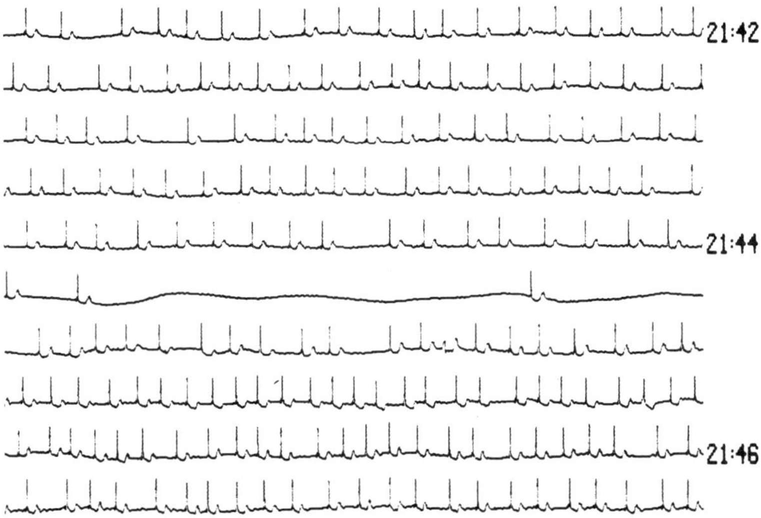

Fig. 4-2. Segment of 24-hour recording of a patient in atrial fibrillation with unexplained syncope. Note the lengthy periods of sinus arrest.

B. QRS complexes are scanned for a period of 24 hours.
C. Abnormalities in rhythm are categorized, and areas of interest printed (Fig. 4-2).
D. As most scanners are programmed to recognize a regular R-R interval, the normal sinus arrhythmia of most canine patients may be noted as premature atrial contractions.

Indications for Holter Monitoring

When a transient rhythm disturbance is suspected on the basis of either auscultation or history, electrocardiographic evaluation is warranted. When such rhythm disturbances are transient and cannot be documented by office electrocardiography, a Holter recording may be advisable, depending on the clinical circumstances.

I. Syncope
   Many animals have historical findings compatible with syncope, yet the resting electrocardiogram may be unremarkable. In such animals, Holter recordings will help identify periods in which cardiac rhythm is abnormal.

II. Antiarrhythmic therapy
In those animals that have had known life-threatening arrhythmias and that are taking antiarrhythmic medications, Holter recordings may be used to monitor the effectiveness of such therapy.

III. Pacemaker evaluation
In those animals that have already undergone pacemaker implantation yet still experience syncopal episodes or whose owners auscult or palpate pauses in cardiac rhythm, Holter evaluation may substantiate failure of pacemaker function.

ECHOCARDIOGRAPHY

INTRODUCTION

Echocardiography is a completely noninvasive technique that enables the visualization of cardiac chambers, cardiac valves, the great vessels, and the pericardium. This technique provides excellent resolution of both intra- and extracardiac structures.

I. Ultrasound
Electric current is passed across a piezoelectric crystal. The crystal oscillates, converting this electrical energy into high-frequency mechanical vibrations.

II. Ultrasound transmission
Ultrasound in the frequency range of 2 to 5 MHz is directed from the transducer toward the heart.
   A. As the ultrasound travels through the structures in the chest, a portion of the sound beam is reflected back toward the transducer each time the ultrasound beam strikes an interface between tissues of differing impedance.
   B. The reflected ultrasound is detected by the same crystal, which also serves as a receiver. The returning echos are then processed and displayed as either a one-dimensional or two-dimensional representation of the heart.

FORMAT AND DISPLAY

Depending on the instrumentation, the returning echos are displayed in different formats, each format provides varying degrees of resolution:

I. A-mode

Amplitude mode provides a graphic representation of the distance from the transducer, represented by the horizontal axis, and the amplitude of returning echos on the vertical axis. It has little practical use in evaluating cardiac anatomy but is frequently used to adjust the gain control for other formats.

II. B-mode

Brightness mode is most useful in noncardiac imaging, as the time required to obtain an image exceeds that of the cardiac cycle.

III. M-mode

Motion mode is a biaxial format that displays a unidimensional cardiac image with distance from the transducer on the vertical axis and time on the horizontal axis.

A. Because of its high sampling rate of 1,000 times per second, this technique provides the best resolution of interfaces and is therefore frequently used for cardiac imaging.
B. This method provides superior resolution of wall and valve motion and thereby permits quantification.

IV. Two-dimensional

Two-dimensional, real-time, or cross-sectional echocardiography projects multiple echo beams in an arc to produce a tomographic image at the frame rate fast enough to produce a real time image.

A. Since this method has the ability to represent the heart as a tomographic plane rather than as the unidimensional image of M-mode echocardiography, it has the distinct advantage of displaying lateral relationships directly and thereby can depict cardiac relationships and cardiac anatomy without interference.
B. It also permits better quantification of ventricular function, such as in a patient with asymmetric ventricles or valvular stenosis.
C. This technique also permits superior delineation of intracardiac and pericardial masses.
D. By peripheral injection of a contrast agent such as agitated saline or cardiogreen dye, one can evaluate intracardiac flow.

Doppler Echocardiography

Doppler echocardiography offers an alternative method to M-mode and two-dimensional evaluation of cardiac hemodynamics.

I. According to the Doppler principle, the frequency of transmitted

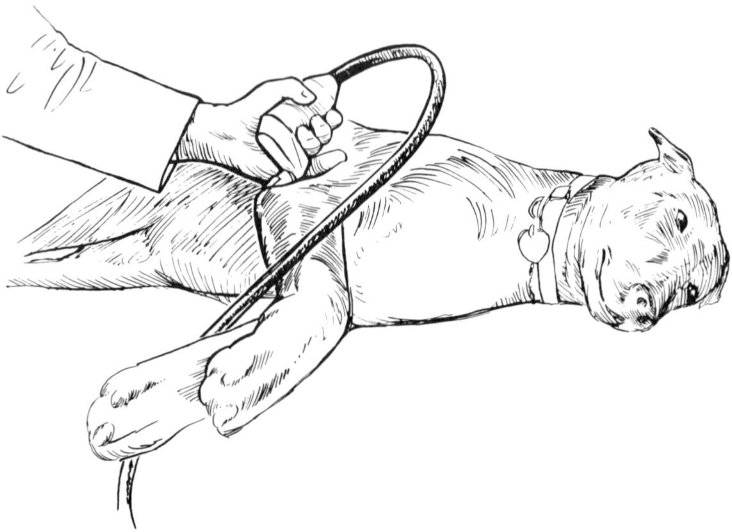

Fig. 4-3. Most cardiac areas can be obtained from a single right parasternal window. The transducer is positioned for showing a short-axis view of the heart.

sound is altered when the source of sound is moving; hence the relationship of Doppler shift both to the direction of blood flow and to the blood flow velocity.

II. The Doppler shifts obtained by either pulsed- or continuous-wave techniques can be recorded and used as an index of blood flow velocity characterizing either normal laminar blood flow or flow disturbances secondary to valvular lesions.

Acquisition of the Echocardiogram

To perform an echocardiogram, the precordium is initially palpated to find the point of maximal cardiac impulse—generally the areas in which acceptable acoustic windows are available. In a thick-haired animal, the precordium is clipped and transmission jelly is applied to provide a good cutaneous transducer interface.

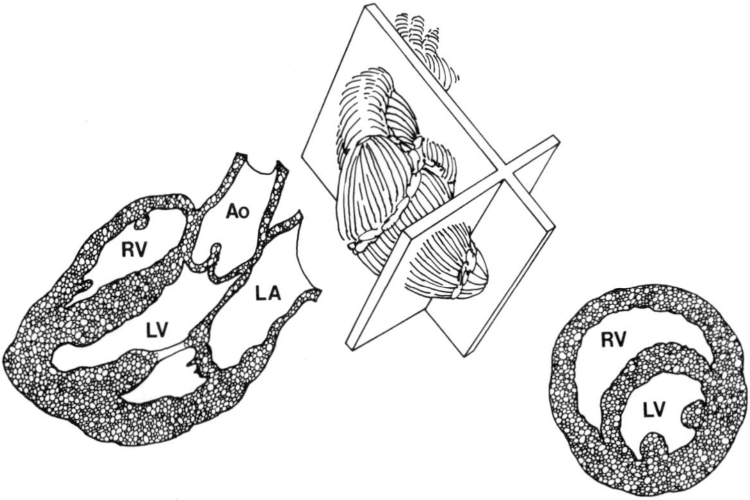

Fig. 4-4. Long- and short-axis views of the heart from the right parasternal window. RV, right ventricle; AO, aorta; LV, left ventricle; LA, left atrium.

I. Acoustic windows

Cardiac anatomy can be best visualized from the right parasternal windows (Fig. 4-3).

A. Animals are most comfortable either standing or in sternal recumbency. The pericardium is then placed close to the chest wall, which is important since the lung provides a poor interface for the transmission of high- frequency sound.

B. In an animal with a deep chest or significant cardiac enlargement, diagnostic studies can be obtained in lateral recumbency with greater ease.

C. In the occasional animal for which it is difficult to obtain an image, greater chest wall to cardiac contact can be gained by imaging from the dependent side (e.g., from between two tables or through a window cut in a special table).

II. Evaluation of cardiac anatomy

A. Frequently, all areas can be obtained from a single right parasternal window, using a combinatior of long- and short-axis views (Fig. 4-4).

B. Other windows, such as from the left parasternal region, may be needed for complete evaluation of the cardiac structures at the heart base. In certain animals, all structures cannot be adequately evaluated.

C. A complete study of cardiac structure consists of evaluating seven basic anatomic regions:
   1. Pericardium
   2. Aortic root, outflow, and valves
   3. Left atrium and mitral valve
   4. Left ventricle, papillary muscles, and chordae tendineae
   5. Right ventricle, papillary muscles, and chordae tendineae
   6. Right atrium and tricuspid valve
   7. Pulmonic valve and outflow tract

Indications for Echocardiographic Evaluation

Since echocardiography is the most valuable noninvasive means available for evaluating cardiac anatomy and function, the indications for obtaining a study are broad.

I. Cardiac valves

Echocardiography is most helpful in the assessment of valvular anatomy and function.

A. Both M-mode and two-dimensional studies permit direct visualization of valves for possible stenosis, congenital and acquired malformations, or other abnormalities such as endocarditis.

B. These techniques also permit indirect assessment of valvular disease by evaluation of chamber size and function (e.g., in an animal with aortic insufficiency, one might expect a volume overloaded left ventricle if the aortic insufficiency were severe).

C. Finally, through the use of Doppler echocardiography, direct assessment of valvular stenosis or insufficiency is possible.

II. Myocardium

Echocardiography is essential in the assessment of myocardial anatomy and function.

A. It provides a method for differentiation of primary myocardial disorders from other concurrent disorders (e.g., the presence of mitral regurgitation associated with cardiomyopathy).

B. It also provides a method of differentiation of the primary myocardial disorders. For example, echocardiography easily distinguishes dilated cardiomyopathy from hypertrophic cardiomyopathy. Regional as well as global wall motion abnormalities can be detected through this diagnostic mode.

III. Pericardium

Echocardiography is the only method available for direct imaging of pericardial effusions (see Chapter 9). This technique permits qualitative assessment of the size of the pericardial effusion, as well as evaluation of hemodynamic sequelae of pericardial effusions.

A. In the presence of cardiac tamponade, it it not uncommon to find evidence of either right atrial or right ventricular diastolic collapse.

B. This technique is superior to pneumopericardiography for the evaluation of pericardial masses.

C. Not only can this technique evaluate pericardial disorders, but echocardiography can detect extrapericardial fluids such as pleural effusions or ascites.

IV. Congenital heart disease

Two-dimensional and M-mode echocardiography are helpful in the evaluation of an animal with suspected congenital heart disease.

A. This technique permits direct evaluation of the cardiac abnormalities as well as the interrelationship of the cardiac chambers.

B. The hemodynamic sequelae of a cardiac anomaly can be observed, such as cardiac chamber enlargement or myocardial hypertrophy.

C. Through the use of noninvasive contrast studies, one is able to evaluate not only the presence or absence of an intracardiac shunt, but also the location of the lesion.

V. Intracardiac masses

Aside from the above uses of echocardiography, M-mode and two-dimensional studies can directly visualize intracardiac mass lesions. Echocardiography can also be used to subjectively differentiate neoplasia from thrombi.

Advantages and Limitations of Echocardiography

Echocardiography has several advantages and disadvantages as compared with other noninvasive and invasive methods of evaluating cardiac structure.

I. Advantages
   A. It is a totally noninvasive technique with no ionizing radiation and no known long-term sequelae.
   B. Cardiac chambers, cardiac valve structure, and intracardiac relationships may be directly evaluated.
   C. Cardiac hemodynamics can be evaluated with Doppler echocardiography rather than with more invasive intracardiac catheterization.

II. Disadvantage

   The major disadvantage is that diagnostic studies cannot be obtained in all animals. This accounts for probably less than 10 percent of the animals studied.

CARDIAC NUCLEAR IMAGING

Introduction

Cardiac nuclear imaging is a safe, relatively noninvasive technique that permits evaluation of overall and regional left ventricular function, left and right ventricular chamber size, the anatomic relationship of chambers to one another, and myocardial perfusion characteristics.

Technique

Radiopharmaceuticals are injected intravenously and their activity then recorded by radiation detection devices.

I. Radiopharmaceuticals

   The radiopharmaceutical employed is dependent upon the physiologic state under investigation and the type of radiation detection device utilized.

A. Several monovalent cations are concentrated in the myocardium and thereby are useful for imaging the myocardium. Technetium-99m and thallium-201 are the most common radiopharmaceuticals employed today for clinical evaluation.
B. These radiopharmaceuticals are attached to a vehicle for insertion into the blood pool. Commonly, the vehicle is either albumin or red blood cells that can be labeled either in vivo or in vitro.

II. Radiation-detection devices

The most frequently used radiation-detection devices are able to determine both the quantity and location of the radionuclide activity in the heart. A gamma camera with a scintillation crystal is the most commonly used instrument, which is then linked to a computer programmed to sample multiple cardiac cycles and areas of interest.

Indications for Cardiac Nuclear Imaging

The most common use of radionuclide imaging is the assessment of cardiac systolic function.

I. Gated studies

Technetium-99m-labeled red blood cells are injected into the blood pool; images are then recorded throughout the cardiac cycle. Multiple images are recorded by a computer and are synchronized to the R wave of the electrocardiogram. All blood pool activity that occurs during the beginning of the cardiac cycle (after the onset of the R wave) is stored collectively. Counts obtained in diastole are likewise processed and stored.

A. This gating technique allows multiple observations to be made from a single injection over time. The end result is an image that represents an average cardiac cycle.
B. Because the data are collected over multiple cardiac cycles, this technique produces a higher number of counts than a first-pass study, which collects counts only during one cardiac cycle. This technique thereby permits greater resolution of the blood pool from the background.
C. The blood pool images are commonly collected in several perspectives, such as anterior, left anterior oblique, and left posterior

oblique. This technique permits qualitative assessment of chamber size, of systolic ventricular contraction, and of the anatomic relationship of cardiac chambers.

D. A gated pool image can be used to measure the ejection fraction of both the right and left ventricle directly from the changes in the blood pool activity through the cardiac cycle.

II. First pass

A second radionuclide technique records the passage of a radiopharmaceutical bollus through the heart.

A. This technique does not require electrocardiographic gating and permits evaluation of time activity in the cardiac chambers and great vessels.

B. By means of evaluating the anatomic and temporal relations of the cardiac chambers, this technique has proved useful in the detection and localization of intracardiac shunts.

III. Thallium-201 myocardial imaging

This technique demonstrates blood flow patterns to the heart through the coronary arteries and is therefore useful in evaluating myocardial perfusion. Thallium-201 is taken up by normally perfused myocardium. Thus, an area of myocardial scar or ischemia would be devoid of thallium uptake, whereas the surrounding normal myocardium would be recorded by the radiation-detection device.

Advantages and Limitations of Radionuclide Studies

Radionuclide ventriculography has both advantages and disadvantages as compared with traditional contrast ventriculography.

I. Radionuclide imaging is relatively noninvasive and has none of the risks of anesthesia, hypotension, or the induction of arrhythmias commonly seen with contrast ventriculography.

II. The radiation exposure is less than that encountered with traditional contrast ventriculography.

III. This technique is only available in a limited number of teaching hospitals and research institutions that have gamma cameras. This technique also does not have the resolution of contrast ventriculography and therefore cannot define valvular, pericardial, or intracardiac anatomy to the extent of traditional cardiac catheterization or echocardiography.

CARDIAC CATHETERIZATION

Cardiac catheterization is generally a procedure whereby both angiographic and hemodynamic assessments are undertaken to assess cardiovascular disease. Nonselective angiography is discussed in Chapter 2.

INDICATIONS

The indications for cardiac catheterization have some variability, depending upon the institution or cardiologist consulted. The following reflect both the general considerations as well as the authors' personal philosophy.

I. Establishing the diagnosis.
   In most circumstances, the nature of the animal's disorder has provided clinical clues to its identity. In certain complicated congenital lesions or multiple acquired lesions (e.g., combination of mitral regurgitation and tricuspid regurgitation), the precise nature of the disease may be in doubt. In such cases, the intent is to establish the definitive nature of the cardiovascular lesion.

II. Quantifying the cardiovascular lesion
   This is probably the most frequent reason for undertaking cardiac catheterization. Measurement of valvular or subvalvular gradients, magnitude of intracardiac shunts, or evaluation of cardiac performance may all be derived from cardiac catheterization.

III. Collecting data for research purposes
   Data derived from the cardiac catheterization laboratory are an important part of describing and categorizing groups of disorders. Complete assessment of cardiovascular disease in a controlled manner will ultimately provide more accurate information.

IV. Valvular heart disease
   In general, those animals that are undergoing elective catheterization are those that have significant complications of their disease (e.g., recurrent unexplained cardiac failure). This study is done

usually to rule out other unrecognized valvular lesions as well as to define the hemodynamics. In the future, those animals being considered for valvular replacement or repair will also fall into this category.

V. Congenital heart disease
Cardiac catheterization is performed in suspected or confirmed congenital heart disease to establish the diagnosis, for the localization of shunts and their quantification, and to determine the need for or ability to correct them surgically.

VI. Pacemaker implantations
Both temporary and permanent transvenous pacing is accomplished by catheterization of the right heart with the appropriate pacing wire.

VII. Therapeutic
Pulmonary artery catheterization with a balloon tipped, flow directed (Swan-Ganz) catheter will allow continuous evaluation of right atrial and pulmonary artery pressure. Thermodilution cardiac output as well as pulmonary "wedge" pressure can be measured. These parameters when measured directly, are of great benefit in managing animals with cardiac disorders or whose volume states are difficult to balance.

Risks

Mortality

Unfortunately, there are no known nationwide statistics available to evaluate the morbidity and mortality associated with veterinary cardiac catheterization. In the human population, the annual mortality is around 0.14 percent. The overall mortality is low, and the patients at greatest risk are those that are critically ill.

Morbidity

When studies are undertaken by trained individuals in a properly equipped cardiac catheterization laboratory, the incidence of serious complications should be low. When they occur, early recognition and rapid intervention will minimize the risk.

I. Arrhythmias

In the setting of the cardiac catheterization laboratory, the full gamut of atrial and ventricular arrhythmias is observed.

A. When ventricular tachycardia or fibrillation occurs, it is most frequently secondary to manipulation of catheters within the ventricular chambers. Ventricular arrhythmias may also be observed following injection of contrast for ventriculography or aortography.

B. Premature atrial beats, supraventricular tachycardia, atrial tachycardia, and atrial fibrillation are more frequently observed in animals with disorders producing large atrial volumes (i.e., tricuspid regurgitation, mitral regurgitation, atrial septal defect, or hypertrophic obstructive cardiomyopathy).

C. In most cases arrhythmias are self-limiting and require no pharmacologic intervention. When they are persistent and responsible for hemodynamic deterioration, pharmacologic or electrical intervention is indicated.

D. Left bundle branch block, right bundle branch block, high second-degree block, or complete heart block are uncommon. The consequence of these arrhythmias, when encountered, is usually bradycardia. As such, temporary transvenous pacing may be required in rare instances.

II. Cardiac perforation

Perforation of the heart or great vessels is not uncommon. The most frequently perforated chamber in our experience is the right ventricle (usually the free wall).

A. The most common setting for cardiac perforation appears to be a combination of an inexperienced operator catheterizing a young animal with a thin and soft myocardium.

B. Rarely, the left ventricle or right ventricle are perforated during power injections. This can be minimized by making sure that the catheter is freely placed within the ventricular cavity. Multiple sidehole angiographic catheters (such as the NIH angiographic catheter) will also reduce catheter recoil during injection. A test hand injection should always precede power injection to minimize the risk of catheter entrapment.

C. Right atrial perforation will occasionally be encountered in attempts at transseptal catheterization.

D. The major sequelae of cardiac perforation are hemopericardium and tamponade. If hypotension occurs following suspected perforation, pericardiocentesis should be undertaken without delay. Rarely is significant blood loss encountered with cardiac perforation.

III. Arterial embolization

There appears to be a relatively low incidence of clinically apparent embolism, either systemic, cerebrovascular, or coronary.

IV. Pulmonary complications

Clinically significant pulmonary embolism and thrombosis are an unusual occurrence in patients free of pulmonary vascular disease. Significant problems may arise in patients undergoing pulmonary arteriography when preexisting embolism or thrombosis is present.

A. Thrombus movement from the main pulmonary artery to the periphery may follow catheter manipulation and pressure injection.
B. Pulmonary edema may occur following injections of large volumes of contrast in patients with reduced cardiac reserve.

V. Hypotension

Hypotension may be observed under a number of circumstances during catheterization. Systemic arterial pressure should therefore, be continuously monitored.

A. Blood loss from either faulty surgical technique, perforation of the great vessels or myocardium, and overzealous sampling for blood gas evaluation may result in hypotension.
B. The overuse of diuretics prior to catheterization can result in hypovolemia. Early evaluation of central venous pressure and pulmonary arterial pressure in combination with systemic arterial pressure should be used as guidelines for the administration of fluid during the procedure.
C. Primary tachyarrhythmias or bradyarrhythmias with subsequent hypotension are not frequent, but are easily recognized. Bradycardia is usually seen secondary to hypotension and is not the initiating cause of low blood pressure.
D. Hypotension can occur after an injection of contrast for ventriculography. This is due to the vasodilatory properties of the contrast. Hypotension is usually transient and lasts 30 to 60 seconds.
E. Anesthesia-related hypotension is always a consideration, requiring constant evaluation of anesthetic depth and gas concentration.

ANESTHESIA

As most animals are not cooperative enough to tolerate cardiac catheterization awake, anesthesia becomes a necessary aspect of the procedure. The decision of whether to use sedation with regional anesthesia depends on the animal's temperament and the proposed procedure at hand.

I. General anesthesia

   There are numerous routes and agents for both induction and maintenance of general anesthesia. The employment of both narcotic analgesia and neuromuscular blockade with mechanical ventilation provides excellent relaxation, oxygenation, and the least myocardial depression. When this is not possible, the combination of narcotic induction with methoxyfluorane maintenance has been recommended.

II. Sedation with regional anesthesia

   In animals unable to withstand general anesthesia that must undergo cardiac catheterization (e.g., pulmonary embolus), the combination of narcotic sedation and regional anesthesia may be used. This is most effective when gaining access to the external jugular vein for right heart catheterization or when catheterizing the femoral artery. Deep dissection of the carotid artery may be prohibitive with this technique.

CATHETERIZATION PROCEDURE

In general, the catheterization procedure includes the following sequence of events: (1) Introduce catheters, right heart first, left heart second. The right heart catheter is placed first, as it carries the lowest risk and provides a route for drug administration if emergencies arise; (2) pressure measurement; (3) cardiac output and other quantitative measurements; (4) angiography.

I. Vascular access

   Most procedures use one of two approaches: (1) cutdown with direct visualization or (2) percutaneous technique.

II. Catheters

   A. Catheters with single end holes are not suitable for injection of large volumes under high pressure. The recoil of such catheters

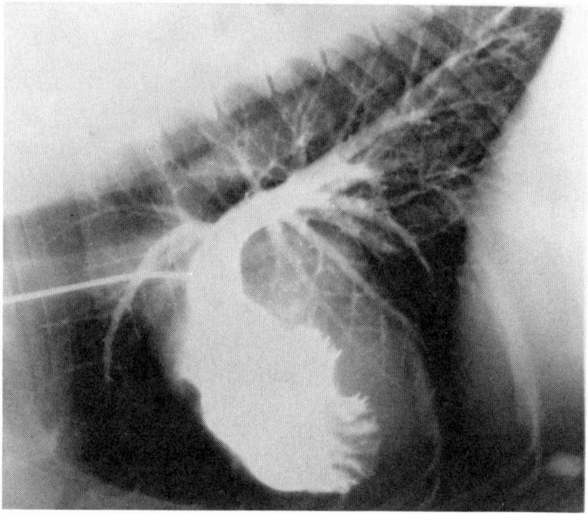

Fig. 4-5. Normal right ventriculogram obtained by selective catheterization.

may injure the myocardium and may predispose myocardial injection of contrast.

B. The NIH or pigtail-type multiple-hole catheters are best suited for right heart or pulmonary artery injections. Such catheters may also be used for left ventricular injections, however, the contour of the catheter tip may preclude easy retrograde passage across the aortic valve.

C. Before a power injection through any catheter is used, the position of the tip and its freedom within the chamber must be determined by hand-test injection.

III. Right heart catheterization

Entrance to either superficial neck veins or femoral veins will provide access to the right heart or pulmonary vasculature.

IV. Left ventricular retrograde catheterization

The carotid or femoral artery is entered. The catheter is threaded retrograde to a position above the coronary sinus. Entrance is gained by threading the catheter gently between the aortic valve cusps during systole.

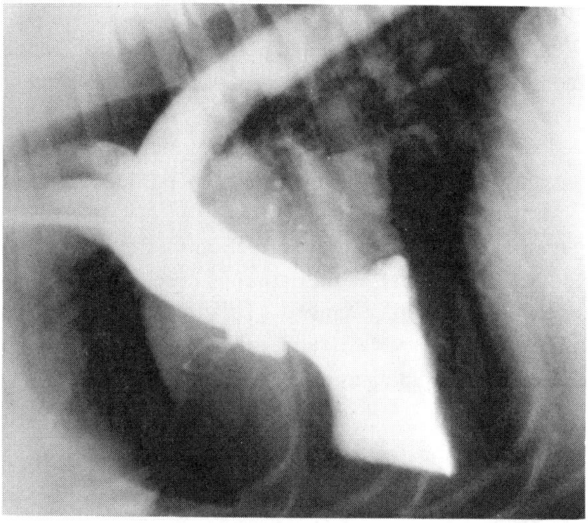

Fig. 4-6. Normal left ventriculogram obtained by selective catheterization.

ANGIOGRAPHY

Angiocardiography is the radiographic filming of the cardiac chambers and of the adjacent great vessels during the injection of radiopaque contrast material (Figs. 4-5 and 4-6).

I. Four methods of recording cardiac events:
  A. Rapid film changers using roll film or individual cassettes: Exposures are rapidly obtained to record the passage of contrast within the heart and vasculature.
  B. Cineradiography: 16mm or 35mm movies are obtained off the output screen of the image intensifier.
  C. Biplane cineradiography: Rapid-sequence serial films are simultaneously exposed at right angles to each other.
  D. Videotape: As with cineradiography, the images are recorded from the output of the image intensifier. Chamber volumes and mass can be calculated by either cineradiography or a biplane cineradiography, however, the biplane method is simpler and more accurate. In addition, the image is larger and provides greater resolution and detail.

II. Contrast media

Both Renografin-76 and Hypaque M-75% (brands of sodium and meglumine diatrizoate) are relatively low in toxicity and have good radiodensity properties.

A. The dosage of contrast is concentration dependent. For the above agents, a dose of 0.5 ml/lb will usually produce high-quality ventriculograms.

B. Contrast agents have a direct effect on the myocardium as well as provoking peripheral vasodilation. These factors do not pose a problem to the healthy cardiovascular system; however, with myocardial failure or with fixed cardiac output (i.e., valvular stenosis), transient hypotension may occur.

Approaches to the Evaluation of Common Problems

I. Aortic regurgitation

A qualitative evaluation of aortic regurgitation and valvular anatomy can be obtained by supravalvular aortography.

II. Aortic or subaortic stenosis

The diagnosis is established by measuring the systolic gradient across the aortic valve. Ventriculography will define the lesion's anatomy. (Similar technique is used to evaluate pulmonic stenosis.)

III. Mitral regurgitation

Quantitative measurement of mitral regurgitation requires measurement of left ventricular volumes by biplane cineangiography. Qualitative estimates can be made from left ventriculograms. It is frequently easier to gain retrograde access to the left atrium from the femoral rather than the carotid artery, if direct left atrial access is not possible, pulmonary wedge pressure should be obtained, as it is a direct reflection of left atrial pressure.

IV. Hypertrophic obstructive cardiomyopathy

When this condition is suspected rather than congenital valvular or subvalvular stenosis, it is especially important to eliminate catheter entrapment. In order to define the hemodynamics, simultaneous recordings are made from the left ventricular inflow area and the aorta or a peripheral artery. Ventriculography will define the anatomy and associated mitral regurgitation if present.

V. Congenital heart disease

In most cases, the diagnosis of congenital lesions are made by radiologic evaluation. Hemodynamic evaluation helps describe and quantify the defect (e.g., measurement of obstructive gradients). The combination of angiography, intracardiac blood gas determination, and hemodynamic evaluation should be systematically carried out.

FUTURE DEVELOPMENTS IN CARDIAC DIAGNOSIS

Computed Tomography

Computed tomography (CT) is a relatively new, noninvasive method for cardiac imaging. The CT scanners use computer technology to produce thin cross sections of cardiac structure. This is accomplished by image reconstruction of information collected by directing radiation through a selected slice of the body from multiple angles.

I. Resolution

Through the use of contrast agents, cardiac chambers can be differentiated from their lumens. CT scanning can be used to display a three-dimensional reconstruction of cardiac structures with excellent spatial resolution. At this time, resolution of fine structure, such as valvular anatomy, is somewhat limited.

II. Clinical application

Clinical application of CT scanning has been for the evaluation of congenital abnormalities of the great vessels and venous structures, cardiac masses including ventricular thrombi, and pericardial abnormalities.

III. Limitations

The present major limitation of CT scanning is that the present scanners are too slow to fully explore cardiac anatomy. The recent development of a new millisecond and simultaneous multislice CT scanner will greatly increase the resolution, and hence, capabilities of this diagnostic tool.

Nuclear Magnetic Resonance

Nuclear magnetic resonance (NMR) is a noninvasive imaging technique that does not involve ionizing radiation. Images of the heart and surrounding tissues are obtained by applying fluctuating radiofrequency impulses across a static magnetic field. This technique depicts organs in relation to the interaction of their compositional nuclei.

I. Resolution

Since blood flow in a normal vessel or within the cardiac chambers produces little signal, NMR produces a clear distinction between vessel walls and blood flow. Because NMR also estimates blood flow velocity, this imaging modality is helpful in assessing both physiologic and anatomic abnormalities. In addition, this technique is also useful in tissue characterization.

II. Limitations

NMR is now available only in research facilities. There is too little clinical experience to predict its future role in the diagnosis of cardiovascular disorders. NMR may prove to be an exciting tool in cardiovascular imaging because of its ability to perform tissue characterization, measurement of blood flow, and chemical and metabolic imaging.

Positron Emission Tomography

Recent advances in radionuclide imaging permit cross-sectional evaluation of the heart by positron emission tomography (PET).

I. Camera

The positron camera consists of an array of detectors used to record scintillations produced by positrons.

A. Annihilation of a positron produces two gamma rays that move in opposite directions; only those emissions that strike opposite detectors simultaneously will register, permitting reconstruction of acecurate three-dimensional images.

B. Thus, the images quantitatively reflect the distribution of radioactivity within the heart and quantifies regional myocardial metabolism and perfusion.

II. Radiopharmaceuticals

This approach commonly uses rubidium-82 and nitrogen-13-labeled ammonia as positron-emitting pharmaceuticals.

III. Limitations.

As with other cardiac nuclear imaging techniques, the resolution is less than with traditional contrast angiography or echocardiography.

SUGGESTED READINGS

Braunwald, E: Heart Disease, A Textbook of Cardiovascular Medicine. WB Saunders, Philadelphia, 1980.

Ettinger, SJ, Suter, PF: Canine Cardiology, WB Saunders, Philadelphia, 1970.

Feigenbaum, H: Echocardiography. ed 3. Lea & Febiger, Philadelphia, 1981.

Hurst, JW: The Heart, McGraw-Hill, New York, 1979.

Mason, DT: Congestive Heart Failure: Mechanisms, Evaluation and Treatment. Dunn-Donnelley, 1976.

Tilley LP: Essentials of Canine and Feline Electrocardiography. Interpretation and Treatment. ed 2. Lea & Febiger. Philadelphia, 1985.

Tilley, LP (ed): Symposium on Cardiopulmonary Diagnostic Techniques. Vet Clin North Am (Small Animal Pract), Vol. 13, 1983.

Section II
DISEASES OF THE HEART

5

Acquired Valvular Heart Disease

Larry Patrick Tilley

INTRODUCTION

General Features

I. Valvular heart disease can be either congenital or acquired. Valvular defects are common congenital heart abnormalities and are described in Chapter 10.

II. Chronic atrioventricular valvular fibrosis is the most common cardiovascular lesion of the dog; it is also a major cause of congestive heart failure in older dogs. This chapter deals primarily with chronic mitral valvular fibrosis in association with mitral valvular insufficiency.

III. Atrioventricular valvular insufficiency is a clinical term that refers to a functional abnormality of the atrioventricular valve leaflets that results in regurgitation of blood from the ventricle into the atrium during ventricular systole. The terms regurgitation or incompetence can also be used for the term insufficiency.

IV. Atrioventricular valvular fibrosis is rare in the cat and usually does not produce major cardiovascular signs.

Heart Failure

I. Mitral valvular insufficiency is a common cause of left-sided heart failure.

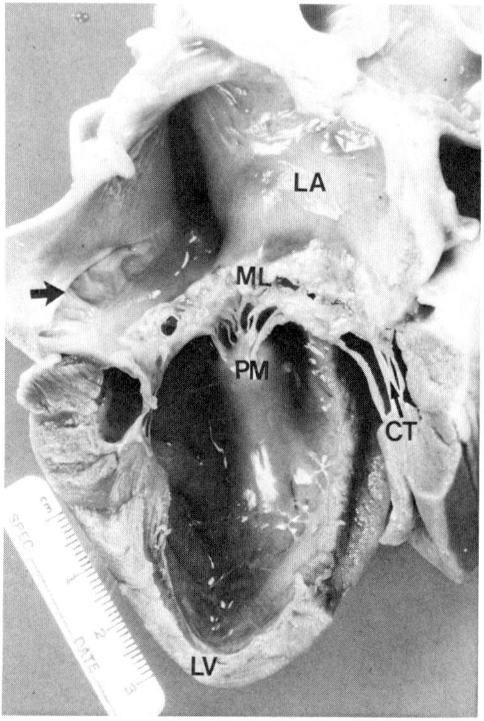

Fig. 5-1. Functional anatomy of the abnormal mitral valve apparatus in a dog that died from severe left-sided heart failure. ML, mitral valve leaflets, grossly thickened and contracted; CT, chordae tendineae; PM, papillary muscle; LV, dilated left ventricular muscle wall. Mitral valvular regurgitation has resulted in severe left atrial enlargement (LA) and subsequent increase in size of the annulus. Rupture of the left atrial wall (arrow) occurs at the site of a jet lesion resulting from regurgitant streams of blood from the left ventricle continuously striking the atrial wall.

II. Ascites and other clinical signs of right ventricular failure often seem to be secondary to left-sided heart failure. Right-sided failure is most likely related to the increased pressure work necessary to pump blood against a hypertensive pulmonary venous circulation. In some dogs with severe tricuspid regurgitation from tricuspid valvular fibrosis severe right ventricular failure can develop.

III. Mitral valvular fibrosis is sometimes associated with ruptured chordae tendineae and left atrial tear. Acute congestive heart failure is the result.

Other Valvular Disorders

I. Dilatation of the left atrium and left ventricle in cardiomyopathy and in congenital heart disease can result in secondary atrioventricular valvular insufficiency.
II. Acquired valvular heart disease can also be associated with bacterial endocarditis. Mitral valvular insufficiency and aortic valvular insufficiency can result.
III. Pulmonic valvular insufficiency is a rare condition that can occur secondary to heartworm disease.
IV. Traumatic disruption of a valve is quite rare in the dog and cat.

MITRAL VALVULAR INSUFFICIENCY

Mitral Valvular Apparatus

The anatomy of the mitral valve complex or apparatus is important to understand in explaining the multiple etiologies of mitral regurgitation (Fig. 5-1). Damage to any of the following structures can lead to regurgitation of blood from the left atrium:

I. Valve leaflets
II. Size and function of annulus
III. Chordae tendineae
IV. Papillary muscles
V. Left ventricular muscle wall

Incidence and Etiology

I. Incidence
   A. Chronic mitral valvular fibrosis and subsequent mitral valvular insufficiency is the most frequent cause of congestive heart failure in the dog. Various studies have estimated the overall incidence as from 8 to 42 percent.

B. Males are affected more often than females.
C. Small breeds have a higher incidence than that of large-breed dogs.
D. The incidence of chronic valvular fibrosis increases with age. The lesions of valvular fibrosis are degenerative and predominantly affect the mitral valve.
E. Approximately one-third of dogs have both mitral and tricuspid valvular disease. The mitral valve leaflets are grossly thickened and contracted, with grayish white nodules rolling in the free edges of the cusps.
F. The chordae tendineae are sometimes affected and may rupture resulting in a sudden onset of severe congestive heart failure.

II. Etiology
A. The etiology of chronic valvular fibrosis in dogs is still unknown. Numerous correlative pathologic studies have been done, but no clues to the exact etiology have been found.
B. As discussed in the previous section, distortion of any of the structures of the mitral valve apparatus can result in mitral regurgitation. For example, the anatomic relationship of the papillary muscles, chordae tendineae, and mitral valve leaflets can be distorted from left ventricular dilatation secondary to other cardiac disorders.
C. Mitral valvular regurgitation can be the result of many different disorders:
1. Chronic mitral valvular fibrosis resulting in valvular insufficiency
2. Severe left ventricular dilatation secondary to cardiomyopathy or congenital heart disease; resulting in dilatation of the mitral valve annulus
3. Bacterial endocarditis
4. Hypertrophic obstructive cardiomyopathy
5. Ruptured chordae tendineae
6. Atrial and ventricular arrhythmias
7. Miscellaneous: tumor, chest trauma

Pathophysiology

I. Mitral valvular regurgitation produces left atrial and left ventricular enlargement. Blood regurgitating from the left ventricle into the left atrium during systole causes the left atrium to dilate. Hypertrophy eventually occurs as a compensatory response so that the large volume of blood can be propelled back to the left ventricle. The work of the left ventricle is increased because of energy used to propel blood into the left atrium through the abnormal mitral valve, as well as work needed to propel sufficient bood into the aorta and the rest of the body.

II. Left atrial dilatation causes displacement of the mitral valve leaflets, increasing the degree of mitral regurgitation. Pulmonary edema often occurs from increased pulmonary venous pressure secondary to a rise in left atrial pressure.

III. As pulmonary arterial pressure rises, right ventricular enlargement may also occur. Right ventricular failure with secondary tricuspid regurgitation occurs. Severe biventricular failure is the result, pulmonary edema and ascites being most common.

IV. Increased vascular resistance or hypertension increases the regurgitation of blood into the left atrium. Vasodilator drugs can be very effective in decreasing peripheral resistance and subsequently decreasing the volume of regurgitation.

V. As the left atrium dilates, atrial tachyarrhythmias occur, especially atrial fibrillation. Syncope may occur from paroxysmal cardiac arrhythmias, decreased ventricular output during exercise, and from coughing episodes.

Diagnosis (The Four Phases)

There are four generally accepted phases or stages of heart disease in dogs (Table 5-1). The four-phase outline provides a fairly reliable guide. The classification is according to clinical signs, radiography, and electrocardiographic findings. It must be remembered that the phases are arbitrary and that most animals gradually move from one phase to another as the disease progresses.

Phase I

I. The dog is generally asymptomatic. Normal activity does not produce undue fatigue, dyspnea, or coughing.

TABLE 5-1. PHASES OF CARDIAC DISEASE

Phase	Clinical Signs	Thoracic Radiographs	Electrocardiogram
I	None (cardiac murmur only)	Normal (sometimes left atrial enlargment)	Normal
II	Usually none; slight cough with severe stress, normal at rest	Left ventricular enlargement and mild left atrial enlargement Lung fields normal	Normal or left ventricular enlargement
III	Coughing, decreased exercise tolerance, enlarging abdomen, fainting, nocturnal cough	Biventricular enlargement, left atrial enlargement Pulmonary congestion (sometimes pulmonary edema)	Biventricular enlargement, left atrial enlargement Cardiac arrhythmias
IV	Signs listed in phase III plus dyspnea at rest; congestive heart failure	Severe biventricular enlargement; moderate to severe left atrial enlargement Pulmonary edema, pleural effusion	As in phase III, but greater frequency of arrhythmias

II. The condition is not serious at this point, and the prognosis is good. This phase often goes undiagnosed.
III. Radiographs may reveal slight left atrial enlargement.
IV. The electrocardiogram is normal.

Phase II

I. The pet's owner generally complains that the dog coughs, especially at night, or has trouble breathing during excitement or exercise; however, he acts normal when at rest.
II. This phase is not serious, and the prognosis is good. Often it will be diagnosed incidentally when the owner brings the dog in for other reasons.
III. Radiographs may exhibit left atrial and slight left ventricular enlargement. In this stage, the heart is usually well compensated.
IV. The heart rate may be elevated. The electrocardiogram may show left heart enlargement.

Phase III

I. The common complaint is that the dog coughs while sleeping or when in a recumbent position. Minimal exercise and/or excitement may produce fatigue, dyspnea, or coughing. These cases are usually comfortable at rest.
II. Prognosis is generally good at this stage. Diagnosis may be made incidental to other reasons for a visit or the owner may bring the animal in for this specific reason.
III. Radiographs usually reveal generalized heart enlargement along with some evidence of pulmonary congestion. Pulmonary edema may also be present.
IV. The ECG usually reveals biventricular enlargement and cardiac arrhythmias.

Phase IV

I. Congestive heart failure is actually present. Dyspnea and coughing are present when the dog is at rest, and the signs may be exaggerated by physical activity. Ascites may also be present. Immediate treatment is required if a dog in this category is to be saved.
II. Prognosis in phase IV can range from fair with therapy to guarded despite therapy.
III. Life-threatening heart failure is sometimes classified as phase V (see Chapter 12).
IV. The electrocardiogram is similar to that in phase III, but with a greater frequency of cardiac arrhythmias. Heart rate is usually very rapid (> 180 beats/min, bpm).
V. Radiographs show generalized heart enlargement and pulmonary edema. Small amounts of pleural effusion are frequently identified.

History

I. Animals with chronic mitral valvular regurgitation may remain asymptomatic for many years. Valvular fibrosis can begin early in life with a murmur audible by 6 to 8 years of age.

II. Early signs of cardiac failure can occur before 10 years of age, with generalized congestive heart failure often occurring between 10 and 12 years of age.
III. Dilatation or hypertrophy of the left ventricle will take place as a compensatory mechanism secondary to the volume overload. In most cases, left ventricular failure eventually develops. Right ventricular failure develops as a result of left ventricular failure with secondary pulmonary hypertension.
IV. Acute mitral valvular regurgitation can occur as a result of a ruptured chordae tendineae with severe left ventricular failure and pulmonary edema present. In these patients, medical therapy is usually not successful.
V. Atrial arrhythmias, especially atrial fibrillation, are relatively common after a long history of mitral valvular insufficiency.

Physical Examination

The diagnostic features of chronic mitral valvular fibrosis vary with the severity of the lesion.

I. Palpation
   A. On palpation of the thorax, a precordial thrill is felt when the intensity of the murmur is high.
   B. The apical impulse (left ventricular thrust) is large at the ventral fourth to sixth intercostal space in advanced mitral valvular insufficiency.
II. Clinical signs
   A. With left-sided heart failure, dyspnea and coughing are present when the dog is at rest; the signs are exaggerated by physical activity.
   B. With right-sided heart failure, ascites and hepatic enlargement are frequently found.
   C. Arterial pulses are usually normal. Pulse deficits occur with many cardiac arrhythmias (e.g., ventricular premature complexes, atrial fibrillation).
III. Auscultation
   A. The typical murmur of mitral valvular regurgitation is heard best at the left fifth intercostal space, with radiation dorsal, cranial, or

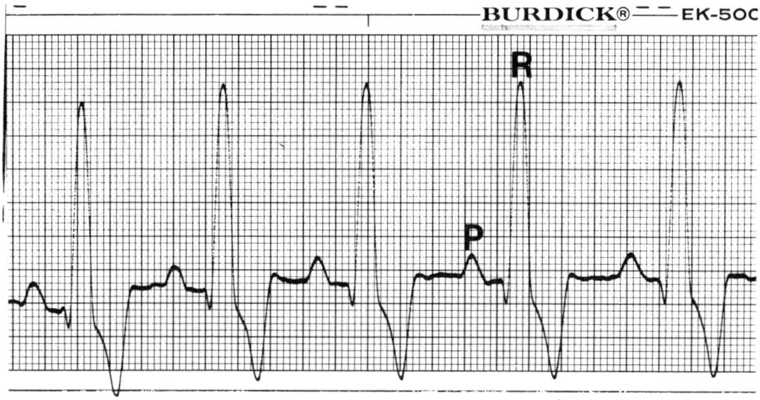

Fig. 5-2. Left ventricular enlargement in a dog with chronic mitral valvular insufficiency. The QRS complexes are wide (0.09-second). The S-T segment coving also reflects left heart enlargement. The P waves are wide (0.06-sec), suggesting left atrial enlargement.

caudal. The typical systolic murmur is holosystolic. A decrescendo systolic murmur is typical of mild mitral valvular regurgitation.

B. The loudness of the murmur can cover the entire range from grade I to grade VI. In most cases there is no relationship between the intensity of the murmur and the magnitude of the regurgitation.

C. In moderately severe or severe mitral valvular regurgitation, an S_3 or gallop sound may be present. The S_3 in mitral regurgitation is often the result of a large amount of blood entering the left ventricle during early diastole from a dilated left atrium.

Electrocardiogram

A wide range of findings can be found (Table 5-1). The electrocardiogram can also be normal, since the lesion may be mild and the early stages of mitral valvular regurgitation are present. Electrocardiographic findings in most dogs with mitral valvular regurgitation include the following:

I. Left ventricular hypertrophy with left axis deviation, although the mean electrical axis is frequently normal

II. Left atrial enlargement (wide P waves) (Fig. 5-2)

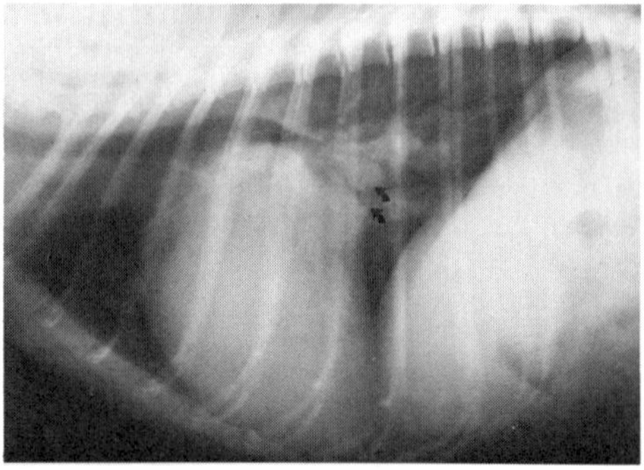

Fig. 5-3. Mitral valvular insufficiency. Lateral projection. The left ventricular border is straightened and there is loss of the caudal waist. There is moderate left atrial dilation (arrows).

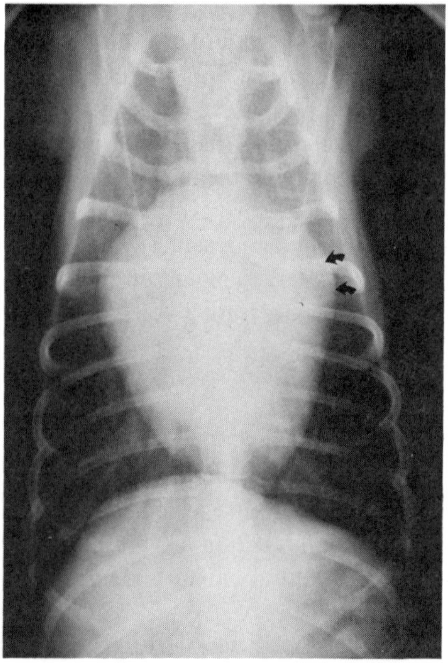

Fig. 5-4. Mitral valvular insufficiency. Dorsoventral projection. The dilated left auricle extends beyond the cardiac border (arrows).

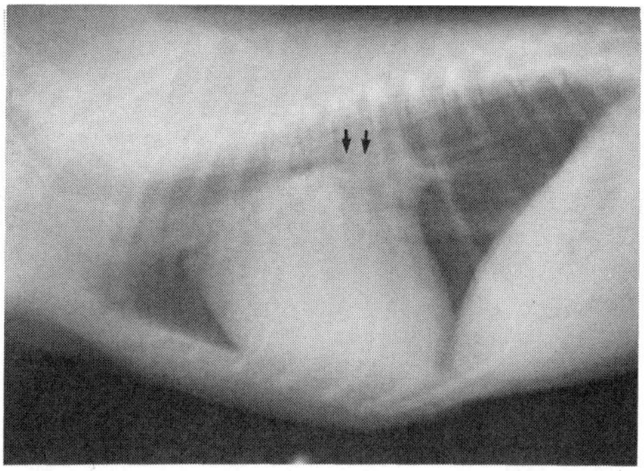

Fig. 5-5. Generalized cardiomegaly. Lateral projection. There is biventricular enlargement and left atrial dilation with elevation and compression of the left mainstem bronchus (arrows).

III. Prolongation of the QRS complex (Fig. 5-2) and increased amplitude of the QRS complex; compatible with left ventricular enlargement. Even with marked cardiomegaly, it is common for the electrocardiogram to have no increased QRS voltage.
IV. Sinus tachycardia
V. Supraventricular arrhythmias, suggestive of underlying atrial enlargement
VI. Ventricular premature complexes, possibly due to myocardial ischemia, ventricular dilatation, or hypoxia

Thoracic Radiography

I. The radiographic signs of chronic mitral valvular fibrosis vary according to the severity of the condition (Table 5-1) (Figs. 5-3 through 5-6).
II. Usually the first chamber to enlarge is the left atrium. With marked enlargement of the left atrium, compression of the left main stem bronchus may occur.
III. Left ventricular enlargement and hypertrophy occurs as a compensation of the mitral valvular regurgitation.
IV. Right ventricular enlargement is common and results from tricuspid regurgitation, pulmonary venous hypertension from mitral regurgitation, or concurrent chronic obstructive pulmonary disease.

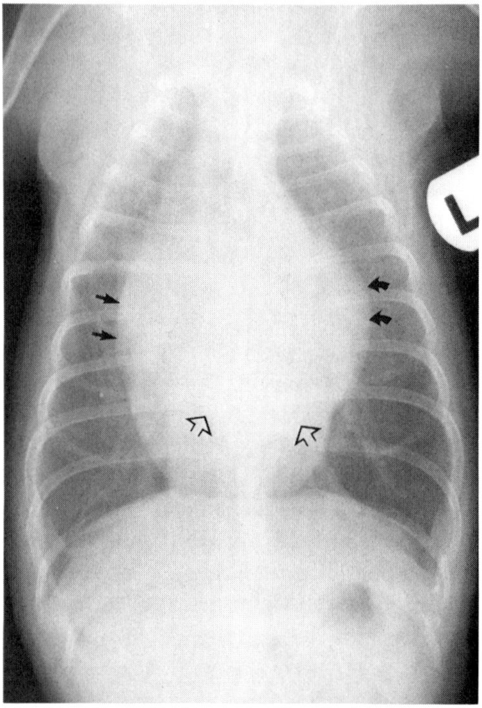

Fig. 5-6. Generalized cardiomegaly. Dorsoventral projection. The marked left atrial dilation is noted by protrusion of the left auricular border beyond the lateral cardiac border (curved arrows) and a double density of the enlarged left atrium caudal to the heart base separating the caudal lobar bronchi (open arrows). There is rounding of the right ventricle and bulging of the right atrium (small arrows).

V. In left ventricular failure there is pulmonary venous distention and pulmonary edema.

VI. In right ventricular failure there is pleural effusion, enlargement of the caudal vena cava, ascites, and frequently hepatomegaly.

Other Laboratory Studies

I. Other studies useful in the diagnosis and assessment of dogs with chronic valvular fibrosis include serum biochemistry blood profiles, echocardiography, and angiocardiography.

A. Angiocardiography and echocardiography can be useful in the identification of structural lesions of severe valvular fibrosis. In most instances this extensive evaluation is not needed.
B. Biochemistry blood profiles are usually necessary especially when a cardiac therapeutic regimen is being established. Hypokalemia and renal failure can promote digitalis toxicity. Anemia, hypothyroidism, and infections can also complicate the congestive heart failure state.

Differential Diagnosis

I. Chronic pulmonary diseases
  A. Respiratory diseases should always be considered in any dog that has dyspnea, coughing, or pulmonary rales.
  B. A cardiac murmur of mitral valvular regurgitation may just be an incidental finding.
  C. Causes of pulmonary diseases include chronic bronchitis, collapsed trachea, collapsed bronchi, pneumonia, heartworm disease, pulmonary neoplasia, and systemic mycosis.
  D. In general, dyspnea secondary to pulmonary disease is more gradual than dyspnea due to cardiac dysfunction.
II. Tricuspid insufficiency
  A. Tricuspid valvular fibrosis can often coexist with mitral valvular fibrosis.
  B. When the murmur of triscuspid insufficiency is severe, it may radiate to the left side of the thorax and be confused with mitral regurgitation.
  C. In most dogs, severe tricuspid valvular insufficiency will be associated with right-sided heart failure.
III. Functional systolic murmur
  A. Functional murmurs and anemic murmurs are rarely holosystolic.
  B. The thoracic radiographs and electrocardiogram are usually normal.
IV. Ventricular septal defect
  A. The murmur is usually holosystolic and can be similar to that of mitral valvular insufficiency. However, the murmur tends to extend to the right of the sternum.

TABLE 5-2. PHASES OF CARDIAC DISEASES WITH APPROPRIATE TREATMENT

Phase	Initial Treatment	Maintenance Treatment[a]	First Follow-up Examination
I	None	None Client education	6 to 12 months
II	Outpatient Low-sodium diet Restricted exercise	Low-sodium diet Low-dose diuretics if near phase III Restricted exercise Client education	3 to 4 months
III	Hospitalize or as outpatient Digitalization (slow oral if possible) Diuretics Restricted exercise Vasodilators?	Maintenance digitalis Low-sodium diet Diuretics as needed Vasodilators? Restricted exercise Client education	1 to 2 weeks
IV	Inhospital emergency Cage rest, O_2 cage "Rapid" digitalization, oral (refractory heart failure) or IV (atrial tachyarrhythmias) Intravenous diuretics Vasodilators	Maintenace digitalis Maintenance diuretics Vasodilators Restricted activity Client education	1 to 2 weeks

B. A history of a murmur as a puppy favors ventricular septal defect.

V. Cardiomyopathy

A. Mitral regurgitation can be either secondary to cardiomyopathy or be a coexistent abnormality.

B. Dogs with hypertrophic or dilated cardiomyopathy can present with a systolic murmur that may mimic mitral regurgitation.

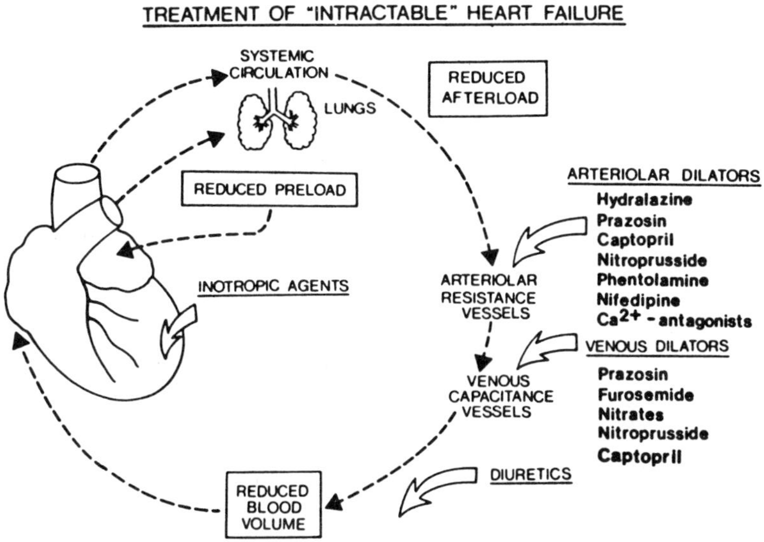

Fig. 5-7. Agents used in the treatment of severe heart failure. (Reproduced by permission from Opie LH (ed.): Drugs for the Heart. Grune & Stratton, New York, 1983.)

C. Most dogs with cardiomyopathy are usually young, are large breeds, and often have atrial fibrillation at the time of examination.

Therapeutic Approach

I. When congestive heart failure occurs, the usual treatment consists of a low-sodium diet, digitalis, and diuretics (see the discussion on treatment of heart failure in Chapter 12). Vasodilator therapy is often very helpful in the treatment of heart failure (Chapter 12).

II. Congestive heart failure represents one of the most challenging problems to the clinician. The therapy of congestive heart failure involves essentially three steps (Table 5-2):

A. Initiation of treatment: According to the phase determined after the evaluation of all of the factors involved in a given case (e.g. clinical signs, radiographs, electrocardiogram) (see Tables 5-1 and 5-2).

B. Maintenance therapy: Adjusted periodically according to the animal's response.

C. Client education

III. Medical therapy for the treatment of heart failure is to improve ventricular function. Three basic types of pharmacologic therapy are available to improve ventricular function and heart failure:

A. Decrease of excessive retention of fluids (diuretics)

B. Augmentation of myocardial contraction (digitalis, dopamine, dobutamine, and catecholamines)

C. Decrease of cardiac workload (vasodilators, restricted activity, low-sodium diet)

IV. Figure 5-7 illustrates the agents used in congestive heart failure.

BACTERIAL ENDOCARDITIS

General Features

I. Infective endocarditis represents an acute or subacute disease of the endocardium and heart valves, almost always caused by invasion and growth of bacterial organisms.

II. Pathogens most frequently found include strains of streptococci, *Staphylococcus aureus, Aerobacter aerogenes, Escherichia coli, Pseudomonas aeruginosa, Erysipelothrix rhusiopathiae,* and *Corynebacterium* sp.

III. Male dogs of large to medium-size breeds are most often affected, with the German Shepherd most commonly affected.

IV. Possible predisposing conditions include various diseases causing severe debilitation, previous use of intravenous catheters, previous surgery, immunosuppresive drug therapy, and congenital cardiac defects such as cardiac lesions associated with turbulent flow (e.g., aortic stenosis).

V. The pathologic picture of endocarditis involves inflammatory vegetations that consist of fibrinous structures mixed with blood cell aggregation and the pathogenic organisms. The localization of the vegetations is most common on the mitral and aortic valves. The vegetations are often friable and tend to embolize.

VI. The results of the endocarditis process can either be its effect upon the valve structure and function or the secondary effects of embolism.
   A. Aortic regurgitation or mitral regurgitation can be produced due to destruction and perforation of the valve leaflets.
   B. Secondary lesions related to embolization can include: myocarditis, glomerulonephritis, myocardial infarction, and peripheral arterial emboli.

VII. The prognosis is guarded in the majority of cases.

Diagnosis

I. Clinical signs
   A. Clinical signs of bacterial endocarditis are related to cardiac lesions, bacteremia, arterial embolization, and host response to infection.
   B. The clinical signs of bacterial endocarditis vary greatly, and include
      1. Fever
      2. Anemia
      3. Shaking
      4. Muscle stiffness
      5. Lameness
      6. Hemorrhages
      7. Seizures
      8. Dyspnea

II. Auscultation–palpation
   A. A cardiac murmur is not always detected. A systolic murmur associated with mitral regurgitation or a diastolic murmur of aortic regurgitation can sometimes be heard.
   B. Cardiac arrhythmias can sometimes also be auscultated, secondary to an infection extending into the other cardiac structures.
   C. A bounding arterial pulse can sometimes be palpated.

III. Electrocardiogram
   A. Atrioventricular block on the electrocardiogram can often be present in a patient with a septal abscess.
   B. It is not uncommon to have atrial and ventricular arrhythmias, es-

pecially when the infection has extended into the myocardium or when a coronary artery has been embolized.

C. Left ventricular enlargement may also be present.

IV. Other diagnostic techniques

A. Thoracic radiographs

Depending on the nature and severity of the infectious process and on the preexisting cardiac disease, left ventricular enlargement and/or pulmonary edema may be recognized.

B. Laboratory tests

A positive blood culture obviously confirms the diagnosis and guides appropriate therapy. Many cases can have repeatedly negative blood cultures, sometimes as a result of previous antibiotic treatment. At least four to six serial blood cultures should be taken and incubated in an aerobic media. Anemia is not uncommon. The white blood cell count may be elevated, normal, or low. Urinalysis may sometimes indicate albuminuria and hematuria.

C. Echocardiographic examination

Moderate-size to large vegetations can be identified.

Therapeutic Approach

I. Prevention

A. Antibiotics should be used during procedures known to be associated with infectious endocarditis.

B. Animals with various cardiac murmurs, especially congenital defects, should be placed on antibiotics when a bacteremia is possible.

II. Antibiotics

A. Animals with bacterial endocarditis should receive a long course of intravenous antibiotics, to which the infective organisms are sensitive.

B. The antibiotic dosage should be high, sufficient to achieve a serum concentration four times greater than the concentration that killed the infective organism in vitro. Bactericidal agents should be administered, if possible.

C. Standard therapy of bacterial endocarditis in animals with an unknown pathogen consists of:
   1. Parenteral therapy with doses of penicillin for at least 2 weeks (sodium or potassium penicillin G 40-60,000 units per kilogram, procaine penicillin G 40-80,000 units per kilogram, or ampicillin 20 to 40 mg/kg)
   2. The addition of an aminoglycoside such as streptomycin or gentamicin (2 mg/kg TID)
   3. An oral antibiotic such as ampicillin or Keflex (20 mg/kg TID) can be used orally for another 2 to 4 weeks.

III. Cardiac failure
   A. Animals that have heart failure as a result of bacterial endocarditis are treated with digitalis, diuretics, and afterload-reducing agents as required.

SUGGESTED READINGS

Alpert JS, Rippe JM: Manual of Cardiovascular Diagnosis and Therapy. Little, Brown, Boston, 1980

Bonagura JD: Bacterial endocarditis. p. 1052. In Ettinger SJ (ed): Textbook of Veterinary Internal Medicine. ed 2. WB Saunders, Philadelphia, 1983

Edwards NJ: Canine mitral valve disease. p. 367. In Kirk RW (ed): Current Veterinary Therapy: Small Animal Practice. Vol. 6. WB Saunders, Philadelphia, 1983

Ettinger SJ: Valvular heart disease. p. 959. In Ettinger SJ (ed): Textbook of Veterinary Internal Medicine. ed 2. WB Saunders, Philadelphia, 1983

Ettinger SJ, Suter PF: Canine Cardiology. WB Saunders, Philadelphia, 1970

Fox PR, Tilley LP, Liu S-K: The cardiovascular system. p. 249. In Pratt PW (ed): Feline Medicine. American Veterinary Publication, Santa Barbara, Calif, 1983

Goldberger E: Textbook of Clinical Cardiology. CV Mosby, St. Louis, 1982

Humphries J O'Neal, Hopkins CB: Valvular heart disease. p. 204. In Selzer A (ed): Principles and Practice of Clinical Cardiology. WB Saunders, Philadelphia, 1983

Keene BW, Bonagura JD: Valvular heart disease. p. 311. In Kirk RW (ed): Current Veterinary Therapy: Small Animal Practice. Vol. 8. WB Saunders, Philadelphia, 1983

Kittleson MD, Eyster GE, Knowlen GG, et al: Myocardial function in small dogs with chronic mitral regurgitation and severe congestive heart failure. J Am Vet Med Assoc 184:455, 1984

Kittleson MD, Eyster GE, Oliver NB, Anderson LK: Oral hydralazine therapy for chronic mitral regurgitation in the dog. J Am Vet Med Assoc 182:1205, 1983

Opie LH, Harrison DC: Vasodilating drugs. p. 129. In Opie LH (ed): Drugs for the Heart. Grune & Stratton, New York, 1983

Sisson D, Thomas WP: Endocarditis of the aortic valve in the dog. J Am Vet Med Assoc 184:570, 1984

6

Cardiomyopathy

Betsy R. Bond

INTRODUCTION

Definition

The term cardiomyopathy is used to designate a disease of the heart muscle as opposed to a disease involving other cardiac structures, such as valves or coronary arteries. Cardiomyopathies may be divided according to underlying etiology:

I. Idiopathic or primary—unknown etiology.
II. Secondary—i.e., metabolic, infectious, toxic, or neoplastic process (Table 6-1).

Classification

Primary cardiomyopathies may be further classified according to hemodynamic and structural differences (Fig. 6-1). Four types of primary cardiomyopathy will be discussed:

I. Hypertrophic cardiomyopathy
II. Dilated (congestive) cardiomyopathy
III. Restrictive cardiomyopathy
IV. Excessive left ventricular moderator bands

Diagnosis

I. Typical findings in the history and physical examination should alert the clinician to the possibility of cardiomyopathy. The most common owner complaints include:

TABLE 6-1. CAUSES OF SECONDARY CARDIOMYOPATHY

1. Infectious (bacterial, viral, fungal, rickettsial, protozoal)
2. Metabolic (hyperthyroidism, hypothyroidism, electrolyte disturbances, uremia, pheochromocytoma)
3. Infiltrative (neoplasia, amyloidosis)
4. Genetic, unproved (hypertrophic cardiomyopathy)
5. Toxic (doxorubricin, heavy metals)
6. Inflammatory (toxins, immune reactions)
7. Nutritional
8. Physical agents (heat stroke, hypothermia, chest trauma)

A. Cough (dogs only)
B. Dyspnea
C. Abdominal distention
D. Weakness, lethargy, or exercise intolerance
E. Collapse or syncope
F. Anorexia
G. Acute onset of posterior paresis (cats)

II. Additional findings on physical examination that support the diagnosis of cardiomyopathy include:
A. Murmur or gallop rhythm
B. Harsh lung sounds
C. Muffled heart and lung sounds
D. Ascites
E. Arrhythmias
F. Absence of femoral pulses, cold hind limbs (cats)

III. Confirmation of the presence of myocardial disease and differentiation into specific type is based on the results of fluid analysis, electrocardiography, thoracic radiography, echocardiography, and angiography.

IV. Blood tests elucidate metabolic changes that may occur secondary to the myocardial disease (e.g., prerenal azotemia).

Therapy

I. Medical therapy may be divided into acute and chronic phases. Emphasis in the acute phase is placed on the management of life threatening consequences of heart failure. General measures are aimed at

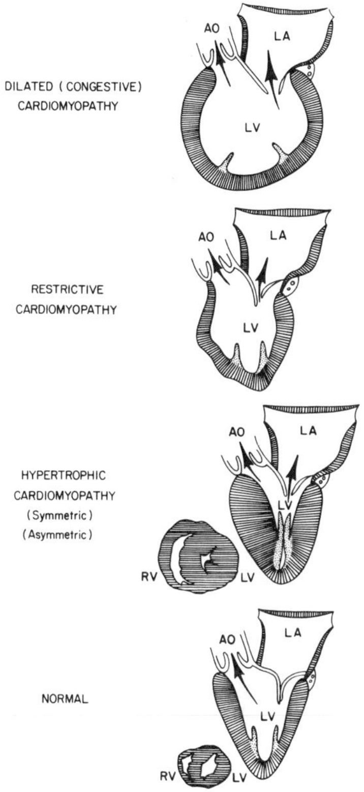

Fig. 6-1. Three types of cardiomyopathy, classified according to hemodynamic and structural changes. Normal left ventricle and a transverse section illustrating both ventricular chambers is show for comparison. LV, left ventricle; AO, aorta; LA, left atrium; RV, right ventricle.

providing support and relieving symptoms without additional stress to the animal.

II. Chronic therapy has a threefold purpose:
   A. Control fluid accumulation
   B. Enhance cardiac output
   C. Control arrhythmias

Feline Cardiomyopathy

I. Cardiomyopathy is the most frequently diagnosed cardiac disease in the cat. Primary cardiomyopathy is extremely varied, with all forms being represented.

II. Secondary cardiomyopathy is rare with the exception of the cardiac manifestations of hyperthyroidism. Feline hyperthyroidism is being recognized with increasing frequency in elderly cats and is becoming a significant part of feline heart disease.

Canine Cardiomyopathy

I. Dilated cardiomyopathy is the type of primary myocardial disease diagnosed most commonly in the dog. The hypertrophic form is rare, and restrictive cardiomyopathy and excessive left ventricular moderator bands have not yet been identified.
II. Secondary cardiomyopathies are uncommon in the dog.

PATHOPHYSIOLOGY

Inasmuch as each type of cardiomyopathy has specific hemodynamic consequences, a complete understanding of the structure and function will enhance the clinician's ability to diagnose and treat the disease.

Hypertrophic Cardiomyopathy

I. Caused by a pathologic hypertrophy of the left ventricle, hypertrophic cardiomyopathy is common in the cat but rare in the dog.
II. If the septum and left ventricle are hypertrophied to an equal degree, the term symmetric hypertrophic cardiomyopathy is used. In asymmetric septal hypertrophy, the septum is thicker than the left ventricular free wall. Outflow obstruction of the left ventricle occurs for two reasons:
  A. Encroachment of the hypertrophied septum on the left ventricular free wall
  B. Systolic anterior motion of the mitral valve, which moves into the aortic outflow tract during systole
III. Consequences of hypertrophied free wall and septum:
  A. A smaller left ventricular cavity

B. Decreased left ventricular compliance
C. Distortion of the mitral valve apparatus
D. Diastolic dysfunction and resistance to ventricular filling as the end result and the combination of abnormal ventricular filling and mitral valve distortion leading to mitral regurgitation, left atrial dilatation, and pulmonary venous congestion and edema

Dilated (Congestive) Cardiomyopathy

I. Dilated cardiomyopathy is characterized by a thin-walled flabby left ventricle with severe systolic dysfunction.
II. This form of cardiomyopathy may actually be the end stage of various other cardiac diseases that are not apparent at the time the animal is examined for heart failure.
III. Because of biventricular pump failure, clinical signs are consistent with low cardiac output and right- and left-sided heart failure.

Restrictive Cardiomyopathy

I. The hallmark of restrictive cardiomyopathy is endomyocardial fibrosis, which causes severe restriction of normal ventricular function and decreased left ventricular compliance. The primary hemodynamic consequence is impaired ventricular filling and elevated left ventricular end diastolic pressure.
II. If the fibrosis is severe enough, it may obliterate the left ventricle or interfere with systolic function.

Excessive Left Ventricular Moderator Bands

I. This type of cardiomyopathy is characterized by excessive moderator bands bridging the septum and left ventricle. This disease is only now being recognized; pressure studies to elucidate the hemodynamics have not yet been undertaken.

II. Clinical correlations are complicated by the fact that excessive left ventricular moderator bands may also be seen in a hypertrophied or dilated left ventricle.

CANINE CARDIOMYOPATHY

Canine Dilated Cardiomyopathy

Introduction

This is the most common form of cardiomyopathy in dogs.

Diagnosis

I. Age, breed, and sex characteristics
  A. Dilated cardiomyopathy generally affects large-breed males, 3 to 7 years of age.
  B. The etiology is unknown, although genetic or nutritional factors may be involved.

II. History
  A. The history is usually short, of approximately 1 to 3 weeks' duration.
  B. Animals usually are examined because of lethargy, cough, exercise intolerance, anorexia, or abdominal swelling.

III. Physical examination
  A. Palpation
    1. Pulses are usually weak and rapid. A pulse deficit may be present due to:
      a) Atrial fibrillation
      b) Atrial premature complexes
      c) Ventricular premature complexes
    2. The left apex beat may be difficult to palpate due to pleural effusion or poor systolic function. When present, it also tends to be weak and rapid, and it may be irregular.
  B. Clinical signs
    1. The most common findings on physical examination include

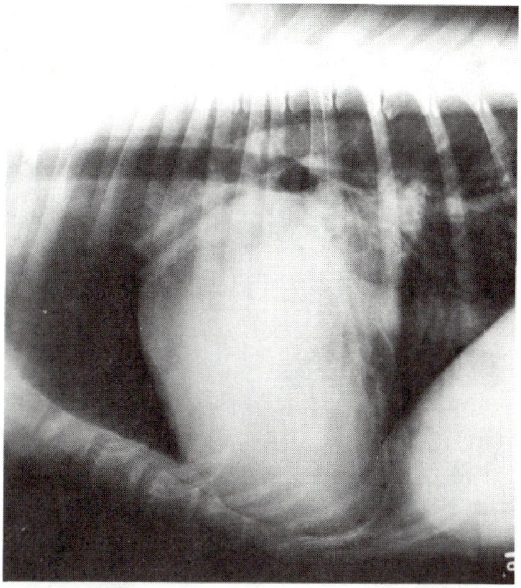

Fig. 6-2. Lateral thoracic radiograph. Eight-year-old Doberman Pinscher with dilated cardiomyopathy. There is mild generalized cardiac enlargement with right and left atrial dilation.

harsh lung sounds, dyspnea, and ascites. Mucous membranes may be pale due to poor perfusion.

2. The presence of cardiac cachexia or extreme muscle wasting is a poor prognostic sign.

C. Auscultation

1. The heart rate is rapid, and a soft, systolic murmur of mitral regurgitation is frequently present.
2. If atrial fibrillation is present, the heart rate may be over 200 beats/min (bpm) with an irregular rhythm. In addition, a varying intensity to the beats that is characteristic of atrial fibrillation is easily auscultated.
3. Lung sounds may be harsh from pulmonary edema, or heart and lung sounds may be muffled secondary to pleural effusion.

IV. Electrocardiogram

A. The most common findings are tall wide QRS complexes, tachycardia, and wide P waves.

B. There is a high degree of association between atrial fibrillation

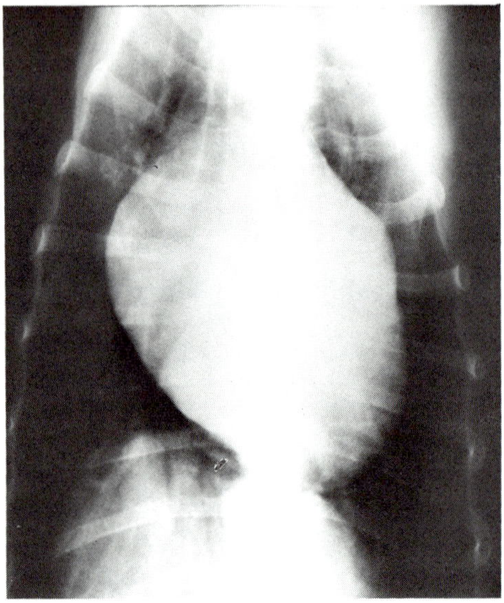

Fig. 6-3. Dorsoventral thoracic radiograph, dog in Fig. 6-2. There is generalized cardiac enlargement. Both right atrial and left auricular enlargement is seen.

and canine primary myocardial disease. Atrial fibrillation is not present in all cases.

C. Ventricular premature complexes are common, and frequent atrial premature complexes may indicate impending atrial fibrillation.

V. Thoracic radiographs (Figs. 6-2 and 6-3)

A. The most consistent feature is generalized cardiomegaly with moderate to marked left atrial dilation.

B. Most dogs will have pulmonary edema and congestion indicative of left heart failure. Pleural effusion may also be present.

VI. Echocardiogram

A. The advent of ultrasound has been of tremendous benefit in the diagnosis of this disease, and helps to differentiate cardiomyopathy from severe mitral regurgitation and secondary atrial fibrillation.

B. Characteristically, cardiomyopathy leads to severe failure of myocardial function, and there is a concomitant and parallel decrease in indices of systolic function. The left ventricle is extremely dilated, and there is a lack of left ventricular hypertrophy to help offset the dilatation.

C. The left atrium is dilated in cases of cardiomyopathy, but not as much as in chronic mitral regurgitation.

VII. Other diagnostic techniques

A. Mild increases in blood urea nitrogen and creatinine resulting from prerenal azotemia are frequently seen. Restoration of renal blood flow by medical therapy will usually lower these values to normal, but a urinalysis should be done to identify underlying primary kidney disease. A hypothyroid state may represent a complicating factor (especially in Doberman Pinschers).

B. Mild liver enzyme elevations secondary to chronic passive congestion also may be present.

Therapy and Prognosis

I. Digoxin and furosemide continue to be the mainstays of therapy, especially in cases in which atrial fibrillation is present.

A. Digoxin. In severe cases of rapid atrial fibrillation, two partial loading doses of digoxin are given 12 hours apart. Thereafter, an average maintenance dosage of 0.50 to 0.75 mg divided twice daily (> 100 lb) is administered.

B. Furosemide is given by injection (2 to 4 mg/kg, TID) until acute symptoms of heart failure have resolved. Thereafter, it is given orally at a dosage of 2 mg/kg BID.

C. Propranolol is recommended to help control rapid heart rates secondary to atrial fibrillation after heart failure has resolved and the patient has had sufficient time to become fully digitalized. The dosage is broad, 10 to 40 mg, BID–TID to effect.

D. Vasodilators. Vasodilators along with digoxin and furosemide can be effective. The most commonly used are prazosin, hydralazine, and captopril. A thorough knowledge of the actions, pharmacology, and side effects of these medications is recommended before use.

II. Prognosis for idiopathic cardiomyopathy must remain guarded, even with the excellent results that have been obtained in some animals. Survival times of two to four years may be seen, however, sudden death does occur in some patients. The average life span is 6 months to 2 years after diagnosis. Severe weight loss indicates a poor prognosis. Doberman Pinschers in general have a more grave prognosis than other canine breeds.

Canine Hypertrophic Cardiomyopathy

Introduction

I. Unlike dilated cardiomyopathy, hypertrophic cardiomyopathy is rare in the dog.
II. Sudden death is a common feature, and may or may not be preceded by heart failure.

Diagnosis

I. Age, breed, and sex characteristics
  A. One report of 10 dogs diagnosed at necropsy listed the German Shepherd as the most common breed affected, with ages in all breeds ranging from 1 to 13 years.
  B. Males were predominantly affected in the above study.
II. History
  A. A large percentage of dogs have no antecedent sign of any cardiac abnormality, and are diagnosed after anesthetic death or sudden death of unknown cause.
  B. In those dogs that are symptomatic, left-sided heart failure is more common than right-sided.
III. Physical examination
  Little is known about findings on physical examinations because of the small number of symptomatic dogs.
  A. Dogs in heart failure may have a systolic murmur of mitral regurgitation and moist rales of pulmonary edema.
  B. Dyspnea and ascites caused by right-sided heart failure may also be present.
  C. If a conduction disturbance is present, the arrhythmia may be easily auscultable.
  D. Unfortunately, there may be no abnormalities to lead the clinician to suspect underlying cardiac disease.
IV. Electrocardiogram
  A. Conduction disturbances such as third-degree heart block, bifasci-

cular block, and first-degree heart block are the most common findings.

B. The electrocardiogram may be normal.

V. Thoracic radiographs

Cardiomegaly with left- or right-sided failure may be present.

VI. Echocardiogram

This is one diagnostic procedure that can allow early diagnosis of canine hypertrophic cardiomyopathy. The criteria are the same as in the cat and human—a thickened left ventricular free wall and septum and a small left ventricular cavity.

VII. Angiocardiogram

Selective catheterization of the left ventricle is beneficial for two reasons:

A. It permits visualization of the left ventricle via angiography, which demonstrates:
   1. Left ventricular dynamics and outflow obstruction.
   2. The presence of hypertrophic cardiomyopathy versus discrete fibrous subaortic stenosis.

B. Left ventricular pressure studies may be performed to elucidate
   1. Left ventricular hemodynamics at rest and during pharmacologic intervention.
   2. The presence of a systolic gradient from the left ventricle to the aorta.

VIII. Differential diagnosis

Hypertrophic cardiomyopathy mimics valvular diseases that produce left heart failure (e.g., mitral valvular fibrosis) and conduction disturbances of unknown etiology.

Therapy and Prognosis

I. The aim of treating hypertrophic cardiomyopathy is twofold:

A. Prevent sudden death

B. Control heart failure (if present)

II. β-blockers

A. β-blockers such as propranolol may prevent sudden death.

B. These drugs also may improve diastolic filling time.

III. Restriction of exercise, excitement, and stress-related situations is advised.
IV. Heart failure is controlled primarily through the use of diuretics.
V. Digitalis is not indicated since systolic function is usually normal. Positive inotropic agents also may increase outflow obstruction.
VI. Severe conduction disturbances generally require a pacemaker; however, dogs with hypertrophic cardiomyopathy are poor surgical candidates.
VII. Because of the high possibility of sudden death, the prognosis is guarded.

Secondary Cardiomyopathy

Introduction

Myocardial disease secondary to other conditions is relatively rare in veterinary medicine. There are, however, certain conditions that may lead to cardiomyopathy.

Hypothyroidism

Low thyroid hormone concentrations have been noted in some dogs with the dilated form of cardiomyopathy. How much this contributes to the disease is unknown.

Doxorubricin Therapy

This mode of treatment is used with increased frequency in veterinary medicine. Doxorubricin is a well-known myocardial toxin. Dogs with cardiomyopathy secondary to this therapy exhibit clinical and hemodynamic changes equivalent to those seen in dilated cardiomyopathy.

Parvovirus Myocarditis

I. Typically, pups 4 to 8 weeks of age are affected and usually die within minutes to hours after onset of symptoms.

II. Clinical signs include dyspnea, depression, anorexia, crying out, vomiting, or convulsions.

III. Physical examination reveals dyspnea, tachycardia, systolic murmurs, gallop rhythms, arrhythmias, or pink fluid in the nose and mouth.

IV. Survivors of the acute phase may survive but can develop dilated cardiomyopathy.

Boxer Cardiomyopathy

Introduction

I. Cardiomyopathy of unknown etiology has been described in the Boxer breed.

II. It is distinguished by a lack of ventricular dilatation and histologic myocardial alterations.

Diagnosis

I. Age, breed, and sex characteristics
  A. The age range is from 1 to 15 years, although most dogs are above 10 years of age.
  B. Although considered unique to Boxers, a similar condition has been recognized in a small number of Doberman Pinschers.

II. History: Dogs with Boxer cardiomyopathy may be divided into three categories depending on symptoms:
  A. Syncope or weakness
  B. Heart failure
  C. No symptoms related to heart disease

III. Physical examination
  A. Clinical signs
     Physical examination indicates dyspnea, cyanosis, and ascites.
  B. Auscultation and palpation
     1. The most common finding is the presence of cardiac arrhythmias, especially premature beats.
     2. Other findings include tachycardia, murmur, gallop, abnormal lung sounds, and pulse deficits.

IV. Electrocardiogram
   A. Ventricular premature beats singly, in pairs, and in runs (ventricular tachycardia) are extremely common.
   B. Supraventricular arrhythmias, prolongation of the QRS complex, and left ventricular hypertrophy occur with less frequency.
V. Thoracic radiographs
   A. Radiographs are usually normal in dogs that are asymptomatic or showing signs of weakness or syncope.
   B. Varying degrees of left ventricular and left atrial enlargement, pulmonary congestion and pulmonary edema may be seen in dogs with clinical signs of heart failure.
VI. Echocardiogram
   Objective data concerning results of ultrasound evaluation are not available.

Therapy and Prognosis

I. Medical management
   A. Asymptomatic dogs are managed with antiarrhythmic therapy if the frequency of extrasystoles exceeds 20 to 30 per minute, or if pairs, runs, or sustained tachyarrhythmia is present. Antiarrhythmic agents include
      1. Quinidine
      2. Procainamide
      3. Propranolol
   B. Syncope and weakness are usually secondary to ventricular arrhythmias. If no heart failure is present, ventricular antiarrhythmic therapy is instituted.
      1. In acute situations, intravenous lidocaine is used as an intravenous bolus, then as a constant rate infusion.
      2. Maintenance therapy with antiarrhythmics may be used as previously described.
   C. Dogs with simultaneous heart failure and arrhythmias are treated depending on the type of arrhythmia and severity of heart failure.
      1. Supraventricular arrhythmias are treated with a combination of digoxin and diuretics. Ventricular rates that continue to be excessively rapid are treated with propranolol.

2. Ventricular arrhythmias and simultaneous heart failure are difficult to manage.
    a) Lower doses of antiarrhythmics should be used to minimize myocardial depressant effects.
    b) Low-maintenance digoxin may be added cautiously. Close monitoring of the electrocardiogram is indicated.

II. Prognosis
  A. Long-term prognosis is poor, but dogs without heart failure have a better prognosis.
  B. Death is usually due to sudden fatal arrhythmia or to inability to control heart failure.

FELINE CARDIOMYOPATHY

FELINE Hypertrophic CARDIOMYOPATHY

Introduction

I. Hypertrophic cardiomyopathy is more frequently diagnosed in the cat than in the dog.
II. It is also associated with sudden death in the cat.
III. Left-sided heart failure is more prevalent than right-sided heart failure.

Diagnosis

I. Age, breed, and sex characteristics
  A. Middle-aged to older cats are primarily affected, and males more commonly than females.
  B. Persian cats may be more susceptible to hypertrophic than to other forms of cardiomyopathy.

II. History
  A. Most cats are examined because of acute onset of dyspnea, lethargy, or anorexia.
  B. Coughing secondary to heart disease is rare in the cat.

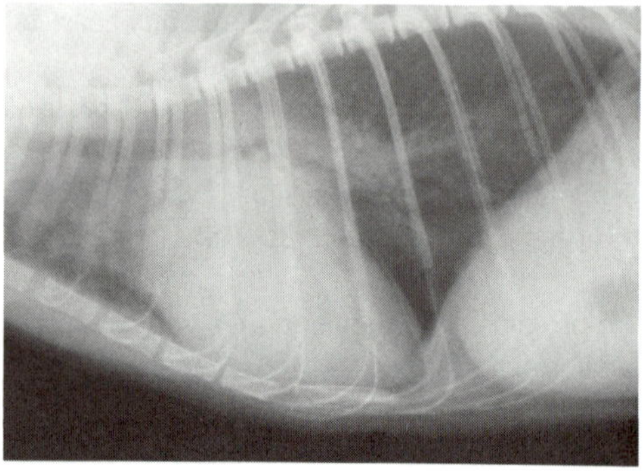

Fig. 6-4. Hypertrophic feline cardiomyopathy. Lateral thoracic radiograph. There is generalized cardiac enlargement. The pulmonary vasculature is engorged and increased interstitial and alveolar infiltrate due to pulmonary edema.

III. Physical examination
  A. Clinical signs
    1. Dyspnea is the most obvious symptom and some cats may exhibit open-mouth breathing.
    2. If heart failure is severe, cyanosis may be present.
  B. Auscultation
    1. Moist rales are usually heard in all lung fields.
    2. A gallop rhythm or systolic murmur may be present but may also be obscured by the rales.
    3. Many cat murmurs are frequently missed since they are very localized. Auscultating low on the left side near the sternum will provide greater success in finding murmurs.
IV. Electrocardiogram
  A. As with all feline cardiac disease, the ECG may be normal, and this should not lead the clinician to eliminate the possibility of cardiomyopathy if all else is compatible with the diagnosis.
  B. ECG features
    1. P waves and QRS complexes may be increased in amplitude and duration.
    2. Atrial and ventricular premature complexes are common.
    3. Conduction disturbances may also be present.
    4. Although not seen in all cases, a left anterior fascicular block may be peculiar to hypertrophic cardiomyopathy.

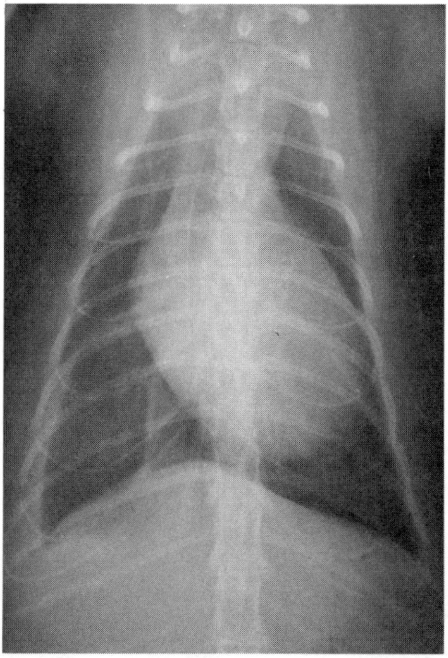

Fig. 6-5. Dorsoventral thoracic radiograph, cat in Fig. 6-4. There is generalized cardiac enlargement and the dilated atria cause the shape of the heart to assume a "valentine" appearance. Interstitial and faint alveolar infiltrate due to pulmonary edema is noted in both lungs.

V. Thoracic radiographs (Figs. 6-4 and 6-5)

A. Biatrial enlargement with a seemingly normal left ventricular apex or generalized cardiomegaly is seen. This typical valentine-shaped heart is not diagnostic of hypertrophic cardiomyopathy, thus one should avoid making a specific morphologic diagnosis based solely on the shape of the cardiac silhouette on the radiograph.

B. Pulmonary venous congestion and edema are usually present.

C. Mild pleural effusion may exist but is usually not the major abnormality.

D. Long-standing cases may develop pleural effusion secondary to chronically elevated left ventricular end-diastolic pressures.

VI. Echocardiogram

Echocardiography is an excellent tool for noninvasively distinguishing between the different types of cardiomyopathy.

A. Cats with hypertrophic cardiomyopathy have extremely thick left ventricular and septal walls, a dilated left atrium, and a small left ventricular cavity.

B. Echocardiography has the added advantage of giving more specific information regarding left ventricular function and the size of the right ventricle, which may be dilated secondary to long-standing hypertrophic cardiomyopathy.

VII. Angiography

Nonselective angiography may not be necessary if the diagnosis has been established by echocardiography.

A. Nonselective angiography usually indicates a hypertrophied left ventricular wall, enlarged papillary muscles, a small left ventricular cavity, and tortuous pulmonary veins.

B. Circulation time is normal.

VIII. Other diagnostic techniques

Results of blood tests are usually normal, although a mild prerenal azotemia may be present.

IX. Differential diagnosis

Hypertrophic cardiomyopathy, restrictive cardiomyopathy, and excessive left ventricular moderator bands may be clinically similar. The final diagnosis is frequently not made until postmortem examination.

Therapy and Prognosis

I. Therapy

A. In the acute stages, cage rest, oxygen, and administration of furosemide are the sole requirements.

B. Because of their sensitivity to the diuretic effects of furosemide, cats should be given no more than 1 to 2 mg/kg IV or IM once as an initial dose. Thereafter, a dosage of 1 mg/kg BID to TID is administered.

C. Once the patient has stabilized and failure has resolved, propranolol therapy (2.5 mg TID for cats less than 6 kg, 5.0 mg BID to TID for cats weighing more than 6 kg) is instituted.

D. Furosemide is continued at a dosage of 1 mg/kg orally once to twice daily. For cats that are refractory, this amount may be increased gradually to the level that controls edema.

E. If atrial fibrillation or right-sided heart failure occurs as a sequela, digoxin therapy at a dosage of 0.007 to 0.015 mg/kg tablet daily or every other day may be added to the regimen.

F. A vasodilator such as nitroglycerin paste or captopril may also prove beneficial.

II. Prognosis

A. Long-term prognosis of hypertrophic cardiomyopathy is generally more favorable than other forms of cardiomyopathy in cats.

B. Sudden death is always a possibility, however.

Feline Dilated (Congestive) Cardiomyopathy

Introduction

This form of cardiomyopathy is also very common, and is easily distinguished from other types of cardiomyopathy.

Diagnosis

I. Age, breed, and sex characteristics

A. Age and sex (middle-aged to older males) is the same as for hypertrophic cardiomyopathy.

B. Siamese, Burmese, and Abyssinians seem to be predisposed to dilated cardiomyopathy.

II. History

A. Cats with dilated cardiomyopathy usually have a relatively short history of only 1 to 3 days prior to examination.

B. Signs are nonspecific:

1. Anorexia
2. Lethargy
3. Dyspnea.
4. Occasional vomiting is frequently noted.

III. Physical examination

A. Clinical signs

Typical findings include

1. Hypothermia

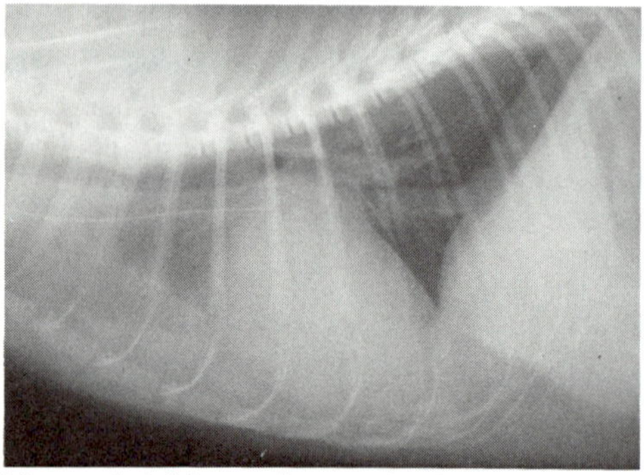

Fig. 6-6. Dilated (congestive) feline cardiomyopathy. Lateral thoracic radiograph. There is generalized cardiac enlargement with rounding of the cardiac silhouette. Mild pleural effusion due to right heart failure is noted.

2. Depression
3. Dehydration
4. Pallor
5. Dyspnea

B. Auscultation and palpation
1. Heart and lung sounds are usually muffled, and a murmur or gallop may be heard.
2. Pulses are usually weak.

IV. Electrocardiogram
A. Sinus bradycardia with wide and tall QRS complexes (lead II) are the most common findings.
B. First-degree heart block and ventricular arrhythmias are also common.

V. Thoracic radiographs (Figs. 6-6 and 6-7)
A. Generalized cardiomegaly with a rounded left ventricular apex is visualized, unless obscured by pleural effusion.
B. Ascites is rare in the cat.
C. The pleural effusion often needs to be withdrawn via thoracocentesis before the size of the cardiac silhouette can be appreciated.
D. Pulmonary edema may be present but is usually overshadowed by pleural effusion.

VI. Echocardiogram
Dilated cardiomyopathy presents one of the most dramatic echocardiographic pictures.

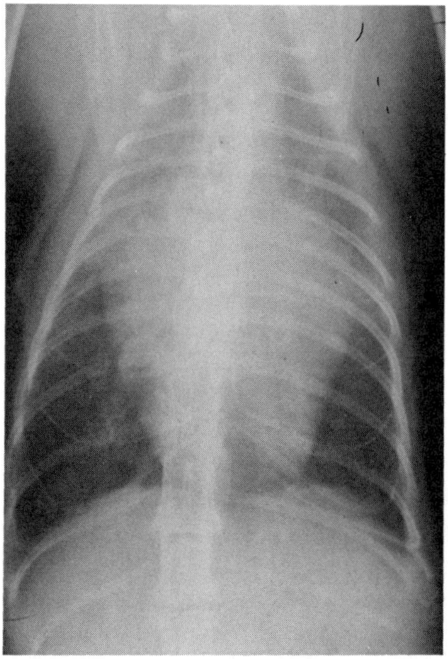

Fig. 6-7. Ventrodorsal projection, cat in Fig. 6-6. There is generalized cardiac enlargement. Mild pleural effusion due to right heart failure is seen in the right thorax within the lobar fissures and separating the visceral surface of the lung from the thoracic wall.

A. Both the septum and left ventricular free wall are thin and poorly contractile.

B. The left ventricle is severely dilated.

C. There is moderate left atrial dilatation, a normal to small aortic root diameter, and poor aortic root motion.

VII. Angiogram

A. Because of the stressful nature of angiography, extreme caution must be observed in selecting those patients to be studied. Only those cats whose diagnosis is in doubt should be chosen.

B. The hallmark of dilated cardiomyopathy is an extremely slow circulation time, accompanied by a dilated, thin-walled left ventricle and a poorly opacified aorta.

VIII. Other diagnostic tests. Because of cardiac insufficiency, most cats show a moderate prerenal azotemia.

IX. Differential diagnosis. Although more distinctive than other types of cardiomyopathy, the dilated form must still be distinguished from other forms. Any other cause of severe pleural effusion must also be considered (e.g. hemothorax, pyothorax, feline infectious peritonitis).

Therapy

I. Acute therapy

Cardiogenic shock may be a significant contributing factor in cats with dilated cardiomyopathy. Initial therapy should include:

A. Thoracocentesis
B. Oxygen
C. Intravenous fluids, 20 to 35 ml/kg-day
D. Furosemide, 1 mg/kg BID to TID
E. Heat lamp as needed
F. Intravenous digoxin (optional)
G. Vasodilators (optional)
H. For those with the capability of administering small volumes at a constant rate infusion, dopamine (1 to 10 μg/kg-min) or dobutamine (5 to 20 μg/kg-min) for 24 to 48 hours

II. Maintenance therapy

Cats recovering from the acute stages are discharged on digoxin, furosemide, and captopril.

III. Prognosis

Although this form of cardiomyopathy carries the poorest prognosis (average survival time 1 month from onset of clinical signs) there are documented cases of cats with dilated cardiomyopathy surviving more than 1 year.

Restrictive Cardiomyopathy

Introduction

Although less common than the other types of cardiomyopathy, restrictive cardiomyopathy is being diagnosed with increasing frequency.

Diagnosis

I. Age, breed, and sex characteristics
There are no distinguishing characteristics for restrictive cardiomyopathy.

II. History
Recent onset of lethargy, anorexia, and dyspnea are the usual complaints by the owner.

III. Physical examination
- A. Clinical signs. In general, cats with restrictive cardiomyopathy are more alert and less hypothermic than cats with dilated cardiomyopathy.
- B. Auscultation. Dyspnea, muffled lung sounds, and the presence of a murmur or gallop are common.

IV. Electrocardiogram
- A. Atrial fibrillation is occasionally seen due to marked left atrial dilatation.
- B. Ventricular arrhythmias may be seen; there also may be no abnormal findings.

V. Thoracic radiographs
- A. Generalized cardiomegaly with an enlarged left atrium is observed.
- B. Pulmonary edema or pleural effusion is present.

VI. Echocardiogram
Objective studies have not been undertaken to elucidate specific changes, but some general comments may be made:
- A. The left atrium is extremely dilated.
- B. The left ventricular diastolic diameter may be normal or slightly dilated.
- C. The left ventricular free wall may be normal or thick.
- D. Contractility may be normal or slightly diminished.

VII. Angiogram
- A. Nonselective angiography is very beneficial and frequently reveals an irregular left ventricular cavity with filling defects.
- B. The left atrium is extremely dilated and pulmonary veins are tortuous.

VIII. Differential diagnosis
Restrictive cardiomyopathy must be distinguished from other types of feline myocardial disease.

Therapy and Prognosis

I. Therapy
   A. If severe pleural effusion is present, thoracocentesis and oxygen are the most important early therapeutic measures.
   B. Several maintenance regimens have been employed using diuretics, digoxin, and vasodilators, all with limited success.
   C. The most useful drug seems to be furosemide, and much higher doses than expected have been administered. The amount in some cats has been increased in degrees to doses as high as 12.5 mg two times daily, and cats have often tolerated this amount well.

II. Prognosis

   Survival times fall between those of the dilated and hypertrophic form, although monitoring and control of the pleural effusion may prolong survival to a year or more.

Excessive Left Ventricular Moderator Bands

Introduction

This type of cardiomyopathy may exist as a single entity that resembles restrictive cardiomyopathy clinically, electrocardiographically, radiographically, or echocardiographically, or it may exist concurrently with hypertrophic or dilated cardiomyopathy.

Diagnosis

I. There are no distinctive characteristics of excessive moderator bands that distinguish it from other feline primary myocardial diseases.
II. Occasionally, fine, linear filling defects are visible on nonselective angiography, but they are not visible on the echocardiogram.

Therapy and Prognosis

I. Therapy depends on type of heart failure and on underlying hemodynamic abnormalities.
II. Prognosis is related to other underlying myopathic processes.

Arterial Thromboembolism

Introduction

Any cat affected with cardiomyopathy may have thromboembolism as the primary abnormality causing clinical signs. Thromoembolism arises from atrial thrombi or from atrial lesions and usually lodges in the iliac artery bifurcation, although it may affect any other area, (e.g., brachial, artery, celiac artery).

Diagnosis

I. History
   Acute onset of posterior paresis with associated dragging of the rear legs and crying is the hallmark of thromboembolism.
II. Physical examination
   A. Clinical signs
      Findings include
      1. Crying
      2. Panting
      3. Dyspnea
      4. Inability to use the hind legs
      5. Cyanotic nail beds
      6. Lower motor neuron paralysis
   B. Palpation
      1. Cool to cold rear limbs and diminished or absent femoral pulses.
      2. In the acute stages, limb muscles are soft but painful, progressing to firm or hard muscles during the first 24 hours. Pain in the limbs is transient.

III. Electrocardiography, radiography, and echocardiography vary depending on the associated type of cardiomyopathy.

IV. Angiogram

Nonselective angiography is helpful both in revealing the location of the clot and in diagnosing the type of cardiomyopathy.

V. Other diagnostic tests

A. Results of laboratory testing are consistent with severe muscle damage, and include greatly elevated serum lactic acid dehydrogenase, creatine phosphokinase, and asparate aminotransferase.

B. Clotting times may also be prolonged, indicating chronic disseminated intravascular coagulopathy.

C. Severe blood urea nitrogen and creatine elevations indicate the clot is lodged cranial to the renal arteries.

VI. Differential diagnosis

Acute injury to the spinal cord from trauma, tumors, or hemorrhage may be confused with arterial thromboembolism. Two findings that assist diagnosis are:

A. Acuteness of the paresis

B. Typical findings of cold limbs and absence of pulses

Therapy and Prognosis

I. Therapy

A. Acute arterial thromboembolism can be managed either medically or surgically.

B. Surgical intervention is no longer widely advocated; for two reasons:

1. Most cats are in heart failure.
2. Ischemic neuromyopathy is usually present, primarily as a result of vasoactive substances elaborated by the clot.

C. Rational medical regimens must include the use of appropriate agents specific for the two types of thrombosis:

1. Intravenous thrombosis (rare in the cat) consists primarily of fibrin clots. Drugs used include heparin and coumarin.
2. Intraarterial thrombosis is initiated by platelet aggregation, with secondary fibrin deposits. Platetet antiaggregates include aspirin, dipyrimadole, and propranolol. A dosage of 25 mg 1 kg of as-

pirin with an antacid (Ascriptin-Rorer) may be given every third to fourth day to an average-size cat.

D. Spontaneous recanalization of the thrombus may occur without drug therapy.

II. Prognosis

A. Collateral circulation around the clot and recanalization have been demonstrated angiographically 2 to 4 days after formation, resulting in returning of warm extremities, pink nail beds, and pulses.

B. Return to partial function is common within 2 to 3 weeks, with maximum recovery taking 4 to 6 weeks.

C. Prognosis is much better if only one front leg is affected and is much worse if the vessels of three or more legs are occluded.

D. Thromboemboli proximal to the renal arteries carry an extremely grave prognosis, and in such cases euthanasia should be considered.

E. Although recovery from aortic thromboembolism is usually good, many cats succumb to either heart failure or a repeat episode in a few months.

Hyperthyroid Heart Disease (See also Chapter 11)

Introduction

Most secondary cardiomyopathies in the cat are rare and will probably never be encountered in general practice. The exception is hyperthyroidism, which, because of its increasing frequency, will be discussed as a singular disease entity. Hyperthyroidism is caused by functional adenomas of the thyroid gland that produce excessive thyroid hormone.

Diagnosis

I. Age, breed, and sex characteristics

A. Affected cats are elderly.

B. There is no sex or breed predilection.

II. History
  A. The typical history is usually one of weight loss, hyperactivity, polyphagia, polydipsia, and bulky stools.
  B. Less commonly seen are clinical signs of lethargy and anorexia
III. Physical examination
  A. Clinical signs
    1. Cats affected by hyperthyroidism are usually thin; some are emaciated.
    2. Most are elderly and tend to be hyperactive.
  B. Auscultation and palpation
    1. Auscultation frequently reveals a systolic murmur heard best at the left apex, and a hyperdynamic apex beat is palpated easily.
    2. Unilateral or bilateral thyroid nodules can usually be palpated in the cervical region.
IV. Electrocardiogram
  A. Increased R-wave amplitude and sinus tachycardia are the most common abnormalities.
  B. Various atrial and ventricular arrhythmias and intraventricular conduction disturbances are not as common.
V. Thoracic radiographs
  A. Cardiac enlargement, especially of the left atrium and ventricle, are not unusual.
  B. Some cats will have radiographic changes of left or right heart failure.
VI. Echocardiogram
  Left ventricular hypertrophy, increased diastolic dimensions, left atrial dilatation, and increased indices of contractility are present in most cats with hyperthyroidism.
VII. Other diagnostic tests
  A. Diagnosis is confirmed by elevated serum thyroxine (T4) and/or triiodothyronine (T3) levels.
  B. Mild to moderate liver enzyme elevations are sometimes present.
  C. Radionuclide scanning using radioactive Technetium 99m or Iodine 131 can aid in the diagnosis and determine if one or both thyroid glands is affected, and the location of the thyroid glands.
VIII. Differential diagnosis
  A. Thyrotoxic heart disease must be differentiated from primary cardiomyopathy, especially the hypertrophic form.

B. Elevated serum thyroxine levels may exacerbate compensated mild myocardial disease.

Therapy and Prognosis

I. Medical therapy
   A. Propranolol: Hyperthyroidism is probably one of the best indications for the use of β-blockers because of the presence of tachycardia. Administration of propranolol is continued until the time of surgery.
   B. Furosemide: Diuretics are necessary only in the presence of heart failure.
   C. Propylthiouracil: This antithyroid drug has been used to lower thyroid concentrations prior to surgery. It is given at a dosage of 50 mg TID. Extended use has been associated with immune-mediated anemias.
   D. Methimazole: Another antithyroid drug currently being used is methimazole (5 mg TID). Extended use is reserved for those animals who are not able to undergo surgery.

II. Surgical therapy
   A. Removal of the thyroid gland is the most common method of treating this disease.
   B. If all precautions are taken beforehand (controlling cardiac abnormalities and lowering T_3 and T_4 to normal), results are usually favorable.

III. Prognosis
   A. Most cats respond extremely well to surgery.
   B. Serial radiographs and ECGs often show a diminution in cardiac size over time.

Summary—Feline Cardiomyopathy

I. There are four distinct types of feline cardiomyopathy, but the associated clinical findings frequently overlap, and it is not always easy to make an exact diagnosis. Even with the advent of echocardiography,

TABLE 6-2. COMMON CHARACTERISTICS OF FELINE CARDIOMYOPATHY[a]

Type	Breed	Hemodynamics	Pathology	ECG Features	Radiographic Features	Echocardiographic Features
Hypertrophic	Persians?	Impaired diastolic filling, decreased compliance	LVH, LAD	LAFB, Tall R, arrhythmias	Pulmonary edema, biatrial enlargement	Normal contractility, LAD, small LV cavity
Dilated (congestive)	Siamese Burmese Abyssinians	Systolic dysfunction, low output heart failure	LVH, LAD, thin LV wall	Bradycardia, tall wide R wave, arrhythmias	Pleural effusion, rounded LV apex	Severe LVD, thin LV and septal walls, mild LAD, poor contractility
Restrictive	No breed predisposition	Impaired diastolic filling, decreased compliance	Endomyocardial fibrosis, LAD		Pleural effusion or pulmonary edema, cardiomegaly	Normal to thick LV free wall and septum, mild decrease in contractility, LAD
Excessive moderator bands	No breed predisposition	Unknown	Excessive moderator bands in LV, LVH or LVD, LAD	Unknown	Pleural effusion or pulmonary edema, cardiomegaly	Variable
Hyperthyroid	No breed predisposition	High output heart failure, hypercontractile	LVH	Tall R wave Sinus tachycardia	LV enlargement	Mild LVD, LAD, LVH, increased contractility

[a]These characteristics should be used only as a guide in the differentiation of feline cardiomyopathy; they are not exclusively associated with the type listed, nor is the list exhaustive for each type.

LAD, left atrial dilatation,
LAFB, left anterior fascicular block,
LV, left ventricle,
LVD, left ventricular dilatation
LVH, left ventricular hypertrophy.

distinctions are often blurred. Therapy is sometimes selected more on the basis of type of heart failure and on what medications are effective in the individual animal than on underlying morphology.

II. Several generalizations can be made.

A. Left-sided heart failure is usually associated with hypertrophic cardiomyopathy. Furosemide and propranolol are the medications of choice.

B. Any cat examined because of severe hypothermia and signs compatible with cardiogenic shock should be considered to have dilated cardiomyopathy and treated as such.

C. Cats with right-sided heart failure are always treated with diuretics, but digoxin and/or vasodilators may be added.

D. Any aged cat diagnosed as having cardiomyopathy should have a thyroid concentration (T4) determined to rule out underlying hyperthyroidism as a contributing or primary cause.

SUGGESTED READINGS

Fox PR, Tilley LP, Liu S–K: Feline Medicine. p. 282. American Veterinary Publication, Santa Barbara, Calif. 1983

Harpster NK: Boxer cardiomyopathy. p. 329. In Kirk RW (ed): Current Veterinary Therapy. VIII. WB Saunders, Philadelphia, 1983

Kittleson M: Drugs used in the management of heart failure. p. 285. In Kirk RW (ed): Current Veterinary Therapy. VIII. WB Saunders, Philadelphia, 1983

Kittleson M: Concepts and the therapeutic strategies in the management of heart failure. p. 279. In Kirk RW (ed): Current Veterinary Therapy. VIII. WB Saunders, Philadelphia, 1983

Liu S–K, Tilley LP, Maron BJ: Canine hypertrophic cardiomyopathy. J Am Vet Med Assoc 174:708, 1979

Liu S–K, Fox PR, Tilley LP: Excessive moderator bands in the left ventricle of 21 cats. J Am Bet Med Assoc 180: 1215, 1982

Tilley LP, Liu S–K, Fox PR: Myocardial disease. p. 1029. In Ettinger SJ (ed): Textbook of Veterinary Internal Medicine, WB Saunders, Philadelphia, 1983

Wood GL: Canine myocardial disease. p. 321. In Kirk RW (ed): Current Veterinary Therapy. VIII. WB Saunders, Philadelphia, 1983

7

Cor Pulmonale

Glen L. Spaulding
Jerry M. Owens

INTRODUCTION

Definition

Cor pulmonale, also referred to as pulmonary heart disease, is defined as alterations occurring in the structure and/or function of the right ventricle induced by pulmonary hypertension secondary to primary diseases of the lung or pulmonary vasculature. Right ventricular changes and pulmonary hypertension secondary to congenital cardiac defects or diseases of the left side of the heart do not constitute cor pulmonale.

ETIOLOGY

I. Acute cor pulmonale usually occurs as a result of pulmonary thromboembolism. Some causes of acute cor pulmonale are listed in Table 7-1. In the dog, most clinical cases of pulmonary thromboembolism have been observed in animals with heartworm infestations, chronic renal diseases, glomeronephritis, hyperadrenocorticism, and pancreatitis.
II. Chronic cor pulmonale can develop as a result of a variety of conditions with a combination of factors most often involved in its development. (See Table 7-2.)
III. Hypoxia-induced vasoconstriction further contributes to the severity of this condition.

TABLE 7-1. SOME ETIOLOGIES OF ACUTE COR PULMONALE

Pulmonary thromboembolization
Heartworm infestation
Trauma
Surgical procedures (including cryosurgery)
Air contrast radiographic diagnostic procedures (especially pneumocystograms)
Septicemia
Neoplasia
Blood clotting abnormalities
Hyperviscosity states (paraneoplastic syndrome)
Amyloidosis
Pancreatitis
Hyperadrenocorticism
Hypothyroidism
ARDS (shock lung syndrome)
Severe hypoxia states
Upper airway obstruction
Trauma (e.g., pneumothorax and atelectasis)
Aspiration pneumonia
Inhalation of smoke and toxic gases
High altitude and low ambient O_2 environments
Inadequate ventilatory drive (e.g., anesthesia and coma)
Miscellaneous (and iatrogenic)
Positive-end expiratory ventilation during anesthesia
Drug-induced pulmonary hypertension (e.g., aspirin and ketamine)

IV. Exercise, respiratory infections, concurrent heart disease, and some medications, (e.g., aspirin and ketamine anesthesia) can aggravate pulmonary hypertension.

Incidence

I. The actual incidence of cor pulmonale in the dog and cat is unknown. It is probably not uncommon, but is only occasionally identified.

II. Heartworm infection (dirofilariasis) is probably the most common cause of both acute and chronic cor pulmonale in the dog.

III. Acute cor pulmonale due to thromboembolism is often fatal and not clinically diagnosed. In nonfatal thromboembolism, the diagnosis of embolism is usually not made.

IV. Chronic cor pulmonale is probably common as a sequel to chronic

TABLE 7-2. SOME ETIOLOGIES OF CHRONIC COR PULMONALE

Disorders of the pulmonary parenchyma and intrathoracic airways
Chronic bronchitis and bronchiectasis
Restrictive lung disease
Pulmonary fibrosis
Infiltrative lung disease (e.g., neoplasia and infection)
Allergic pulmonary disease
Upper airway obstruction
Collapsing trachea
Laryngeal paralysis and collapse
Redundant soft palate
Pulmonary vascular diseases
Heartworm infestations
Recurring thromboembolization
Lungworms
Abnormalities of chest wall structure and/or function
Thoracic deformities (e.g., pectus excavatum)
Obesity
Neuromuscular dysfunction of the chest wall and/or diaphragm

respiratory diseases in the dog and cat; however, it is frequently silent and not identified. Chronic cor pulmonale probably complicates the diagnosis and therapy of many pulmonary diseases due to the lack of recognition of its existence and the complexity of many pulmonary diseases.

PATHOPHYSIOLOGY

I. The development of pulmonary hypertension is the essential feature of cor pulmonale. A reduction of more than 50 percent of the cross-sectioned area of the pulmonary vasculature must occur, before pulmonary hypertension will occur. This decreased pulmonary vascular patency may be due to intraluminal obstruction, vasoconstriction, and extraluminal compression.
   A. Alveolar hypoxia or hypoventilation owing to respiratory disease results in hypoxemia, hypercapnia, and acidemia. These abnormalities, especially chronic hypoxia, are potent stimuli for pulmonary vasoconstriction.
   B. Pulmonary infections and inflammatory diseases are especially

deleterious because they contribute to the development of hypoxia and provide substrate for local production of prostaglandins and leukotrienes, which are potent mediators of vasoconstriction.

C. Pulmonary hypertension tends to become self-perpetuating as reversible medial hypertrophy of the pulmonary arteries develops. Cats apparently are highly predisposed to developing medial hypertrophy of the pulmonary arteries. Often a underlying cause for its development cannot be identified.

II. The right ventricle dilates, hypertrophies, or fails in response to pulmonary hypertension. Fluid retention and right-sided congestive heart failure may develop as the right heart fails. However, right ventricular failure is uncommon and is not an essential feature of cor pulmonale.

DIAGNOSIS

History

I. Acute cor pulmonale

A. The onset of cardiopulmonary signs may be acute or gradual and may be preceded by signs of weakness, depression, panting, anorexia, or trembling.

B. If the pulmonary thrombosis is severe, the patient may show severe inspiratory and expiratory distress, orthopnea, tachypnea, open mouth breathing and cyanosis. Sudden death may occur, usually because of circulatory failure and shock.

C. Coughing is uncommon. Hemoptysis and syncope are rarely observed.

II. Chronic cor pulmonale

A. This form of cor pulmonale is usually associated with chronic respiratory signs. The clinical signs referable to the underlying respiratory disease may include difficult or labored breathing, tachypnea, wheezing or chronic cough.

B. Certain canine breeds are more prone to chronic respiratory disease. Toy breed dogs are predisposed to tracheal collapse; small breed dogs commonly have chronic bronchitis and chronic mitral valve diseases. Brachycephalic breed dogs are more susceptible to obstructive upper airway disease.

C. The geographic background of the animal should also be considered as a predilection for chronic respiratory disease:
   1. Systemic mycosis infection in the River valleys and Southwest United States
   2. Dirofilariasis as an endemic disease in warm climate regions.

D. Exertional dyspnea, weakness, cachexia, and syncope may occur as the animal becomes progressively hypoxic.

E. Further hypoxia may be induced by infection or transiently by exercise.

Physical Examination

I. Tachypnea is the most common clinical sign associated with acute or chronic cor pulmonale.

II. The severity of the respiratory distress is variable. In patients with severe thromboembolism, rest and oxygen therapy usually fail to improve the clinical condition.

III. A fever is usually absent, unless the clinical problem is complicated by infection.

IV. Many affected animals may show compensatory conformational or postural changes, such as a barrel chest, abducted forelimbs, reluctance to lie down, and abdominal respirations.

V. The mucous membranes are sometimes cyanotic, but are usually discolored due to poor tissue perfusion.

VI. On thoracic auscultation, tachycardia, a gallop rhythm, a prominent or split second heart sound, or a soft systolic murmur due to tricuspid insufficiency may be heard. In addition, abnormal lung sounds associated with concurrent respiratory disease may be heard.

VII. If right-sided congestive heart failure is present, the physical findings may include distention of the jugular veins with jugular pulses, muffled heart and lung sounds due to pleural and/or pericardial effusion, ascites, hepatosplenomegaly, or peripheral edema.

VIII. In chronic cor pulmonale, the animal may show signs relative to progressive dyspnea, weakness, and cachexia.

Electrocardiographic Findings

I. No consistent electrocardiographic abnormalities are associated with acute or chronic cor pulmonale. However, abnormalities frequently are associated with the condition.
  A. P pulmonale (tall P waves) may be present in chronic cor pulmonale.
  B. Electrocardiographic evidence of right ventricular enlargement may be absent, but when present, it is usually indicated by a right axis deviation (S waves present in leads I, II, III, and AVF). Frequently deep Q waves are present.
  C. Alterations in the size and configuration of the T wave and S-T segment depression may reflect a hypoxic state.
  D. Arrhythmias are uncommon but include atrial premature complexes, atrial fibrillation, and ventricular premature complexes.

II. Conduction disturbances resulting in right or left axis deviation, marked ST-T changes, and arrhythmias occur more frequently when pulmonary thrombolization has occurred and severe hypoxemia is present.

III. Electrocardiographic examination may be useful in differentiating cor pulmonale with congestive heart failure from congestive cardiomyopathy, pericardial diseases, chronic valvular disease, and congenital heart disease.

Radiographic Examination

I. In acute cor pulmonale, the thoracic radiographs may appear normal or may show abnormalities that are highly suggestive of thromboembolism, including:
  A. Normal to reduced lung volume associated with lobar or sublobar hyperlucency.
  B. Hypoperfusion indicated by a reduced size of the peripheral lung vessels in the involved areas.
  C. The main pulmonary arteries may be normal sized or enlarged.
  D. Small amounts of pleural effusion may be present.

E. Right ventricular enlargement may be noted.
F. There is usually an absence of consolidation, atelectasis, or edema.

II. In dogs with heartworm infection, the radiographic features of pulmonary arterial disease include:
A. Enlargement of the right ventricle.
B. Enlargement of the pulmonary artery segment.
C. Enlarged, tortuous and pruned pulmonary arteries.
D. If pulmonary infarction has occurred, focal ill-defined regions of pulmonary consolidation may be seen.
E. In the regions of thromboembolism without infarction, the peripheral portions of the affected lung lobes may appear underperfused and more radiolucent than normal.
F. If right heart failure has occurred, pleural effusion, hepatomegaly and ascites may be identified. Pericardial effusion may be suspected if the cardiac silhouette appears more rounded and globular than normal.

III. In animals with chronic cor pulmonale due to other respiratory diseases, the radiographs may show associated abnormalities such as chronic airway disease, and pulmonary fibrosis.

IV. In animals suspected of having pulmonary thromboembolism, the definitive diagnosis can be made via pulmonary angiography.
A. Selective pulmonary angiography is the procedure of choice in which contrast media is infused directly into the pulmonary trunk. The size and degree of filling of the pulmonary arteries can be directly and clearly evaluated.
B. Nonselective angiography may be substituted for a selective technique with reasonable opacification of the pulmonary circulation. This is a practical technique and easily employed in a private practice. A bolus of iodinated contrast media (e.g., Renografin 76) is injected into the jugular vein at a dose of .25 ml/kg. A dorsoventral projection of the thorax is exposed 2 to 4 seconds after the injection is made.

V. Nuclear imaging of pulmonary perfusion is available at some institutions. It is a noninvasive procedure with a good assessment of lung perfusion and will readily demonstrate patency of the pulmonary circulation.

Clinical Pathologic Evaluation

I. The hematologic evaluation may be helpful in some cases of cor pulmonale.

A. If pulmonary embolism has occurred, the platelet count is sometimes decreased and the serum fibrin-split products is sometimes elevated.

B. In acute thromboembolism, the PCV and fibrinogen levels are frequently abnormal and can either be increased or decreased.

C. Polycythemia rarely develops as a result of chronic cor pulmonale.

II. A biochemical evaluation is of limited diagnostic value except in the identification of coexistent underlying disease.

III. Arterial blood gas abnormalities of hypoxemia ($PaO_2 < 80$ mm Hg), hypercapnia ($PaCO_2 > 40$ mm Hg), and acidosis ($pH < 7.4$) are frequently present in cor pulmonale.

A. Hypocapnia may develop secondary to hyperventilation, if arterio-venous shunting is not severe.

B. Monitoring blood gases may be helpful in determining the response to therapy and in establishing an accurate prognosis.

IV. A microfilaria examination should be done. If negative for microfilaria, and if heartworm disease is clinically suspected, an occult antibody test should be done.

V. If lungworms are suspected, a fecal examination for lungworm larvae should be performed.

Special Diagnostic Techniques

I. Elevations in central venous pressure (CVP), an easily measured parameter may be a good indicator that cor pulmonale is present. However, it does not provide an accurate estimate of pulmonary artery pressure.

II. Direct pulmonary arterial pressure measurements are not routinely performed in clinical small animal practice. When measured, however, greater than eightfold increases in mean arterial pressures have been observed in cor pulmonale due to pulmonary thrombosis and heartworm disease.

III. Echocardiography can be useful in differentiating chronic cor pulmonale from dilated cardiomyopathy and pericardial disease.

IV. In animals with chronic cor pulmonale additional diagnostic tests that may provide useful information include:
   A. Aspiration of pulmonary fluid, exudate or cells via tracheal or bronchial lavage for cytological evaluation and bacterial culture.
   B. Analysis of free pleural effusions
   C. Bronchoscopy to assess directly the internal anatomy of the trachea and major bronchi: also helpful in evaluating tracheal and bronchial collapse
   D. Fluoroscopically evaluating pulmonary and cardiac movements during respiration: helpful in observing tracheal collapse, bronchial collapse, and diaphragmatic movements.

Differential Diagnosis

I. Acute cor pulmonale and pulmonary arterial thromboembolization must be differentiated from other causes of acute respiratory distress (e.g., airway obstruction or pneumothorax) and from causes of acute congestive heart failure.

II. Chronic cor pulmonale must be differentiated from other causes of congestive heart failure, such as chronic valvular disease, congestive cardiomyopathy, pericardial disease, and the congenital cardiac defects (regardless of the age of the animal). When right-sided congestive heart failure is present, causes of hypoproteinemic states (e.g., protein-losing nephropathies, enteropathies and hepatic failure) should also be considered in the differential diagnosis.

TREATMENT

I. Early recognition of the problem and initiation of therapy is essential.

II. Correction of hypoxia to reverse the pulmonary vasoconstriction and hypertension should be the immediate aim of therapy. Supplemental oxygen administration and rest can provide some relief.

III. In animals in which pulmonary thromboembolism is either highly suggested or proved to be present on the basis of clinical, historical, and radiographic findings, treatment should consist of the following:

A. Strict rest:
It is imperative to minimize physical activity thus decreasing oxygen demand. At least 1 to 2 weeks is necessary to permit resolution of the pulmonary thrombi.

B. Oxygen therapy:
Increased oxygen should be made available to the patient, either via face mask or oxygen cage.

C. Anticoagulation therapy:
This is done in two phases.

1. Heparin therapy
   a) Heparin is given at doses to effect anticoagulation. The dose of heparin is titrated such that after intravenous infusion of heparin, a 15-minute blood sample shows an activated clotting time (ACT) two to three times normal and the partial thromboplastic time (PTT) is 1.5 to 2.5 times normal. Approximate doses of heparin that have been effective are:
      1) A total 24-hour dose of 100 to 1,200 IU/kg body weight.
      2) Intravenous heparin every 4 hours at 25 to 200 IU/kg body weight.
      3) A subcutaneous dose of 1,000 IU/kg body weight twice daily.
   b) If excessive bleeding occurs due to overdose of heparin therapy, protamine sulfate can be given intravenously to effect to counteract the anticoagulant effect of heparin.
2. Vitamin K antagonists and/or antiplatelet drugs
   a) Warfarin sodium (coumadin)
      1) Warfarin sodium (coumadin) is initially given at a dose of 0.2 mg/kg orally once daily.
      2) Subsequent doses should be 0.05 to 0.1 mg/kg once daily, titrated to achieve a prothrombin time (PT) two times baseline (pretreatment) values.
      3) Coumadin derivatives should be used for 6 weeks to 6

TABLE 7-3. TREATMENT OF COR PULMONALE

Acute cor pulmonale
Oxygen supplementation
Rest
Anticoagulants if thromboembolization suspected
Treat underlying disease(s)
Chronic cor pulmonale
Restricted activity
Treat underlying disease(s)
If complicated by congestive heart failure:
Diuretics
Salt restriction
Nitroglycerin

months or longer, depending on whether the initial problem is self-limiting or recurrent.

4) If excessive bleeding occurs during coumarin therapy, vitamin K_1 is given to effect. Aquamephyton is the injectable form of Vitamin K_1, and is also available in an oral tablet form.

b) Aspirin is an effective antiplatelet drug at doses of approximately 5 gr per 20 kg body weight per day.

1) Aspirin decreases platelet aggregation and is helpful in reducing further thrombosis.
2) It has also been helpful in preventing thromboembolism associated with feline cardiomyopathy and in decreasing pulmonary thromboemboli associated with heartworm therapy.
3) In some patients, aspirin may be contraindicated, as it causes vasoconstriction and increased pulmonary vascular resistance.
4) The therapeutic dose for the cat (4-6 mg/kg q 12h) is less than that of the dog (4-6 mg/kg q 6-12h). For both species, the dose must be titrated to avoid toxicity. Signs of toxicity include cardiac arrhythmias, muscle tremors, and gastrointestinal upset. This medication should be discontinued if it results in adverse reactions.

IV. Specific and supportive therapy should be directed toward the underlying respiratory disease in animals with chronic cor pulmonale.

A. Bronchodilators are frequently helpful (Table 7-3).

B. If pulmonary infections are present, appropriate antibiotic therapy can result in substantial clinical improvement.
C. Corticosteroid therapy is not recommended unless indicated specifically for the underlying respiratory disease. Steroids are sometimes useful in treating the thromboembolic disease associated with the management of heartworm infection.
D. Weight loss should be encouraged for the obese animal.
E. Conformational abnormalities such as the congenital upper respiratory defects in brachycephalic breeds should be corrected if they are significantly contributing to the development of the hypoxia.
F. Phlebotomy to control polycythemia may be necessary if oxygen therapy and rest are insufficient to control this abnormality.
G. If right-sided congestive heart failure develops, administration of diuretics and salt restriction are indicated. The need for diuretic therapy may be transient.

V. The use of digitalis for the treatment of cor pulmonale is controversial, and if it is used, it should be restricted to those animals that have developed congestive heart failure. The dose of digitalis should be carefully titrated, especially in the presence of hypoxemia, acidosis and electrolyte abnormalities, because these factors predispose the animal to the arrhythmogenic effects of digitalis.

VI. Vasodilator therapy may result in severe undesirable effects and should be used very cautiously if at all. Nitroglycerin is the vasodilator of choice for treatment of pulmonary hypertension in the dog.

VII. Excellent client communication is important. Many chronic respiratory conditions cannot be cured but can be potentially controlled.

PROGNOSIS

I. The prognosis for acute cor pulmonale due to pulmonary thromboembolization is favorable if the underlying cause of the embolization can be corrected and the animal responds to supportive therapy.
A. Resolution of the vascular obstruction due to blood clots occurs within hours of embolization with complete resolution usually occurring within 5 to 13 days.
B. Recurring embolization may result in acute death or progressive development of chronic cor pulmonale.

II. The prognosis for chronic cor pulmonale is usually favorable if signs of congestive right heart failure do not develop. Unfortunately, the underlying respiratory diseases often cannot be treated effectively.
  A. If clinical heart disease does occur, the prognosis is guarded.
  B. Control of secondary bacterial respiratory infections as well as exercise restrictions and supportive care are important.

SUGGESTED READINGS

Bishop MJ, Kennard S, Artman LD, Cheney FW: Hydralazine does not inhibit canine hypoxic pulmonary vasoconstriction. Am Rev Respir Dis 128: 998, 1983

Bredenberg CE, Taylor GA, Webb Wr: The effect of thrombocytopenia on the pulmonary and systemic hemodynamics of canine endotoxin shock. Surgery 87:59, 1980

Brewster, RD, Benjamin SA, Thomassen RW: Spontaneous cor pulmonale in laboratory beagles. Lab Anim Sci 33:299, 1983

Burns MG: Pulmonary thromboembolism. p. 257. In Kirk RW (ed): Current Veterinary Therapy. VIII. WB Saunders, Philadelphia, 1983

Fluckinger MA, Gomez JA: Radiographic findings in dogs with spontaneous pulmonary thrombosis or embolism, Vet Radiol 25:124, 1984

Leffler CW, Passmore JC: Contribution of prostaglandins to the regulation of pulmonary vascular resistance in adult cats and dogs. Prostaglandins and Medicine 3:343, 1979

Lombard CW, Buergelt CD: Echocardiographic and clinical findings in dogs with heartworm-induced cor pulmonale. Comp Contin Ed Pract Vet 5:971, 1983

McFadden ER Jr, Braunwald E: Cor pulmonale and pulmonary thromboembolism. p. 1643. In Braunwald E. (ed.): Heart Disease. vol. II. Philadelphia, WB Saunders, 1980.

Marin MB, Dawson CA: Pulmonary venoconstriction caused by elevated cerebrospinal fluid pressure in the dog. J Appl Physiol 49:73, 1980

Malik AG, vanderZee H, Johnson A. Inhibition of micro-embolization-induced pulmonary edema by early heparin treatment in dogs. Thromb Res 18:139, 1980

Molloy WD, Lee KY, Girling L, et al: Treatment of shock in a canine model of pulmonary embolism. Am Rev Respir Dis 130:870, 1984

Pearl RG, Rosenthal MH, Ashton JPA: Pulmonary vasodilator effects of nitroglycerin and sodium nitroprusside in canine oleic acid-induced pulmonary hypertension. Anesthesiology 58:514, 1983

Rawlings CA, Keith JC, Losonsky JM: Aspirin and prednisone modification of postadulticide pulmonary arterial disease in heartworm-infected dogs: Arteriographic study. Am J Vet Res 44:821, 1983

Thayer GW, Carrig CB, Evans AT: Fatal venous air embolism associated with pneumocystography in a cat. J Am Vet Med Assoc 176:643, 1980

8

Canine Heartworm Disease

Clay A. Calvert

INTRODUCTION

Although the dog is the primary host of *Dirofilaria immitis*, the parasite occasionally infects other mammalian species.

INCIDENCE

Dirofilaria immitis has been endemic in the coastal areas of the southeastern and southern United States for at least 50 years. The incidence has gradually spread and increased to include most of the Eastern and Midwestern states. *D. immitis* infects a smaller percentage of dogs in Texas, Oklahoma, Kansas, and Nebraska and is spreading to the western states.

I. *Epizootiology*

   D. immitis infects dogs of all ages but primarily those 4 to 7 years of age. Male and large dogs are more often infected than are female and small dogs. The risk of infection is directly proportional to the amount of time spent out-of-doors.

II. *Infection*

   Infective larvae (L_3) gain access to the subcutaneous and subserosal tissues via the puncture wound made by the mosquito.

   A. The L_3 molt occurs approximately 2 weeks postinfection. At this time, diethylcarbamazine (DEC) can eradicate the infection.
   B. Young adult worms (L_5) arrive in the heart 90 to 100 days postinfection. Eosinophilia first occurs at this time.
   C. Prepatency is usually 6 months, but microfilariae may not be pro-

duced for as long as 8 months. Patent infections may last more than 7 years.

D. Eosinophil counts increase again when microfilariae appear.

Pathophysiology

The time course and severity of pathology elicited by heartworm infection are determined by the number of worms, duration of infection, and parasite–host interaction.

I. Pulmonary artery pathology

The caudal lung lobes receive the heaviest infection. By the time microfilariae appear, arterial lesions are already present and progressing.

A. Platelet-derived growth factor

Adult worms, probably via a released substance, damage arterial endothelium leading to platelet and leukocyte adherence. Activated platelets release a trophic factor that initiates myointimal proliferation.

1. Smooth muscle proliferation: Muscle cells multiply and migrate to the surface, producing villus proliferation. Villi extend from the pulmonic valve to all arteries large enough to accommodate worms.
2. Pulmonary arterial enlargement: Affected arteries dilate, become tortuous, develop aneurysms, and lose their normal tapering and arborization.

B. Blood flow

Decreased or obstructed circulation occurs and focal alveolar consolidation surrounds the affected vessels.

C. Inflammatory reactions

Vascular permeability leads to plasma leakage into interstitial spaces and alveoli. Inflammation triggered by activated leukocytes contributes to edema formation.

D. Pulmonary hypertension

Arterial obstruction, decreased cross-sectional area, loss of dilatation capability, and the inability for collateral recruitment produce pulmonary hypertension and increased right ventricular afterload.

II. Right ventricular function
The increased afterload and inability to maintain a normal ejection fraction causes the right ventricle to dilate.

A. Frank–Starling mechanism
As right ventricular output decreases, left ventricular output also decreases. This incites the renin–angiotensin–aldosterone mechanism, leading to fluid and sodium retention. The expansion of the intravascular compartment increases right ventricular preload and force of contraction.

B. Right ventricular hypertrophy
1. Chronically increased afterload eventually produces increased myocardial mass and an associated decrease in contractile efficiency.
2. Right ventricular hypertrophy is associated with right-sided congestive heart failure.

III. Electrocardiography
During the right ventricular dilatation process, there is no electrocardiographic evidence of hypertrophy.

A. Hypertrophy
Electrocardiographic criteria of right ventricular hypertrophy develop as the ventricular mass increases.

B. Right-sided congestive heart failure
When the electrocardiogram reflects three or more criteria of right ventricular hypertrophy (see chapter 3), heart failure is usually present or probably will soon develop.

IV. Occult infections
The severity and rapidity of progression of pulmonary, cardiac, and clinical pathology are generally greater in dogs in which circulating microfilariae are not present.

A. Incidence
Between 5 and 25 percent of all infections are occult. The incidence varies considerably by geographic area, tending to be higher in some endemic regions.

B. Hypersensitivity
Host immune-mediated responses and resultant inflammation can produce a hypersensitivity reaction in some dogs.
1. Unusually high levels of antibody entrap the microfilariae within the pulmonary capillaries.

2. Activated leukocyte adhesion to microfilariae facilitates microfilarial sequestration.

C. Granulomatous inflammation

As a result of host immune-mediated reactions to microfilariae, a granulomatous inflammation occurs that worsens and accelerates the development of pulmonary hypertension.

D. Clinical signs

Coughing, exercise intolerance, dyspnea, pulmonary arterial obstructive lung disease, and right-sided congestive heart failure are likely to occur when occult disease is due to host–parasite immune-mediated interaction.

E. Unisex infections

Occasionally, occult infections may be due to unisex infections when the adult worm burden is low. Clinical signs therefore develop more slowly and are less severe.

V. Postadulticide pulmonary pathology

After natural or drug-induced death of adult worms, the same processes that initiated arterial damage are exacerbated.

A. Thrombosis and granulomatous inflammation

During the first 3 to 6 weeks after adulticide, severe thrombosis and granulomatous inflammation occur.

1. Myointimal proliferation into rugose villi worsens.
2. Edema develops due to vascular permeability, inflammation, and thrombosis.

B. Intravascular coagulopathy

The coagulation process is activated, leading to secondary fibrinolysis and either local or disseminated intravascular coagulation (DIC)

C. Pulmonary arterial obstructive disease

Pathologic changes begin to resolve in 3 to 6 weeks, pulmonary arterial pressure diminishes in 4 to 8 weeks, and pressures are usually normal within 6 months.

VI. Glomerulopathy

Although glomerulonephritis is a common sequela of heartworm disease, azotemia and severe proteinuria are uncommon.

VII. Amyloidosis

Renal amyloidosis and the nephrotic syndrome are occasionally diagnosed.

TABLE 8-1. CLINICAL PATHOLOGIC ABNORMALITIES ASSOCIATED WITH 193 CASES OF CANINE HEARTWORM DISEASE[a]

Abnormality	Microfilariae Status	Incidence (%)
Anemia (PCV <38%)		10
Neutrophilia		20
Eosinophilia	Microfilaremic	85
	Amicrofilaremic	95
Basophilia	Microfilaremic	50
	Amicrofilaremic	70
Liver enzyme elevation (SGPT, SAP)		10
Increased BSP retention (>5%)[b]		20
Azotemia (BUN >30 mg%)		5
Proteinuria (≥2+)[c]		20
Metabolic acidosis (arterial pH <7.31)		15
Hypoxia (PAO_2 <85)[d]		30

[a]Seen at the University of Georgia Veterinary Medicine Teaching Hospital.
[b]Fifty percent incidence if heart failure present.
[c]Thirty percent incidence in symptomatic infections.
[d]Severe pulmonary arterial pathology present.

Clinical Pathology

In most dogs with *D. immitis* infection, few, if any, laboratory abnormalities develop. Eosinophilia and, less often, basophilia are the most commonly observed abnormalities (Table 8-1).

Modification of Pulmonary Pathology

Myointimal proliferation of the pulmonary arteries begins soon after the arrival of young adult *D. immitis* and progresses during the infection. The process is exacerbated after adulticide therapy and is directly related to platelet and leukocyte adhesion to damaged endothelium and the release of platelet-derived growth factor.

I. Aspirin

Aspirin administered during heartworm infection diminishes pulmonary artery pathology.

A. Dosage

10 mg/kg, once daily.

B. Postadulticide effect

Aspirin given during and for 3 to 4 weeks after thiacetarsamide treatment reduces postadulticide myointimal proliferation and parenchymal lung pathology.

C. Mechanism of action

Less myointimal proliferation and fibrosis result from decreased platelet adhesion and release of platelet-derived growth factor.

II. Glucocorticoid hormones

Glucocorticoid hormones reduce the inflammatory response of heartworm disease pathology.

A. Allergic pneumonitis

Coughing, dyspnea, fever, interstitial inflammation, and alveolar edema are alleviated by short-term use of glucocorticoid hormones.

B. Thromboembolic disease

Both pre- and postadulticide obstructive arterial disease produces inflammation that is lessened by glucocorticoid hormones.

C. Interference with adulticide

1. Glucocorticoid hormones inhibit the killing effect of thiacetarsamide on young adult female *D. immitis*.
2. Do not administer prednisone or other equivalent steroids during and for 1 week after adulticide therapy.

HISTORY

The clinical history of heartworm-infected dogs depends on the duration of infection and on whether the infection is occult.

Asymptomatic Infections

Most dogs tested yearly for microfilariae will be diagnosed early during the course of infection before the onset of clinical signs.

Symptomatic Infections

In dogs with microfilaremic infections that remain undetected for several years or more relatively severe clinical signs may develop. Although dogs with occult infections may be diagnosed before the onset of moderate to severe pulmonary arterial pathology, occult infections are usually associated with a higher incidence of severe pulmonary arterial pathology, right ventricular hypertrophy, and right-sided congestive heart failure.

I. Clinical signs
   Coughing, exercise intolerance, weight loss, syncope, exertional dyspnea, hemoptysis, and abdominal distention develop sequentially.
II. Occult infections
   Advanced clinical signs such as marked weight loss, syncope, exertional dyspnea, or collapse and abdominal distention are most often associated with occult infections. Although the numbers of adult worms are not necessarily greater than in microfilaremic infections, the parasite–host interaction is usually more severe.

PHYSICAL EXAMINATION

The likelihood of detecting physical abnormalities in heartworm-infected dogs is directly related to the severity of pulmonary arterial obstructive lung disease and concomitant pulmonary hypertension.

Asymptomatic Infections

Most dogs examined annually for heartworm infection exhibit no abnormal physical findings; therefore, microfilarial tests are relied upon for diagnosis.

Symptomatic Infections

Dogs not examined annually for heartworm disease and those with occult infections often exhibit abnormal clinical findings.

I. Overt clinical signs
   Dogs with advanced pulmonary pathology may have grossly visible abnormalities. Weight loss, poor hair coat, cough, tachypnea, dyspnea, or distended abdomen may be observed.

II. Auscultation
  A. Splitting of the second heart sound may be detected in approximately 25 percent of symptomatic dogs.
  B. Cardiac murmurs, when present, are usually associated with the caval syndrome or right-sided congestive heart failure and are detected in fewer than 10 percent of all cases.
  C. Moist lung sounds are often auscultable in dogs with allergic pneumonitis or parenchymal lung disease associated with severe arterial obstructive disease.
  D. Gallop rhythms are uncommon but are usually associated with heart failure or the caval syndrome.

III. Palpation
  A. Hepatomegaly is associated with advanced pulmonary hypertension (usually when right-sided congestive heart failure is present) or the caval syndrome.
  B. Abdominal fluid may be balloted in dogs with heart failure.
  C. Jugular pulses or distended jugular veins resulting from elevation of the central venous pressure are often detected in dogs with right-sided congestive heart failure.

IV. Allergic pneumonitis

In some dogs with occult infections, a pulmonary hypersensitivity occurs shortly after the production of microfilariae.

  A. Clinical signs

  Affected dogs are invariably tachypneic or dyspneic, and coughing is usually a prominent component of the syndrome. Low-grade fever is occasionally present, and moist rales are frequently auscultated.

  B. Pulmonary arterial pathology

  The severity of clinical signs is disproportionate to the minor degree of pulmonary arterial changes seen on the survey radiographs. The reaction is predominantly mixed interstitial and alveolar and develops before advanced arterial pathology.

V. Caval syndrome

When large numbers of worms mature during a short period of time, obstruction of the right atrium and caudal vena cava can occur.

  A. Clinical signs

  Affected dogs are weak and dyspneic and have pale mucous membranes and poor capillary refill. Hypotension and tachycardia are usually present. A heart murmur or a gallop rhythm may be auscultated.

B. Hemoglobinuria is usually present.

VI. Right-sided congestive heart failure

Heart failure is a relatively common occurrence in heartworm endemic areas.

A. Clinical signs

Weight loss, dyspnea, ascites, and visible jugular pulses are usually present. Pale mucous membranes and tachycardia may occur if right ventricular output is drastically reduced. Hepatomegaly, gallop rhythm, and splitting of the second heart sound may be present.

B. Data base

A complete blood count, serum chemistry profile, urinalysis, electrocardiogram, and thoracic radiographs are indicated.

VII. Pulmonary thromboembolic disease

Thromboembolic complications may occur before or after adulticide treatment.

A. Clinical signs

Fever, coughing, tachypnea, or hemoptysis are variably present. Moist lung sounds occur if the inflammatory response extends into the lung parenchyma and plasma leaks from affected small arterioles and capillaries.

B. Data base

Thoracic radiographs, an activated clotting time, and platelet count are indicated.

VIII. Disseminated intravascular coagulopathy

Acute DIC is most common 7 to 14 days postadulticide therapy in dogs with severe pulmonary pathology. Occasionally, chronic low-grade DIC, also associated with severe pulmonary pathology, is detected before treatment.

A. Clinical signs

Epistaxis or hemoptysis should alert the clinician to the possibility of DIC. Dyspnea occurs if thromboembolic complications are severe and plasma or blood accumulate in the lung parenchyma.

B. Data base

A platelet count, activated clotting time, fibrinogin, prothrombin

TABLE 8-2. ELECTROCARDIOGRAPHIC ABNORMALITIES DETECTED IN 276 DOGS WITH HEARTWORM DISEASE[a]

Abnormality	Incidence (%)	Association (%)
Extrasystoles	12 (4)	Advanced disease (100)
Ventricular	8	
Supraventricular	4	
Atrial fibrillation	3 (1)	Heart failure (100)
Bundle branch block	3 (1)	
Right	1	
Left anterior fascicle	2	
Right ventricular hypertrophy[b]	48 (17)	Heart failure (85)
Total abnormalities	66 (24)	Heart failure (80)

[a]Seen at the University of Georgia Veterinary Medicine Teaching Hospital.
[b]Three or more electrocardiographic criteria of right ventricular hypertrophy.

time, activated partial thromboplastin time, and determination of fibrin degradation products are indicated.

ELECTROCARDIOGRAPHY

The electrocardiogram of heartworm-infected dogs is usually normal. Electrocardiographic abnormalities are seen in those dogs suffering advanced pulmonary pathology, most often in dogs with occult infections (Table 8-2).

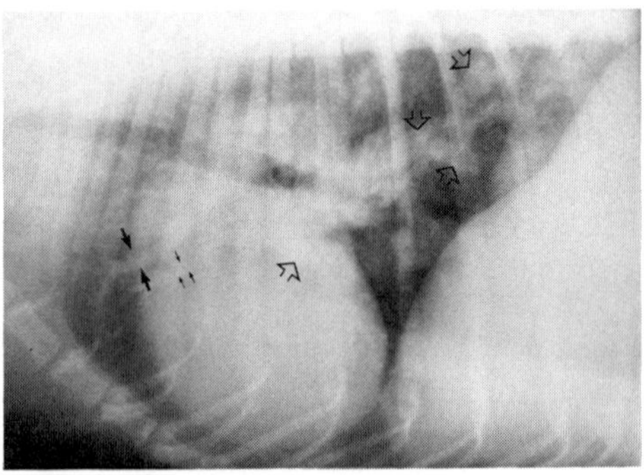

Fig. 8-1. Dirofilariasis in a dog. Lateral thoracic radiograph. There is right heart enlargement. The cranial lobar artery (thick arrows) is larger than its corresponding vein (small arrows), and the caudal lobar arteries are enlarged, tortuous and pruned (open arrows).

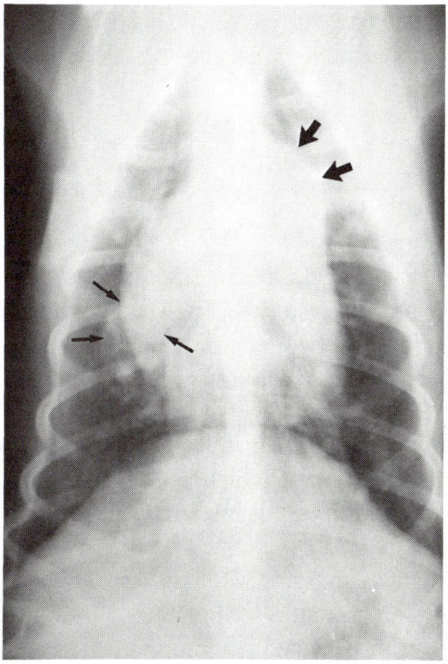

Fig. 8-2. Dorsoventral projection (same dog as in Fig. 8-1). There is right heart enlargement, bulging of the main pulmonary artery (thick arrows) and marked enlargement of the right caudal lobar artery with pruning (small arrows).

I. Right-sided congestive heart failure

In more than 90 percent of instances of right-sided congestive heart failure, the electrocardiogram exhibits three or more criteria of right ventricular hypertrophy. Of the remainder, two criteria are usually present.

II. Electrocardiographic indications

The electrocardiogram, as a component of the data base, may be reserved for those instances wherein right-sided congestive heart failure or severe radiographic pulmonary arterial pathology exists. In all other instances, the electrocardiogram does not exhibit right ventricular enlargement.

THORACIC RADIOGRAPHY (Figs. 8-1 and 8-2)

Almost 90 percent of microfilaremic dogs and more than 90 percent of dogs with occult infections seen at our institution have at least subtle thoracic radiographic changes suggestive of heartworm disease. In nonendemic regions, minimal radiographic lesions may be seen or the radiographs may be normal.

Severity of Disease

Thoracic radiographs are the diagnostic aid most important in the assessment of heartworm disease severity. The complete blood count, serum chemistry profile, and electrocardiogram reveal much less about the severity of cardiopulmonary pathology.

I. Duration of infection
   In general, the number and severity of pulmonary changes correlate directly with the duration of infection. Progression of pulmonary pathology is more rapid in occult infections.
II. Severity of disease
   In heavily infected dogs, survey radiographs can detect vascular changes within 4 to 5 months of infection. Virtually all dogs with advanced heartworm-associated pathology (i.e., heart failure, cor pulmonale, syncope, hemoptysis, exercise intolerance) have characteristic radiographic changes.

Thoracic Radiograph

Indications

Radiographs are indicated for dogs with symptomatic and suspected occult infections. Thoracic radiographs are not a prerequisite for adulticide therapy in every instance.

I. Nonindications
   Asymptomatic microfilaremic dogs, dogs tested yearly for microfilariae, and dogs less than 2 years of age do not require survey radiographs.
II. Indications
   All symptomatic dogs, dogs not tested yearly for microfilariae, dogs with suspected occult infections, and dogs with electrocardiographic evidence of right ventricular hypertrophy should be evaluated with thoracic radiographs.

DIAGNOSTIC TECHNIQUES

The diagnosis of heartworm disease may be based on the identification of *D. immitis* microfilariae, the presence of serum antibodies to microfilarial or adult antigens, or diagnostic thoracic radiographs.

Direct Blood Smear

Although the direct blood smear is an inexpensive, rapid, and useful test, it should not be relied upon as the sole indicator of the absence of infection. The Knott and filter tests are at least 10 percent more sensitive than the direct blood smear.

Knott Test

The modified Knott test is probably the most commonly employed diagnostic test for heartworm disease. The modified Knott test offers the advantage of being less expensive and time consuming than filter tests, and microfilarial morphology is more easily determined.

Filter Tests

The filter tests are at least as sensitive as the modified Knott test and are the tests best suited for fieldwork.

I. Cross-contamination
   Cross-contamination of the lysing solution or dispenser nozzle may result from improper technique.
II. Loss of microfilariae
   Improper assembly or wrinkles in the filter may result in loss of microfilariae.

Indirect Fluorescent Antibody Test

I. The indirect fluorescent antibody test (IFA) detects antibodies to *D. immitis* microfilarial cuticular antigen.
   A. Test of choice for immune-mediated occult heartworm disease.
   B. Test results may remain positive for one year after live adult worms are no longer present.

C. False-negative test results occur in up to 20 percent of all infections and may be due to either antigen excess or early potent infections.

II. The IFA test and enzyme-linked immunosorbent assay (ELISA) for the detection of antibodies to adult *D. immitis.*

A. Very sensitive tests for the detection of heartworm infection in the absence of microfilariemia. Somatic antigens are employed. This IFA test should not be confused with the IFA test for the detection of *D. immitis* microfilarial cuticular antigen.

B. Positive titers occur after day 70 post-L_3 infection. IFA and ELISA titers often decline 6 to 7 months after L_3 infection.

C. IFA and ELISA titers tend to rise and peak approximately 4 weeks post-thiacetersamide and then decrease to non-detectable levels after 6 to 12 months.

D. False-positive test results can occur due to cross reactivity to nematodes, primarily *D. reconditum* and intestinal helminths.

E. A negative IFA or ELISA test almost eliminates the possibility of *D. immitis* infection. The currently available IFA and ELISA tests are of similar sensitivity and specificity.

F. Newer tests for the detection of adult *D. immitis* antigens may be less sensitive and thus reduce the incidence of false-positive results.

Thoracic Radiography

Thoracic radiographs are valuable in the diagnosis of suspected occult infections.

I. Asymptomatic occult infections

Dogs with minimal pulmonary pathology may not have diagnostic radiographic changes.

II. Symptomatic occult infections

Thoracic radiography is a more accurate diagnostic test than the IFA and ELISA tests when clinical signs of advanced disease are present.

PROTOCOL FOR DIAGNOSIS

The recommended minimum data base for heartworm-infected dogs varies with the age of the patient, severity of related pathology, duration of infection, and concomitant problems.

Minimum Data Base

The minimum data base for young to middle aged dogs with no or minimal clinical signs should include

I. Physical examination
II. Hematocrit or complete blood count
III. BUN
IV. Urinalysis

Extended Data Base

Additional diagnostic tests are indicated for older dogs, symptomatic infections, occult infections, in dogs with evidence of major organ failure, and in those not tested yearly for microfilaremia (Table 8-3).

Liver Enzymes

Far too much emphasis is placed on liver enzyme (SGPT, SAP) evaluation.

TABLE 8-3. INDICATION FOR AN EXTENDED DATA BASE

Test	Indication
Thoracic radiographs	Occult infection Symptomatic infection
Electrocardiogram	Heart failure Severe pulmonary pathology
Serum chemistry profile	Symptomatic infection "Old" dog
Platelet count and coagulogram	Hemoptysis Epistaxis Petechiation
BSP test	Hypoalbuminemia Cachexia
Proteinuria quantitation	Proteinuria Hypoalbuminemia Cachexia
Renal biopsy	Severe proteinuria
Transtracheal lavage	Coughing and parenchymal lung disease

I. Pretreatment elevations of SGPT and/or SAP are of little or no prognostic significance.
   A. Adverse reactions to thiacetarsemide are not predicted by liver enzyme elevations.
   B. Treatment associated mortality rates are not higher when SGPT or SAP are elevated.

II. Elevation of SGPT and SAP in response to thiacetarsemide is common.
   A. Treatment-associated enzyme elevations alone are not an indication to abandon adulticide therapy.
   B. Persistent vomiting, anorexia, and icterus are indications to stop therapy.

THERAPEUTIC APPROACH

Proper treatment of heartworm disease depends on the severity of pulmonary arterial pathology and any coexisting related syndromes.

Complicated Heartworm Disease

There are several syndromes that, when present, should be treated before instituting adulticide therapy.

Allergic Pneumonitis

This syndrome occurs in 10 to 15 percent of occult infections seen at our institution and responds dramatically to glucocorticoid hormone therapy. Moist rales, dyspnea, and thoracic radiograph abnormalities diminish within 12 to 24 hours of therapy and are usually resolved within 2 to 3 days.

I. Clinical signs
   Moist rales, coughing, and dyspnea are invariably present. Fever, cyanosis, and slight weight loss may occur.
II. Treatment
   Prednisone (1 to 2 mg/kg-day in single or divided doses) or an equiv-

alent dose of other glucocorticoid hormone should be administered for 5 to 7 days.

III. Precaution
Glucocorticoid hormone therapy should be stopped before adulticide therapy. Relapse of clinical signs usually does not occur during subsequent adulticide therapy.

Pulmonary Arterial Thromboembolic Disease

This syndrome is most often encountered after adulticide therapy, but may be present before any therapy is instituted.

I. Treatment
   A. Cage rest is the most important component of the treatment regimen. Complete inactivity should be maintained for a minimum of 5 to 7 days.
   B. Aspirin (10 mg/kg-day) and glucocorticoid hormones are of value.
   C. Bronchodilators and antibiotics are often prescribed, but without proven benefit.
   D. Arteriolar dilators, such as hydralazine, have been employed by the author as a treatment of pulmonary thromboembolism and/or hypertension. However, no obvious benefits were observed. Furthermore, systemic arteriolar dilatation without an appropriate increase in right ventricular output results in systemic hypotension.

II. Precautions
   A. Aspirin should not be administered if there is clinical or laboratory evidence of a bleeding disorder or if hemoptysis is present.
   B. Adulticide therapy is not given until there is clinical and radiographic evidence of significant resolution of disease.
   C. Glucocorticoid hormones are withdrawn from the therapy regimen before adulticide therapy.

Right-Sided Congestive Heart Failure

This syndrome is relatively common in endemic areas and is usually associated with occult infections.

I. Treatment
   A. Cage rest for at least 7 days before, during, and for 3 to 4 weeks postadulticide therapy.
   B. Aspirin (10 mg/kg-day) for 7 days before, during, and for 3 to 4 weeks postadulticide therapy.
   C. Furosemide (2 mg/kg-day) and a low-sodium diet beginning at the time of diagnosis and continuing for 2 to 3 months.
   D. Adulticide therapy. Thiacetarsamide (2.2 mg/kg bid for 2 days) is administered after 7 to 10 days of cage rest and aspirin therapy.

II. Results
Thirty of 37 dogs (80 percent) treated as outlined survived and returned to functional status. Supportive therapy was required for 2 to 3 months.

III. Complications
Six of 7 dogs not surviving adulticide therapy died 7 to 10 days posttreatment with clinical and laboratory evidence of acute DIC and pulmonary arterial obstructive lung disease.

IV. Conservative treatment
Ten dogs receiving only supportive therapy did not improve and died or were euthanized within 2 to 3 months.

V. Digoxin
Dogs given digoxin in addition to the above protocol did not have a greater survival rate. However, digoxin toxicity was frequently encountered.

Caval Syndrome

This syndrome is relatively common in highly endemic areas and is uniformly fatal unless some adult worms are removed.

I. Treatment
   A. Under local anesthesia, a long alligator forceps is passed, via the right jugular vein, into the right atrium and caudal vena cava.
   B. Multiple attempts are made to remove adult worms. One to four worms are typically removed per attempt. The surgery is terminated when five to six consecutive passages fail to retrieve worms.

C. Fluid therapy (with central venous pressure monitoring) and urine output monitoring are instituted after surgery.

D. Routine adulticide therapy is begun when there is clinical and laboratory evidence of stabilization.

1. Hypotension, tachycardia, dyspnea, and azotemia should be resolved before adulticide therapy.
2. Liver enzyme elevations and excessive BSP retention are slow to resolve and are not contraindications to adulticide therapy.

II. Precaution

Complications such as perforation of the jugular vein, right atrium, or caudal vena cava can occur.

Disseminated Intravascular Coagulopathy

Chronic or subacute low-grade DIC may occasionally be present at the time of diagnosis of severe heartworm disease. Epistaxis, petechiation, or evidence of hemolysis may be detected.

I. Diagnosis

Low-grade DIC is characterized by platelet counts of 75,000 to 150,000/mm^3, normal or slightly prolonged activated clotting time, prothrombin time, and partial thromboplastin time, and the absence of or low levels of fibrin degradation products.

II. Treatment

A. Low-dose heparin (150 to 250 IU/kg, SQ, TID) may reduce the severity of DIC.

B. Cage rest for 7 to 14 days should elapse before adulticide therapy.

III. Precaution

Consultation with a clinician experienced in the treatment of DIC is imperative.

Adulticide Therapy

Thiacetarsamide sodium is the only time-tested treatment for *D. immitis*. The currently recommended protocol has been in use for more than 25 years.

TABLE 8-4. ADULTICIDE TREATMENT REGIMEN

Patient Evaluation	Dosage and Interval
1. Appropriate pretreatment data base	
2. Before each dose fraction:	0.22 ml/kg bid for 2 days
Give physical examination.	Dosage intervals (hours)
Feed patient and determine appetite.	Maximum: 15
	Minimum: 6
Check urine for bilirubinuria.	Optimum: 8–12

I. Protocol

The adulticide regimen is outlined in Table 8-4. Any deviation from this protocol results in decreased efficacy, increased toxicity, or no therapeutic advantage.

II. Method of administration

Thiacetarsamide should be stored under refrigeration and administered carefully to avoid extravasation. Indwelling venous catheters are not necessary and predispose to phlebitis and infection.

A. Thiacetarsamide must not be injected unless there is absolute certainty of proper needle placement.

B. Each injection should be made as peripherally as practical; multiple injections in close proximity are to be avoided.

C. Significant weakening of utilized veins occurs, and at least 1 day should elapse before the same vein is used again.

III. Three-day treatment

Studies performed by Dr. Clarence A. Rawlings at the University of Georgia indicate identical efficacy of 2-day (four-injection) and 3-day (six-injection) treatments.

IV. Extravasation of thiacetarsamide sodium

Pain, heat, and swelling occur within 15 to 60 minutes after drug extravasation. The degree of swelling is directly proportional to the volume of drug extravasated.

A. Treatment

1. DMSO applied topically TID for 3 to 5 days is most effective.
2. Glucocorticoid hormone and saline infiltration of the extravasation site is of unproven value.
3. Whirlpool baths and preventing the dog from licking the area reduce the severity of skin necrosis.

B. Duration of inflammation

The clinical signs of minor extravasations resolve in 5 to 7 days.

Extensive tissue necrosis may require 2 to 3 months for healing of granulation.

V. Liver-sparing drugs

Administration of inositol, choline, and methionine is of no value in preventing or reducing hepatic toxicity associated with thiacetarsamide.

VI. Glucocorticoid hormones

Prednisone and other equivalent drugs should not be administered during or for one week after adulticide treatment. These drugs interfere with the killing effect of thiacetarsamide on young adult female worms.

VII. Indications to stop therapy

It is rare that a 4-week delay in adulticide therapy will adversely affect the animal's prognosis. For that reason, there is no rationale in continuing therapy in the face of certain clinical signs.

A. Gastrointestinal signs

The most common clinical signs necessitating cessation of therapy are anorexia, depression, and persistent vomiting. These signs, when present, usually occur after the first dose.

B. Hepatotoxicity

Icterus at any time or gross bilirubinuria occurring before administration of the second or third dose is an indication to stop therapy.

C. Retreatment

When it is necessary to stop adulticide therapy, restricted activity and a high-carbohydrate diet are prescribed. Adulticide therapy is reinstituted in 4 weeks and is usually completed without further complication.

VIII. Non-indications to stop therapy

A. One or two vomiting episodes following the first treatment

B. Bilirubinuria of any degree occurring after the third dose in an otherwise healthy-appearing dog

C. Elevation of liver enzymes

IX. Postadulticide complications

Serious clinical signs of postadulticide complications are usually limited to dogs with advanced disease and frequently associated with occult infections.

A. Pulmonary arterial thromboembolic disease

This complication is the most common, serious consequence of adulticide and is most often associated with severe pre- and post-treatment radiographic pathology.

1. Life-threatening severity is indicated by dyspnea, hemoptysis, tachycardia, and hypotension. DIC should be suspected.
2. Low-grade fever, coughing, and mild hemoptysis are relatively common clinical signs seen 5 to 21 days postadulticide.
3. Glucocorticoid hormones should not be administered during the first week postadulticide unless absolutely necessary.

B. Azotemia

Renal complications are unusual if renal function is normal before treatment.

1. Azotemia is usually prerenal and associated with vomiting, anorexia, and dehydration.
2. Fluid therapy usually resolves azotemia in 1 to 2 days.

C. Thrombocytopenia

Thrombocytopenia, possibly with additional signs of low-grade DIC, usually develops 7 to 14 days postadulticide in dogs with severe pulmonary arterial pathology.

1. Vincristine (4 mg/m^2, IV): If the platelet count decreases below $50,000/mm^3$ in the absence of clinical or other laboratory evidence of DIC, one dose of vincristine will usually increase the platelet count to more than $150,000/mm^3$ within 3 days.
2. DIC: If evidence of acute DIC is present, vincristine alone is not indicated. Heparin and clotting factors may be given.

D. Acute DIC

Bleeding may occur 7 to 14 days postadulticide in dogs showing severe pulmonary pathology.

1. Diagnosis: Thrombocytopenia (often severe), prolongation of the activated clotting time, prothrombin time, partial thromboplastin time, and the presence of fibrin degradation products.
2. Treatment: Heparin or heparin plus clotting factor replacement is required. Consultation with someone experienced in the treatment of DIC is imperative.
3. Prognosis: Poor.

X. Decreased efficacy of thiacetarsamide sodium

Young adult female *D. immitis* are resistant to thiacetarsamide sodium. Since only 50 percent of 6-month-old female worms are killed, persistent microfilaremia may result.

XI. Window of vulnerability

In endemic areas, it is possible that reinfection by L_3 could occur after adulticide and prior to the initiation of prophylaxis.

A. Decrease adulticide–microfilaricide interval

Microfilaricide may be initiated 4 weeks instead of 6 weeks post-adulticide.

B. Winter adulticide

Adulticide may be planned for colder months if the mosquito population is significantly decreased during that time.

XII. Diethylcarbamazine and microfilaremia

If a dog is found to have heartworm infection while receiving diethylcarbamazine, diethylcarbamazine should be continued throughout adulticide and microfilaricide.

Microfilaricide Therapy

A microfilaricide should be given 4 weeks postadulticide therapy. There are several available microfilaricides; however, of these, only dithiazanine is approved by the Food and Drug Administration.

I. Dithiazanine

This is the most commonly used microfilaricide, but its efficacy is limited.

A. Dosage

Dithiazanine is given at the dose of 6 to 8 mg/kg-day for 7 days. If microfilaremia persists, the dose may be increased to 12 to 14 mg/kg for 7 to 10 additional days.

B. Toxicity

Vomiting is a commonly encountered untoward effect, particularly at higher dose rates. Toxicity may be reduced or avoided by dividing the daily dose and/or by administering the drug after a small meal.

1. Progressive toxicity: If the drug is continued in the face of toxicity, anorexia, depression, and diarrhea occur.
2. Dye stain: The vomitus or diarrhea will impart a purple stain to fabrics.

C. Alternate microfilaricide

If microfilaremia persists after a trial at either dose schedule, an alternate drug may be selected.

II. Levamisole

The therapeutic index of this drug is narrow; therefore, strict adherence to the recommended dose is necessary.

A. Dosage

Levamisole should be administered after a small meal at a dose of 11 mg/kg once daily for 7 days. If microfilaremia persists, the same dosage is continued for 5 additional days.

B. Toxicity

Vomiting is the most commonly encountered side effect. If treatment continues, anorexia, depression, or neurotoxicity may occur.

1. Vomiting: May be avoided by the use of antiemetics.
2. Effective serum level: Due to a short half-life, dividing the daily dose may reduce drug efficacy.

C. Efficacy

Approximately 70 percent of treated dogs are amicrofilaremic after 7 days; more than 80 percent are cleared by 12 days of treatment.

D. Therapeutic index

Increased or decreased dosage schedules result in increased toxicity or decreased efficacy.

III. Fenthion

Although the efficacy of fenthion is as good as or better than that of dithiazanine or levamisole, it is not widely used.

A. Topical dosage

Application of the 13.8 percent or 20 percent solution weekly at a rate of 1 ml/5 kg is effective with minimal toxicity.

B. Subcutaneous injection

The dose of 15 mg/kg once every 2 weeks for two to three treatments is effective.

C. Toxicity

Signs of organophosphate toxicity (salivation, vomiting, weakness, muscle tremors) or other minor reactions may be encountered. Organophosphate or carbamate-containing flea collars, dips, dusts, or sprays should not be administered 2 weeks before, during, or for 2 weeks after fenthion therapy.

D. Efficacy

One subcutaneous injection is effective in more than 50 percent of treated dogs, while 95 percent are cleared of microfilariae after two treatments.

E. Flea control

Since fenthion, as used for flea control, will temporarily eradicate microfilariae, it is possible to produce false negative results on a microfilariae test. Therefore, all dogs given fenthion for flea control should be Knott (or filter) tested and placed on diethylcarbamazine (DEC) therapy.

IV. Ivermectin

A. Dosage

A single oral dose 2 weeks postadulticide is both safe and effective; 0.05 mg/kg.

B. Toxicity

1. Minor side effects are occasionally associated with the drug manufactured for use in dogs.
2. Severe anaphylaxis, often resulting in death, may be encountered when the ivermectin intended for equine use is injected into dogs.
   a) If given orally, there are fewer side effects.
   b) The Collie breed should not be administered this drug by any route.
3. The mechanism of toxicity involves mast cell degranulation, which produces hypotensive shock.

V. Reappearance of microfilariae

If incomplete adulticide occurs, microfilariae may reappear after an initial negative microfilaria concentration test. Therefore, a Knott (or filter) test should be repeated in 4 to 6 weeks.

VI. Microfilaricide preceding adulticide

A. There is no advantage and it is not necessary for asymptomatic and mildly symptomatic cases.

B. In the author's experience, there is no associated improvement in survival or decrease in thiacetarsemide-associated reactions in dogs with advanced disease.

C. Microfilarial death is associated with histopathologic changes in the liver and kidneys:

1. Hepatic microabscesses and granulomas
2. Renal microabscesses and capillary occlusion
3. Unknown clinical significance

Diethylcarbamazine (DEC) Prophylaxis

Daily DEC is effective in killing the larvae of *D. immitis* at the L_3–L_4 molting stage.

I. Time sequence
   In endemic areas, DEC is prescribed year-round. In other areas, DEC is given from the onset of the mosquito season until 2 months after the first frost.
   A. Anaphylaxis
      Acute reactions of variable severity are often encountered when DEC is administered to microfilaremic dogs.
   B. Microfilaremia in dogs receiving DEC
      1. If microfilaremia is detected in a dog currently receiving DEC, the drug can be continued during adulticide and microfilaricide therapy.
      2. If DEC has not been administered for more than a few consecutive days when microfilariae are detected, DEC must not be reinstituted until heartworm treatment is completed.

II. Dosage
   DEC is prescribed at 5.5 to 6.5 mg/kg-day.

III. Prerequisite
   One negative microfilariae test is necessary and adequate for institution of DEC prophylaxis.

IV. DEC prophylaxis is instituted immediately after a successful course of microfilaricide treatment.

V. Toxicity
   Vomiting is an occasional problem that is readily corrected by changing to a different formulation.

VI. Impaired fertility
   Low sperm counts with normal libido have been reported on occasion, especially in the Greyhound. Fertility was reported to return to normal when DEC was withdrawn.

Ivermectin Prophylaxis

This drug is an alternative prophylactic that is both safe and effective. Side effects are uncommon and associated only with supertherapeutic dosages. The primary advantage of ivermectin over DEC is its effectiveness at monthly dosage intervals.

Thiacetarsamide prophylaxis

Thiacetarsamide administered every 6 months will prevent the maturation of *D. immitis* larvae.

PROGNOSIS

In order to justify the treatment of any heartworm-infected dog, there should be a reasonable expectation of significant clinical improvement and long-term survival.

Selection of Patients

Most asymptomatic or mildly symptomatic dogs with no or minimal radiographic changes should be treated. Very old dogs and dogs with severe cachexia, renal failure, hepatic insufficiency, or renal amyloidosis should not be treated.

Routine Infections

Dogs with no or minimal clinical signs and little or no radiographic evidence of pulmonary pathology should have a survival rate approaching 100 percent. Serious treatment-associated complications are usually the result of inadequate or incorrect pretreatment assessment.

Caval Syndrome

The only effective treatment of the caval syndrome is removal of adult worms from the right ventricle and caudal vena cava. When performed by an experienced clinician, this technique can produce a survival rate of up to 85 percent.

Right-Sided Congestive Heart Failure

Thirty of 37 dogs (80 percent) treated in the manner previously outlined survived. Relatively few dogs experienced severe clinical complications. Signs of heart failure resolved in 2 to 3 months.

Disseminated Intravascular Coagulopathy

Dogs with advanced pulmonary pathology with clinical and laboratory evidence of acute DIC have a survival rate of less than 20 percent.

Severe Pulmonary Artery Disease

Dogs with severe pulmonary hypertension and pulmonary arterial obstructive disease, when treated as previously outlined, have a survival rate of more than 75 percent. Insufficient cage rest and possibly failure to administer aspirin reduces the probability of survival.

FELINE HEARTWORM DISEASE

Incidence

Because of the difficulty in diagnosing feline heartworm disease, the incidence is unknown. In general, the prevalence parallels that seen in dogs in a given geographic region, but at a much lower level.

Historical Findings

The most common client observed signs are coughing, lethargy, anorexia, difficulty breathing, and vomiting.

Clinical Signs

Clinical signs of feline heartworm disease tend to fall into three categories.

I. Neurological signs
Seizures, dementia, or coma may result from aberrant adult *D. immitis* in the brain.

II. Cardiovascular signs
Coughing, dyspnea, systolic heart murmur, and gallop rhythm are present in some combination in 60 to 75 percent of affected cats with adult worms in the right ventricle or pulmonary arteries. Ascites and pleural effusion occur with right-sided congestive heart failure.

III. Lethargy and anorexia may be the only obvious clinical signs in some instances.

Thoracic Radiography

Most instances of feline heartworm disease with concomitant cardiovascular signs are associated with subtle thoracic abnormalities detected radiographically.

I. Enlarged caudal lobar pulmonary arteries may be detected, especially on the dorsoventral projection.

II. Right ventricular enlargement may be present.

III. Pleural effusion is seen in approximately one-third to one-fourth of cats.

IV. Pulmonary infiltrates with eosinophilia are seen in approximately one-third of cats.

Electrocardiography

Right ventricular hypertrophy is detected in approximately 25 percent of affected cats with adult worms in the heart and pulmonary arteries. If clinical signs of heart failure are present, right ventricular hypertrophy is detected in more than one-half of the cats.

Clinical Pathology

Eosinophilia, basophilia, and hyperglobulinemia may be present.

I. Eosinophilia and basophilia are not usually present in cats at the time of diagnosis.
II. Hyperglobulinemia is almost always present.
III. Eosinophilia is usually present if there are adult worms in the brain.

Diagnosis

Most cats with heartworm infections do not have microfilaremia at the time of diagnosis.

I. Indirect fluorescent antibody tests may be positive.
  A. False-negative results occur due to the low numbers of adult worms and, thus, the possibility of unisex infections.
  B. Anti-feline globulin serum must be available.
II. Nonselective angiography may better define pulmonary arterial sizes and tortuosity. Linear filling defects created by adult worms in the pulmonary arteries are occasionally detected.
III. Microfilaremia is occasionally detected.
IV. Hyperglobulinemia, eosinophilia, coughing, and cardiac abnormalities in any combination suggest the possibility of heartworm disease, particularly in endemic areas.
V. Echocardiography will rule out hypertrophic and congestive cardiomyopathy.

Treatment

Treatment of feline heartworm disease parallels that of canine heartworm disease except that microfilaricide is usually not required. DEC is seldom prescribed due to the difficulty encountered by clients in administering daily oral medicaments to cats.

Prognosis

Most cats with heartworms in the heart and lungs can be treated successfully. Those with right-sided congestive heart failure are difficult to manage, but most cats seen at our institution have survived. Postadulticide complications such as fever, coughing, dyspnea, and typical thoracic radiograph abnormalities are to be expected. Aspirin (25 mg/kg every 3 to 4 days) may diminish the likelihood of postadulticide pulmonary thromboembolism.

SUGGESTED READINGS

Calvert CA: Management of heartworm disease with concomitant right-side congestive heart failure. Am J Vet Med Assoc 180:1201, 1982

Calvert CA, Rawlings CA: Diagnosis and management of canine heartworm disease. p. 348. In Kirk RW (ed): Current Veterinary Therapy. VIII. WB Saunders, Philadelphia, 1983

Courtney CH, Nachreiner RF: The effect of diethylcarbamazine on fertility in the dog. p. 95. In Otto GF (ed): Proceedings of the Heartworm Symposium '77. Veterinary Medicine Publishing, Bonner Springs, Kansas, 1978

Dillon R: Feline dirofilariasis. Vet Clin North Am (Small Anim Pract) 14:1185, 1984

Howland TP, Todd KS: An evaluation of contamination of the Difil test for *Dirofilaria immitis* microfilariae. p. 31. In Otto GF (ed): Proceedings of the Heartworm Symposium '77. Veterinary Medicine Publishing, Bonner Springs, Kansas, 1978

Jackson RF: The activity of levamisole against the various stages of *Dirofilaria immitis* in the dog. p. 111. In Otto GF (ed): Proceedings of the Heartworm Symposium '77. Veterinary Medicine Publishing, Bonner Springs, Kansas, 1978

Jackson RF, Seymour WG, Growney PJ, et al: Surgical treatment of the caval syndrome of canine heartworm disease. Am J Vet Med Assoc 171:1065, 1977

Keith JC, Schaub RG, Rawlings CA: Early arterial injury-induced myointimal proliferation in canine pulmonary arteries. Am J Vet Res 44:181, 1983

Keith JC, Rawlings CA, Schaub RG: Pulmonary thromboembolism during therapy of dirofilariasis with thiacetarsamide: Modification with aspirin or prednisone. Am J Vet Res 44:1278, 1983

Losonsky JM, Thrall DE, Lewis RE: Thoracic radiographic abnormalities in 200 dogs with spontaneous heartworm infestation. Vet Rad 24:120, 1983

McCall JW, Lindemann BA, Porter CA: Prophylactic activity of ivermectins against experimentally induced *D. immitis* infections in dogs. p. 126. In Morgan DD (ed): Proceedings of the Heartworm Symposium. Veterinary Medicine Publishing, Edwardsville, Kansas, 1981

Palumbo NE, Perri SF, Desowitz RW, et al: Preliminary observations on adverse reactions to diethylcarbamazine (DEC) in dogs infected with *Dirofilaria immitis*. p. 97. In Otto GF (ed): Proceedings of the Heartworm Symposium '77. Veterinary Medicine Publishing, Bonner Springs, Kansas, 1978

Rawlings CA, Losonsky JM, Schaub RG, et al: Postadulticide changes in *Dirofilaria immitis*-infected Beagles. Am J Vet Res 44:8, 1983

Rawlings CA, Keith JC, Losonsky JM, et al: Aspirin and prednisone modification of postadulticide pulmonary arterial disease in heartworm-infected dogs: Arteriographic study. Am J Vet Res 44:821, 1983

Wong MM, Suter PF: Indirect fluorescent antibody test in occult dirofilariasis. Am J Vet Res 40:414, 1979

9

Pericardial Disease

Christophe W. Lombard

INTRODUCTION

General Remarks

The overall incidence of pericardial disease is estimated to represent approximately 1 percent of all cardiac diseases. The recent introduction of echocardiography, an extremely sensitive technique for the recognition of pericardial effusion, is likely to raise the percentage of such clinical diagnoses. The incidence of pericardial disease in the cat is even lower than in the dog. Pericardial diseases recognized in dog and cat include:

I. Congenital diseases of the pericardium: Partial or complete absence, peritoneopericardial diaphragmatic hernia
II. Pericarditis, pericardial effusions of various etiologies: idiopathic, infectious, inflammatory
III. Pericardial mass lesions: heart base tumors, pericardial cysts, mesotheliomas, cardiac hemangiosarcoma, other metastatic or primary neoplasms

Diagnosis

I. Physical examination
  A. The triad of muffled heart sounds, weak arterial pulses, and signs of right heart failure is highly suggestive of pericardial disease and, in particular, pericardial effusion.
  B. Specific physical abnormalities such as a friction murmur are diagnostic for pericarditis.

C. In general, the abnormalities of the physical examination are not sufficient for an etiologic diagnosis of a particular pericardial disease.

II. Electrocardiogram/thoracic radiographs
   A. Abnormalities of the electrocardiogram and thoracic radiographs are fairly specific for pericardial effusion.
   B. Rarely do they permit diagnosis of the underlying cause, however.

III. Laboratory examination
   A. Pericardial fluid analysis including cytology and culture is useful in the presence of a septic exudate, confirming an infectious pericarditis with effusion.
   B. Hemorrhagic effusions, however, are almost never specific enough to confirm an etiologic diagnosis of its three main causes: heart base tumor, right atrial hemangiosarcoma, and idiopathic hemorrhagic effusion.

IV. Special studies
   A. Pneumopericardiography is very helpful in outlining intrapericardial and extracardiac mass lesions such as cysts and heart base tumors.
   B. Two-dimensional echocardiography appears superior even for diagnosing masses with pericardial and intracardiac components, such as hemangiosarcoma, pericardial cysts, mesothelioma, and large thrombi.

THERAPY

I. Diagnostic pericardiocentesis is also palliative therapy (relief of intrapericardial pressure elevation responsible for the clinical signs of low cardiac output and cardiac tamponade). Animals with idiopathic effusion may heal spontaneously after one pericardiocentesis, but recurrence of pericardial effusion is frequent.

II. Concomitant medical therapy of septic or inflammatory processes is indicated.

III. Surgical resection of the pericardium is the treatment of choice in most cases. It is well tolerated and permits inflammatory processes to heal. The greater resorptive surface of the pleural cavity provides

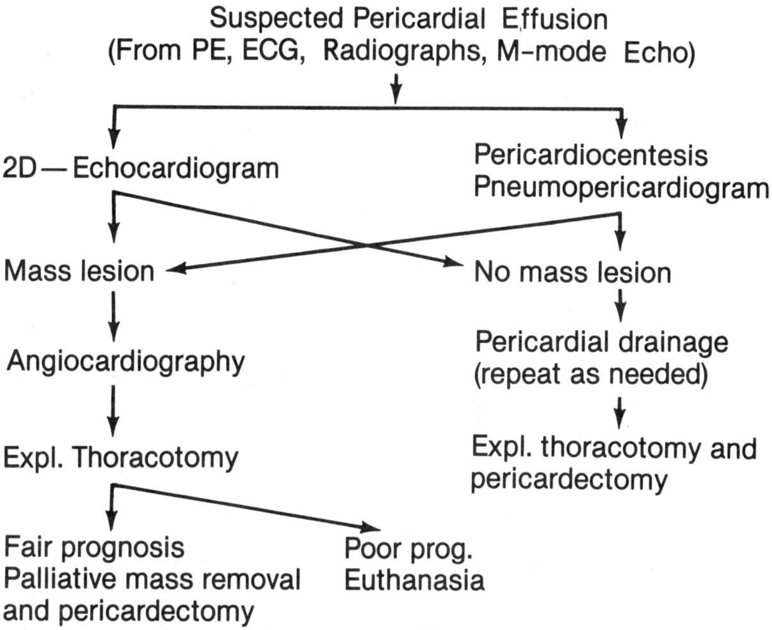

Fig. 9-1. Flow chart for the management of pericardial effusion.

more complete drainage. Figure 9-1 shows a useful flowchart for diagnosis and therapy of pericardial effusion.

PATHOPHYSIOLOGY OF PERICARDIAL DISEASES

The pathophysiologic abnormalities of all subtypes of pericardial diseases are very similar and may be discussed as a group.

I. The pericardial sac is a relatively nondistendible tissue. Any rapid accumulation of fluid or space-occupying mass within the pericardium leads to a rise in intrapericardial pressure.

II. The intrapericardial pressure rise cushions the diastolic excursion and filling of the heart, especially of the low-pressured right atrium and right ventricle. The right heart overcomes the decreased filling with an increase of heart rate and venous pressure, thereby raising the right atrial (central venous pressure) and right ventricular diastolic pressures. Signs of mild venous congestion become evident.

III. Increased central venous pressure reduces the venous return to the heart and therefore stroke volume and cardiac output, unless the increase of the heart rate can fully compensate for the lower stroke volume.

IV. The concomitant rise of the pericardial pressure and venous filling pressures lead to clinical signs of venous congestion (e.g., distention of the jugular veins, hepatic enlargement, and ascites), mimicking right-side congestive heart failure.

V. Slow pericardial fluid accumulations may be compensated for over relatively long periods of time, with considerable stretching of the pericardial sac, leading to a large cardiac silhouette with relatively mild clinical signs. The low cardiac output may only be evident with a decrease in exercise tolerance, with the inability to raise the output much over resting values.

VI. Cardiac tamponade has developed when intrapericardial pressure equals the filling pressures of the atria and both the right and left ventricle. Dangerously low cardiac output and stroke volume, tachycardia, and a very weak arterial pulse, declining excessively during inspiration (pulsus paradoxus) occur and may lead to signs of low output failure and collapse.

VII. The contractile function of the myocardium usually remains normal, unless chronic coronary hypoperfusion and myocardial necrosis with constrictive inflammatory pericarditis have damaged the heart.

CONGENITAL DISEASES OF THE PERICARDIUM

Introduction

I. Pathology

A. Congenital absence of the pericardial sac has been reported as incidental necropsy findings.

B. Peritoneopericardial diaphragmatic hernia (CPDH) results from an open communication between the peritoneal and pericardial cavities, varying in size, and permits protrusion of either liver lobes, bowel loops, omentum, or a combination.

C. A pure to modified transudate of varying amounts is frequently present.

D. Concomitant malformations of the sternebrae (fusion) or of the xyphoid cartilage are frequently present.

II. Etiology

Theories of the embryologic aberrations causing CPDH are multiple, including failure of the pleuroperitoneal folds to meet the ventromedial pars sternalis and faulty development or injury of the dorsolateral septum transversum.

III. Pathophysiology

A. Small CPDH do not cause abnormalities. In large hernias, decreased venous return and right heart filling results from cardiac displacement and compression in diastole. Moderate to marked reduction of the cardiac output is present.

B. Right heart failure or cardiac tamponade rarely occur.

C. Mechanical friction of displaced abdominal organs leads to the accumulation of a pure to modified transudate.

D. Liver lobes, bowel loops or omentum may become incarcerated and eventually necrose.

Diagnosis

I. Predilections

A. Age range at diagnosis varies from birth to old age.

B. There is no known sex or breed predilection.

II. History

A. CPDH is an incidental finding in a small number of asymptomatic dogs and cats.

B. Reduced weight gain, anorexia, vomiting, dyspnea, coughing, and wheezing are common clinical signs.

C. Other signs are nonspecific.

III. Physical examination

A. Depending on the site and amount of herniated organs, a weakened apex beat and muffled heart sounds are present.

B. Gut sounds over the cardiac auscultation field and an empty, tucked-up abdomen are highly suggestive of CPDH.

C. The pulmonary auscultation field may be displaced by large hernias, and disseminated venous distention may occur.

IV. Electrocardiogram

A. The ECG is normal with small hernias.

B. With large hernias, abnormalities include

1. Low voltage, often in some chest leads only

2. Deviation of the mean electrical axis

V. Thoracic radiographs

Abnormal findings vary widely depending on the size of the hernia and the herniated tissue:

A. Severe, generalized cardiac enlargement (pumpkin shape)

B. Dorsal displacement of the trachea

C. Incomplete diaphragmatic outline near the cranioventral sternal attachment

D. Gas-filled bowel loops overlying the cardiac silhouette

E. Malformed fused sternebrae and abnormal xyphoid cartilage

VI. Echocardiogram

Both M-mode and two-dimensional echocardiograms show displacement of the heart, away from the chest wall, by structures with soft tissue density, and effusions.

VII. Laboratory examination

A. Uncomplicated cases have normal blood counts and clinical chemistries.

B. Prerenal azotemia secondary to a low cardiac output may be present.

C. Liver enzymes, total protein, fibrinogen, and white blood cell count may all be elevated with incarcerated liver lobes.

VIII. Special studies

A. Upper gastrointestinal contrast studies may demonstrate herniated portions of the stomach or bowel loops.

B. Pneumoperitoneography allows air to pass through the hernia into the pericardial sac.

C. Positive contrast celiography may demonstrate the presence of a hernia.

D. Venous angiocardiograms show displacement of the heart with large hernias.

IX. Pericardial fluid analysis

A. Pure to modified transudate

B. Clear yellow to hemorrhagic turbid fluid with incarcerated hernias

X. Differential diagnosis

A. A *diaphragmatic hernia* shows discontinuity of the diaphragm and positional changes of abdominal organs; the cardiac silhouette is normal, however.

B. *Dilated cardiomyopathies* have less extreme enlargement of the cardiac silhouette and a less even rounding of its outline. The ECG shows normal voltage and frequent arrhythmias.

C. *Congenital heart defects* have typical heart murmurs and less pronounced cardiomegaly but disproportionate enlargement of either cardiac chamber and/or the great vessels.

D. *Pericardial effusions* rarely have clear transudates, except with hypoproteinemia, overhydration, or congestive heart failure. Also, their diaphragmatic outline is continuous.

E. *Tricuspid insufficiency* with severe cardiomegaly may resemble CPDH. A systolic murmur with maximal intensity over the right apex suggests tricuspid insufficiency.

Therapy and Prognosis

I. Surgery

A. Peritoneopericardial diaphragmatic hernia has a good prognosis after surgical correction.

B. Herniated organs may have been strangulated and need to be resected, with a more guarded prognosis.

C. Neoplastic metaplasia of incarcerated liver lobes may occur.

D. Concomitant other malformations, particularly of the heart, need to be assessed separately.

IDIOPATHIC PERICARDIAL EFFUSIONS

Introduction

I. Pathology

A considerable number of dogs with idiopathic pericardial effusions show only hemorrhage as a gross pathologic finding. The limited

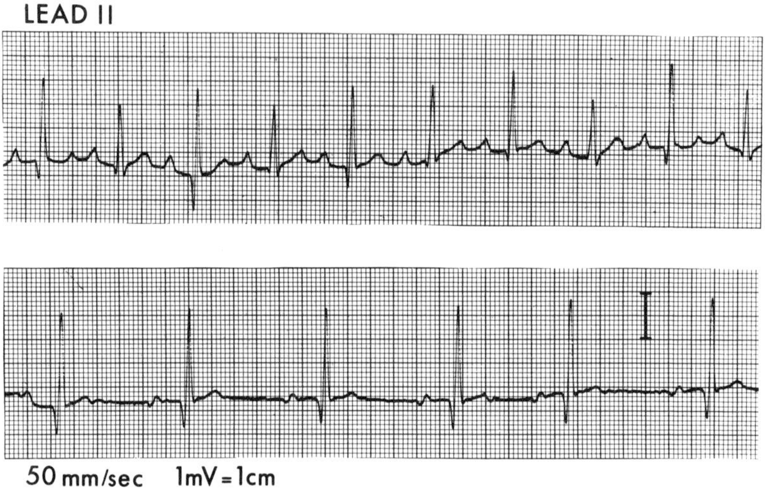

Fig. 9-2. Lead II electrocardiograms from a dog with pericardial effusion. Top tracing shows electrical alternans with normal voltage. Bottom tracing (after pericardiocentesis) has normal QRS complexes.

cases necropsied show the presence of free and clotted blood in the pericardial sac, with secondary fibrous thickening of the epicardium and pericardium. There is no rupture of vessels present. Instead, microscopic inflammation, neovascularization and fibroplasia of the parietal pericardium and the epicardium are seen.

II. Etiology and pathogenesis

Etiology is not clear, due to the limited number of completely worked up cases including necropsy.

III. Pathophysiology

The usual course of the disease is a slow accumulation of blood in the pericardium leading to large effusions and progressing to signs of cardiac tamponade. Rapid hemorrhage and development of acute cardiac tamponade with death of the dogs has been observed in some dogs.

Diagnosis

I. Etiology

The disease affects primarily young to middle-aged large dogs and has not been reported in cats.

II. History
   A. Listlessness, lethargy, decreased exercise tolerance, tachypnea, and coughing are most frequently observed over a period of several weeks.
   B. In more severe cases, abdominal distention (ascites) and syncope may be seen.
   C. A small percentage of dogs present with a sudden onset of signs, suggesting the rapid development of cardiac tamponade.

III. Physical examination
   A. Abnormal findings in cases with congestive heart failure include a normal or subnormal temperature, an elevated respiratory rate, a rapid and weak arterial pulse, and a slow capillary refill time.
   B. The jugular veins are distended and may pulsate.
   C. Prominent X and Y descents may be seen in the jugular groove and recorded on a venous pulse tracing.
   D. Abdominal palpation reveals hepatomegaly, splenomegaly, and ascites.
   E. Cardiac percussion shows excessive dullness over a wider field than usual. The heart sounds are muffled, have a dull character, and may be inaudible.

IV. Electrocardiography
   A. Low voltage and electrical alternans (Fig. 9-2) are present in many cases, depending on the volume of effusion.

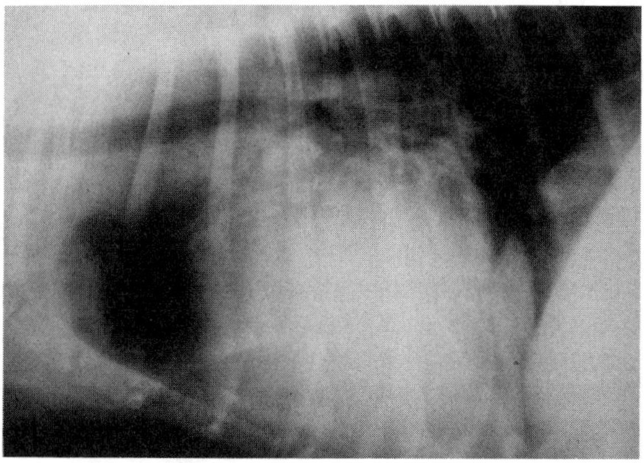

Fig. 9-3. Pericardial effusion, lateral projection. The cardiac silhouette is globular in appearance without delineation of the left ventricular or left atrial border.

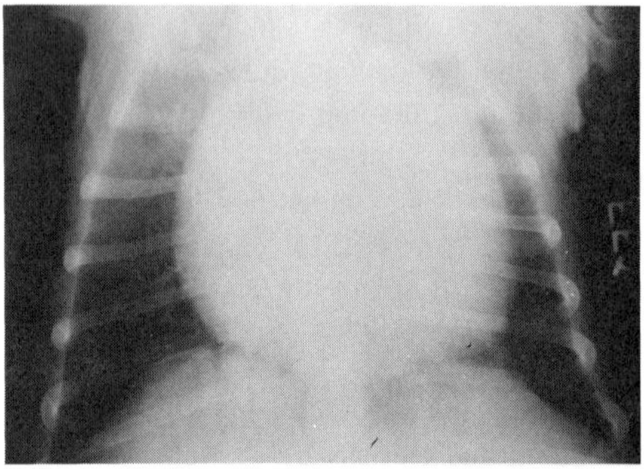

Fig. 9-4. Pericardial effusion, dorsoventral projection. The cardiac silhouette is rounded fairly equally in all directions.

B. The underlying rhythm is sinus tachycardia, with rare ectopic tachyarrhythmias.

V. Radiography (Figs. 9-3 and 9-4)
   A. Enlargement of the cardiac silhouette with a globular shape on both projections.
   B. The trachea is invariably displaced dorsally.
   C. Pleural effusions frequently obscure the heart.
   D. Abdominal radiographs may show hepatomegaly, splenomegaly and ascites.

VI. Echocardiography
   A. Pericardial effusions create an echo-free (fluid) space around the heart (Fig. 9-5).
   B. The heart is displaced away from the chest wall, and the pericardium may be buried in the transducer artifact.
   C. The moving free wall of the left ventricle is separated from the flat, motionless pericardium.
   D. The entire heart typically swings within the pericardial fluid in large effusions with tamponade, and the normal motion patterns of the septum and free walls are no longer recognizable because of the cardiac compression and its swinging motion.
   E. Abnormally large respiratory variations of the right ventricular dimension are present with large effusions.

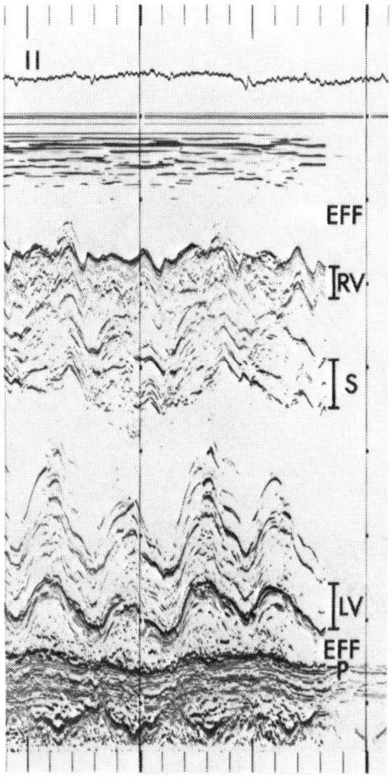

Fig. 9-5. M-mode echocardiogram (ventricular level) of a dog with a large anterior and a smaller posterior pericardial effusion. II, lead II electrocardiogram; EFF, effusion; RV, right ventricular free wall; S, septum; LV, left ventricular free wall; P, pericardium.

F. The echocardiographic abnormalities regress after pericardiocentesis (Fig. 9-6).

VII. Laboratory examination

A complete blood count and serum chemistries usually show no abnormal findings.

VIII. Pericardial fluid analysis

A. It is characterized as a serosanguineous, port-wine colored, nonclotting sterile exudate.

B. There are great variations in the red blood cell count (0.01 to 8.75 $\times$ $10^6/\mu l$), the protein content (0.9 to 5.7 g/dl), and the nucleated cell count (1.1 to 18 $\times$ $10^3/\mu l$).

C. The color varies from blood-tinged to dark red, closely resembling venous blood.

D. The cytologic interpretation varies, is usually that of normal blood elements, and is inconclusive.

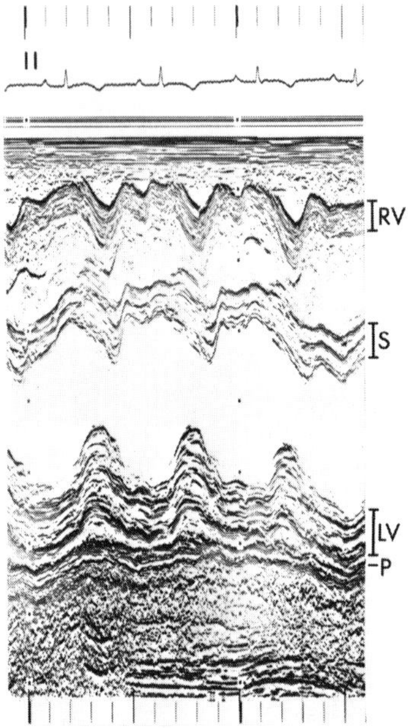

Fig. 9-6. M-Mode echocardiogram (ventricular level) of the same dog from Figure 9-5 after pericardiocentesis. A small anterior and a very small posterior effusion are still present. Abbreviations as in Figure 9-5

IX. Pneumopericardiography
   A. It is negative and rules out masses over the heart base as well as space-occupying lesions within the pericardium.
   B. The pericardial sac is not noticeably thickened.

X. Angiocardiography
   The angiocardiogram is normal and noncontributory.

XI. Differential diagnosis
   A. Signs of primarily right-sided congestive heart failure may be caused by dilated cardiomyopathy and valvular fibrosis. The heart sounds are not muffled, and there is a high incidence of arrhythmias and soft systolic murmurs (from tricuspid and mitral regurgitation) in those patients.
   B. Chronic cor pulmonale with heartworm disease is easily recognized by right cardiac enlargement and tortuosity of the pulmonary arteries on radiographs.

C. Other cardiac disease (e.g., pulmonic stenosis, tricuspid insufficiency) is differentiated by the presence of cardiac murmurs.
D. Dilated cardiomyopathy and CPDH both lack the fluid separation of the pericardium from the epicardium on echocardiography.

Therapy and Prognosis

I. Immediate pericardiocentesis is essential and life saving in cardiac tamponade.
II. Complete fluid drainage should be attempted before pneumopericardiography.
III. Idiopathic hemorrhagic effusions sometimes reoccur and are best treated by subtotal pericardectomy. Their prognosis is fair.

PERICARDIAL EFFUSIONS WITH CARDIAC AND PERICARDIAL NEOPLASIA

Introduction

I. Pathology
  A. Primary pericardial mesothelioma, cysts, or fibroma are very rare. They arise from either the epicardial lining or the free pericardial sac, compress the heart to varying degrees, and cause inflammatory and blood-tinged effusions.
  B. Heart base tumors usually arise from chromaffin cells of the aortic body, infiltrating and encircling the aorta and the pulmonary artery. They are slow growing, but can grow to a large size. They are richly vascularized and cause inflammatory and hemorrhagic effusions. This tumor type has a high incidence in Boxers, Boston Terriers, and other brachycephalic breeds.
  C. Hemangiosarcomas invade the wall of the right atrium and the heart base, leading to thinning of the wall and hemorrhage into the pericardial cavity. They vary in size of their intracardiac and intrapericardial portions. There is a high incidence of this tumor in aged German Shepherd dogs.

D. Metastatic lymphosarcoma (in cats) and other neoplasms occasionally infiltrate the heart and are associated with effusions varying from inflammatory to more hemorrhagic in nature.

II. Pathophysiology

The pathophysiology is very similar to that of idiopathic effusions. The slow tumor growth usually permits slow accumulation of large effusions, with the typical development of chronic cardiac tamponade.

Diagnosis

I. Etiology

See Pathology, above, for the breed predilection for certain neoplasms.

II. History

A. The animal's anamnesis as well as its owner's complaints are similar to those with other pericardial effusions.

B. Shortness of breath and syncope are more frequent because of acute hemorrhage and anemia.

III. Physical examination

A. Dyspnea, weak pulses, venous congestion, pale mucous membranes, and muffling of the heart sounds are the most common clinical signs.

B. Ascites is present in advanced cases.

C. In cats a noncompressibility of the cranial thorax may suggest a mediastinal mass (e.g., lymphosarcoma).

IV. Electrocardiography

A. Low voltage and electrical alternans are usually present with large effusions.

B. Low voltage is difficult to diagnose in cats, because the normal ECG in the cat is of low voltage.

C. Supraventricular and ventricular arrhythmias and conduction defects suggest infiltration of the myocardium with neoplastic cells.

D. Axis deviations can occur with large space-occupying masses.

V. Radiography

A. The cardiac silhouette is large and rounded, and pleural effusions may be observed.

B. Metastatic pulmonary disease occurs frequently with cardiac hemangiosarcoma.
C. Elevation and displacement of the trachea or the great vessels may be visible with very large heart base tumors.
D. Dorsolateral displacement of the trachea, widening of the cranial mediastinum, and pleural effusion are common in feline mediastinal lymphosarcoma.

VI. Echocardiography
A. Two-dimensional echocardiography recognizes masses displacing vascular structures over the heart base and intrapericardial as well as intracardiac masses. It is the best diagnostic technique for these effusions.
B. Marked thickening of the pericardial sac may be caused by mesotheliomas and may be visible on echocardiograms.

VII. Laboratory examination
A. Clinical chemistries are usually normal.
B. Chronic nonregenerative anemias are common with metastatic neoplasia.
C. Cats with mediastinal lymphosarcoma are likely to be FELV-positive, with normal blood counts and differentials.

VIII. Pericardial fluid analysis
A. Nonclotting hemorrhagic effusions with a wide range of red blood cell counts (0.1 to 12 $\times$ $10^6/\mu l$) and protein content (1.3 to 6 g/dl) predominate.
B. The nucleated cell count in the effusions of hemangiosarcoma and heart base tumor is lower than in venous blood.
C. Identification of the tumor type by cytology is rarely possible, with a high incidence of false diagnosis reported.

IX. Pneumopericardiography
A. Failure to outline the origin of the great vessels or suspicious shadows over the cranial heart base in dogs with hemorrhagic pericardial effusions suggest heart base tumors.
B. Right atrial hemangiosarcomas become visible when the extramural mass has reached considerable size and protrudes into the pericardial space.
C. They are best visualized in a left lateral projection, with soft tissue opacities observed over the right heart base.

X. Angiocardiography

A. Leakage of contrast material from the right atrium into the pericardial space may suggest hemangiosarcoma with a small tear of the right atrial wall. It may produce deviation of either vena cava or an abnormal shape of the right atrium, depending on its size and location.
B. Chemodectomas may show up with a "blush" of a suspicious shadow at the heart base in the late arterial phase of the angiogram.
C. Cats with mediastinal lymphosarcoma may show a compression and deviation of the cranial vena cava.
D. When combined with pneumopericardiography, many heart base tumors and atrial tumors are readily visualized.

XI. Differential diagnosis
A. Before a positive pneumopericardiogram or angiocardiogram, all differentials of idiopathic pericardial effusion must be considered.
B. Chronic mitral regurgitation with left atrial tear and hemopericardium is a rare complication of valvular fibrosis in selected breeds such as Cocker Spaniels, Dachshunds, and Poodles.
   1. Typically, the systolic murmur of mitral regurgitation is still audible despite some muffling of the heart sounds.
   2. The left atrial enlargement may still be visible on radiographs, extending dorsocaudally above the globular cardiac silhouette suggestive of pericardial effusion.
   3. The electrocardiogram is likely to show P-mitrale and a decreased voltage and sometimes arrhythmias.
C. Trauma to the chest (e.g., car accident, gunshot wounds) is likely to cause fatal cardiac tamponade from rupture of the heart. Small leaks may be tolerated, and historical and radiographic signs of trauma (e.g., pulmonary contusions, rib fractures) may be present.
D. Chronic uremia and renal failure are a rare cause of small pericardial effusion in dogs, unlikely to cause signs of tamponade.

Therapy and Prognosis

I. The prognosis of intrapericardial masses, prior to exploratory thoracotomy and histopathologic analysis of the tissue, is poor.

II. Pericardiocentesis brings temporary relief of clinical signs.

III. The prognosis of all primary cardiac, pericardial, and metastatic neoplasms is poor.

IV. Pericardectomy may alleviate the tamponade and prolong survival significantly in selected cases.

PERICARDITIS AND CONSTRICTIVE PERICARDIAL DISEASES

INTRODUCTION

I. Pathology

This group of inflammatory effusions is rare in dogs and cats.

A. Mild to severe thickening of epi- and pericardial tissues is present, with fibrinous and fibrous adhesions.

B. The entire pericardium may adhere to the epicardium in chronic cases, with severe constriction of the heart.

C. The overall heart size is normal to slightly enlarged.

II. Etiology

Various etiologies such as trauma (gunshot pellets) and infectious diseases such as feline infectious peritonitis, toxoplasmosis, leptospirosis, and distemper and other viral infections may cause chronic inflammation of the pericardium. The entry of bacteria in septic pericarditis may not be found.

III. Pathophysiology

In contrast to other pericardial diseases, chronic pericarditis frequently has only small volumes of pericardial effusions.

A. Constriction of the heart develops, preventing its diastolic expansion and filling, and caused by adhesions and thickening and stiffening of the epicardium. This may become severe enough to cause signs of mild chronic cardiac tamponade.

B. Characteristically, the early diastolic filling of the ventricles is normal, while expansion of the heart in late diastole is prevented. This leads to typical dip and plateau formation (a square root sign) of the diastolic pressure curves of the atria and ventricles.

DIAGNOSIS

I. History
  A. Nonspecific complaints of lethargy, listlessness, and anorexia predominate.
  B. Frequently, a febrile episode attributable to incompletely diagnosed infectious disease is reported.

II. Physical examination
  A. Sometimes a fever and otherwise nonspecific signs of mild tachycardia, weak pulse, slow capillary refill time, venous distention, and generalized malaise are present.
  B. The heart sounds may be somewhat muffled, and soft pericardial friction rubs occur with serofibrinous effusions. Heart murmurs and arrhythmias are rare.

III. Electrocardiography
  The ECG has nonspecific ST-segment abnormalities and low voltage may be seen in some cases.

IV. Radiography
  The signs vary from a slightly large cardiac silhouette to the even rounding and enlargement diagnostic of pericardial effusion. Foreign bodies (shotgun pellets) or other signs of trauma may be visible.

V. Echocardiography
  A. This technique is most sensitive in detecting these small to moderately large effusions.
  B. The signs are separation of epicardial from pericardial echoes by fluid accumulation.
  C. Echodense structures suggesting fibrin strands may be seen within the effusion. Multiple echoes of a flattened pericardium suggest thickening.

VI. Laboratory examination
  A. A CBC frequently shows leukocytosis with neutrophilia.
  B. The globulin fraction of the total proteins may be elevated in cases of infections and lead to a search for infectious agents by serology (coccidiomycosis, actinomycosis, tuberculosis, feline infectious peritonitis, toxoplasmosis, leptospirosis) or suspect other infectious agents (e.g., distemper, pasteurella).
  C. Other abnormalities are nonspecific.

VII. Pericardial fluid analysis
  A. Typically, an inflammatory exudate with moderately high protein content and a high nucleated cell count ($5 \times 10^3/\mu l$) and a very low red blood cell count ($1.0 \times 10^6/\mu l$) is present, although variations may occur.
  B. Bacterial cultures of septic effusion should grow the causative agent, while some fungal organisms may be difficult to grow.
  C. Special stains on cytology may show the presence of organisms.

VIII. Pneumopericardiography
  The pericardial sac is mildly to moderately thickened.

IX. Differential diagnosis
  A. CPDH has a more transudative effusion and radiographic signs of severe enlargement of the cardiac silhouette.
  B. Hemorrhagic effusions are likely to be caused by neoplasia, with positive pneumopericardiograms, idiopathic hemorrhagic effusions do not have a thickened pericardium.
  C. Pericardial cysts may present with inflammatory exudates, be imaged as multiple small masses on pneumopericardiography and only be recognized on histology after pericardectomy.
  D. With idiopathic pericardial effusion, none of the previously mentioned causes can be found.

Therapy and Prognosis

I. Medical therapy
  A. Pericardial drainage usually is insufficient.
  B. Antibiotics placed in the pericardial sac and systemic antibiotics as well as antiinflammatory drugs are frequently indicated to suppress the underlying disease.
  C. Catheter drainage of the pericardial sac may be attempted.
  D. Combined medical and surgical therapy are most often necessary.

II. Surgical pericardectomy
  A. This operation is indicated in all cases with a thickening of the pericardium on pneumopericardiography.
  B. Stripping of epicardial adhesions (decortication) is technically difficult and should be performed by skilled and experienced surgeons.

C. The prognosis is guarded with severe adhesions and is fair to good after successful surgery.

SUGGESTED READINGS

Berg RJ, Wingfield W: Pericardial effusion in the dog: A review of 42 cases. J Am Anim Hosp Assoc 20:721, 1984

Bonagura JD: Electrical alternans associated with pericardial effusion in the dog. J Am Vet Med Assoc 178:574, 1981

Bonagura JD, Pipers FS: Echocardiographic features of pericardial effusion in dogs. J Am Vet Med Assoc 179:49, 1981

Buchanan JW, Kelly AM: Endocardial splitting of the left atrium in the dog with hemorrhage and hemopericardium. J Am Vet Rad Soc 5:28, 1964

Evans SM, Biery DN: Congenital peritoneopericardial diaphragmatic hernia in the dog and cat: A literature review and 17 additional case histories. Vet Radiol 21:108, 1980

Gibbs C, Gaskell CJ, Darke PG, Wotton PR: Idiopathic pericardial hemorrhage in dogs: A review of fourteen cases. J Small Anim Pract 23:483, 1982

Johnson KH: Aortic body tumors in the dog. J Am Vet Med Assoc 152:154, 1968

Kleine LJ, Zook BC, Munson TO: Primary cardiac hemangiosarcoma in dogs. J Am Vet Med Assoc 157:326, 1970

Lombard CW: Pericardial disease. Vet Clin North Am [Small Anim Pract] 13:337, 1983

Owens JM: Pericardial effusion in the cat. Vet Clin North Am [Small Anim Pract] 7:373, 1977

Reed JR, Thomas WP, Suter PF: Pneumopericardiography in the normal dog. Vet Radiol 24:112, 1983

Shabetai R: The Pericardium. Grune & Stratton, New York, 1981

Sisson D, Thomas WP, Ruehl WW, Zinkl JG: Diagnostic value of pericardial fluid analysis in the dog. J Am Vet Med Assoc 184:51, 1984

Thomas WP: Pericardial disease. p. 1080. In Ettinger SJ (ed): Textbook of Veterinary Internal Medicine. ed 2. Vol. 1. WB Saunders, Philadelphia, 1983

Thomas WP, Reed JR, Gomez JA: Diagnostic pneumopericardiography in dogs with spontaneous pericardial effusion. Vet Radiol 25:2, 1984

Thomas WP, et al: Detection of cardiac masses in dogs by two-dimensional echocardiography. Vet Radiol 25:65, 1984

Thrall DE, Goldschmidt MH: Mesothelioma in the dog: Six case reports. J Am Vet Rad Soc 19:107, 1978

Tilley LP, Bond B, Patnaik AK, Liu SK: Cardiovascular tumors in the cat. J Am Anim Hosp Assoc 17:1009, 1981

Tilley LP: Essentials of Canine and Feline Electrocardiography, Interpretation and Treatment, 2nd Ed. Lea & Febiger, Philadelphia, 1985

10

Congenital Heart Disease

Larry Patrick Tilley
Jerry M. Owens

INTRODUCTION

Hereditary Aspects

I. Congenital heart disease makes up only a small percent (less than 10 percent) of heart disease in dogs and cats.
II. Congenital heart defects are generally recognized in the young animal and usually represent a hereditary trait or a defect originating during gestation. A genetic problem often exists for animals with congenital heart disease.
III. Four common forms of congenital heart disease shown to be inherited in dogs:
   A. Patent ductus arteriosus in the Poodle
   B. Aortic stenosis in the Newfoundland Retriever
   C. Tetralogy of Fallot in the Keeshond
   D. Pulmonic stenosis in the Beagle

Diagnosis

I. The murmurs of congenital cardiac defects are caused either by an abnormal communication between the arterial and venous circuits of the heart and great vessels or by valvular deformities. The presence or absence of cyanosis may be helpful to the clinician in differentiating the various types of congenital heart diseases that present with similar murmurs.

II. For most cases, the final diagnostic impression is based on the results of the electrocardiogram, chest radiograph, angiocardiogram, and sometimes more sophisticated studies such as echocardiography. This chapter emphasizes the differential diagnosis of congenital heart disease in the dog and cat on the basis of results of diagnostic tests available to the average practitioner.

Therapy

I. By identifying a congenital heart defect, a prognosis, genetic basis, and a therapeutic regimen can often be established.
II. Surgical correction is the ideal approach to congenital heart disease, and has been used in some defects such as patent ductus arteriosus and pulmonic stenosis.
III. Medical treatment is primarily for the control or prevention of congestive heart failure and associated arrhythmias. Medical therapy is discussed briefly in this chapter.

Feline

I. Congenital heart disease is less common in cats than dogs. In general, the diagnostic and therapeutic approach to congenital heart disease in the cat is the same as that in the dog. No consistent sex or breed predilection has been adequately demonstrated for congenital feline cardiac anomalies, although familial tendencies have been reported.
II. The most common heart defects in the cat include malformation of the mitral valve complex, tricuspid valve dysplasia, ventricular septal defect, aortic stenosis, persistent common atrioventricular canal, endocardial fibroelastosis, patent ductus arteriosus, and tetralogy of Fallot.
III. Less common defects include incomplete pericardial sac, persistent truncus arteriosus, pulmonic stenosis, atrial septal defect, tricuspid stenosis, and right ventricular hypoplasia, double outlet of the right ventricle, patent foramen ovale, right atrial hypoplasia, and caudal vena cava anomaly. These congenital defects have also been documented in the canine.

CANINE

Tables 10-1 and 10-2 list the most common congenital heart defects in the dog and cat and the typical diagnostic characteristics. Of these congenital heart defects, the five most common defects found in the dog are discussed:

I. Patent ductus arteriosus
II. Pulmonic stenosis
III. Aortic stenosis
IV. Ventricular septal defect
V. Tetralogy of Fallot

Vascular ring anomalies are not discussed here, since the defect does not usually produce significant cardiac disease.

INNOCENT (FUNCTIONAL) MURMUR

INTRODUCTION

Before discussing each of the common congenital heart defects, innocent murmurs should be briefly discussed. A probable significant number of dogs and cats develop an innocent murmur at some time during the early growth stages. The clinician must therefore distinguish between the innocent murmur and the murmur from a congenital heart defect.

AUSCULTATION

I. The innocent murmur is systolic in timing, is usually of short duration and of grade III or less in intensity, it has a low-pitched, vibrating, musical quality to its sound.
II. It is usually loudest along the left sternal border and is poorly transmitted. Its intensity may vary with change and position, with the phase of respiration, with exercise, and from day to day.
III. The most important characteristics of the innocent murmur is that it is heard in the absence of any other demonstrable evidence of cardiovascular disease.

TABLE 10-1. DIAGNOSTIC CHARACTERISTICS OF COMMON CANINE CONGENITAL HEART DEFECTS

Heart Defect	Physical Examination	Electrocardiogram	Thoracic Radiographs	Other Characteristics
Innocent (functional) murmur	Murmur usually soft, <grade 3/6, short, early to mid-systolic, loudest on left side but variable with position, heart rate, etc. All else normal.	Normal	Normal	Common in puppies, kittens, and animals <6 months of age.
Patent ductus arteriosus (PDA)	Continuous murmur loudest in aortic area at left base. May radiate widely; often accompanied by thrill. Exaggerated (bounding, water hammer) arterial pulses. R → L type usually has no murmur, accentuated and split S_2, normal arterial pulses, and differential cyanosis.	LV enlargement patterns (↑ QRS amplitudes with normal mean axis) usually present. Left atrial enlargement pattern (↑ P duration) often present. Advanced cases with heart failure often develop arrhythmias, including atrial fibrillation. RV hypertrophy pattern always present in R → L type.	Enlargement of left atrium, left ventricle, aortic arch, main pulmonary artery, and pulmonary arteries and veins proportional to shunt magnitude. DV view shows dilatation of aorta and main pulmonary artery at site of ductus. R → L type usually shows RV enlargement, prominent main pulmonary artery (±), and normal to slightly enlarged pulmonary arteries.	Polygenic inheritance proven in Poodles. Poodles, Pomeranians, Collies, German Shepherds, and Shelties are predisposed. 2:1 ratio of incidence of females to males.
Pulmonic stenosis	Systolic ejection murmur loudest in pulmonic area near left cranial sternal border or slightly more dorsal. Often equally loud along right cranial sternal border. Arterial pulses normal.	RV hypertrophy pattern nearly always present, even in mild cases (may require thoracic leads to be seen). Right atrial enlargement (↑ P amplitude) is inconsistent.	RV enlargement and post-stenotic dilatation of main pulmonary artery usually seen. Pulmonary vasculature appears normal to slightly diminished.	Polygenic inheritance in Beagles. Beagles, Bulldogs, Fox Terriers, Miniature Schnauzers, Chihuahuas, and Samoyeds predisposed.

Subaortic stenosis	Systolic ejection murmur loudest in aortic area at left base and/or cranial right thorax. May radiate cranially to thoracic inlet and carotid arteries in neck. Arterial pulses have diminished amplitude and delayed upstroke.	May be normal. LV enlargement pattern often present but not striking. ST depression may be present at rest or postexercise. Ventricular premature beats are common in severe cases.	May be normal. LV enlargement often present but not striking. Poststenotic dilatation of aorta may be visible in lateral view, especially in dogs >6 months of age. Left atrial enlargement is variable. Pulmonary vasculature is normal.	Polygenic inheritance in Newfoundlands, Retrievers. Newfoundlands, Boxers, German Shepherds, German Short-Haired Pointers, and Golden Retrievers predisposed. Syncope and sudden death are common sequelae.
Ventricular septal defect (VSD)	Harsh, regurgitant holosystolic murmur loudest in right 2 to 4 intercostal spaces. Often heard well on cranial left thorax. Arterial pulses are normal or brisk and short with larger shunts.	May be normal with small shunts. LV enlargement pattern may develop with larger shunts. Partial or complete right bundle branch block may occur.	May be normal with small shunts. Enlargement of left atrium, left and right ventricles, and pulmonary vasculature proportional to shunt magnitude.	Small defects may close within the first year of life. English Bulldogs predisposed.
Atrial septal defect (ASD)	Soft, mid systolic ejection murmur loudest in pulmonic area on left cranial thorax. Split S_2 is audible and helps distinguish ASD from pulmonic stenosis. Arterial pulses are normal in most cases.	May be normal. Partial or complete right bundle branch block is common and may be confused with RV hypertrophy.	May be normal with small shunts. Left and right atrial, right ventricular, and pulmonary vascular enlargement proportional to shunt magnitude. Left ventricle is normal, and left atrium may also appear normal in some cases.	This defect is infrequently diagnosed in the dog. Samoyeds may be predisposed.
Mitral valve dysplasia	Harsh, regurgitant holosystolic murmur loudest in mitral area at left apex. Arterial pulses are normal or brisk with significant regurgitation.	Left atrial enlargement pattern (↑ P wave duration) is almost always present. LV enlargement pattern varies with severity.	Moderate to marked left atrial enlargement is consistently present. Left ventricular enlargement usually present. Pulmonary veins often enlarged, but pulmonary arteries are normal.	Medium to giant breeds most often affected. Great Danes and German Shepherds predisposed. Higher incidence in males.

(*Continued*)

TABLE 10-1. DIAGNOSTIC CHARACTERISTICS OF COMMON CANINE CONGENITAL HEART DEFECTS (*Continued*)

Heart Defect	Physical Examination	Electrocardiogram	Thoracic Radiographs	Other Characteristics
Tricuspid valve dysplasia	Harsh, regurgitant holosystolic murmur loudest over tricuspid area on right mid thorax. May radiate well to left side. Arterial pulses are usually normal. Jugular distention and pulse may occur with significant regurgitation.	Right atrial enlargement pattern (↑ P wave amplitude and often duration) usually present. RV enlargement pattern variable and inconsistent.	Moderate to marked right atrial enlargement and right ventricular enlargement consistently present and may produce ovoid or globular cardiac silhouette. Left atrium and ventricle are normal. Pulmonary vasculature normal or slightly diminished. Caudal vena cava often enlarged.	Medium to giant breeds most often affected. Great Danes, German Shepherds, and Weimaraners predisposed. Higher incidence in males.
Tetralogy of Fallot	Systolic ejection murmur of pulmonic stenosis loudest in pulmonic area. Murmur may diminish in intensity with pulmonary hypoplasia. Symmetric cyanosis at rest or after exercise. Arterial pulses are usually normal.	RV hypertrophy pattern is always present.	Cardiac size is often normal and may appear small due to lucent, hyperinflated lungs. RV enlargement usually recognized. Main pulmonary artery may or may not show poststenotic dilatation. Pulmonary vasculature consistently diminished Malpositioned aorta.	Polygenic inheritance in Keeshonds. Keeshonds and English Bulldogs predisposed.

From Thomas WP: Congenital heart disease. In Kirk RW (ed): Current Veterinary Therapy—Small Animal Practice. Vol. 8. WB Saunders, Philadelphia, 1983, with permission.

PATENT DUCTUS ARTERIOSUS

INTRODUCTION

I. Anatomy

Patent ductus arteriosus represents persistence of the fetal communication between the aorta and the pulmonary artery. The ductus arteriosus shunts oxygenated blood during fetal life from the nonfunctional pulmonary system to the systemic circulation and normally closes shortly after birth.

II. Etiology

The mechanism of closure is regulated by prostaglandin synthetase inhibition and is probably a combination of hemodynamic, neurologic, and oxygen tension effect. Normally, the ductus closes the first few days to 2 weeks after birth, becoming the ligamentum arteriosum, a fibrous band. When the vessel fails to close beyond this period of time, it is called a patent ductus arteriosus.

III. Pathophysiology

A. With a small ductus, there are no significant hemodynamic changes. As the size of the ductus increases, there is a volume overload of the left ventricle, often with resultant left ventricular failure.

B. With large shunts through a patent ductus arteriosus, pulmonary hypertension frequently occurs. If the pulmonary vasculature resistance exceeds the systemic vascular resistance, then the shunt will reverse and go from right to left. A right-to-left shunt is not common with patent ductus arteriosus. Right ventricular failure can result from the increased afterload imposed upon it by pulmonary hypertension.

DIAGNOSIS

I. Etiology and breed disposition

Patent ductus arteriosus occurs in both the dog and cat with the frequency higher in the dog.

A. The defect is more common in the female and in the following breeds:

TABLE 10-2. DIAGNOSTIC CHARACTERISTICS OF COMMON FELINE CONGENITAL HEART DEFECTS

Heart Defect	Physical Examination	Electrocardiogram	Thoracic Radiographs
Ventricular septal defect (VSD)	Holosystolic murmur is loudest on the right cranial thorax or is equal bilaterally.	Frequently normal with small defects. With larger shunts LV enlargement pattern may develop.	Generalized cardiomegaly, left atrial enlargement, and prominent pulmonary vasculature proportional to shunt magnitude.
Aortic stenosis	Ejection systolic murmur at the heart base, loudest on the left or bilaterally. S_4 may be audible. The femoral pulse strength is diminished.	Increased QRS amplitudes (LV enlargement) are common but variable.	Mild to moderate cardiomegaly with LV and left arterial enlargement. Poststenotic dilatation of aorta is often difficult to recognize. Pulmonary vasculature normal.
Patent ductus arteriosus (PDA)	Continuous murmur loudest at the heart base bilaterally and often widespread. Femoral pulses are brisk and bounding.	LV enlargement consistently present with significant shunts. Increased P wave duration (left atrial enlargement) variable.	Cardiomegaly with left atrial and ventricular enlargement and pulmonary hypervascularity proportional to shunt magnitude. On DV view the heart may appear elongated and prominent pulmonary artery and aortoductal aneurysms are visible.
Endocardial fibroelastosis	Signs of dyspnea and heart failure usually occur at an early age ($<$16 weeks). Tachycardia and mitral systolic murmur most common.	Variable. LV enlargement (increased QRS amplitude and duration) is common.	Generalized, marked cardiomegaly without pulmonary hypervascularity. Pulmonary edema and pleural effusion are often present.
Tetralogy of Fallot	Fatigue, tachypnea, and cyanosis are common, but congestive heart failure is rare. Systolic ejection murmur audible at left base.	Right ventricular hypertrophy pattern usually present.	Cardiomegaly is usually mild. Right ventricular enlargement and pulmonary hypovascularity common. Poststenotic dilation of pulmonary artery may not be obvious.

Mitral and tricuspid valve dysplasias	Systolic murmurs over left and/or right thorax consistently present. Advanced tricuspid insufficiency may cause jugular vein distention and ascites.	Variable. Enlarged P waves often found. The signs of ventricular enlargement are inconsistent.	Mitral: left atrial enlargement consistently present; more difficult to recognize than in dogs. Cardiomegaly may be slight to severe. Tricuspid: marked right atrial enlargement often appears as generalized cardiomegaly with normal pulmonary vasculature. Caudal vena cava often enlarged.
Endocardial cushion defect (atrial septal defect or atrioventricular canal)	Fatigue and dyspnea often occur at an early age. Loud systolic murmur over left thorax from mitral insufficiency or VSD.	Variable. Atrial enlargement common. QRS changes of ventricular enlargement or partial or complete right bundle branch block often present.	Cardiomegaly is usually marked and generalized. Pulmonary hypervascularity helps distinguish this defect from other nonshunting defects.

From Thomas WP: Congenital heart disease. In Kirk RW (ed): Current Veterinary Therapy—Small Animal Practice. Vol. 8. WB Saunders, Philadelphia, 1983, with permission.

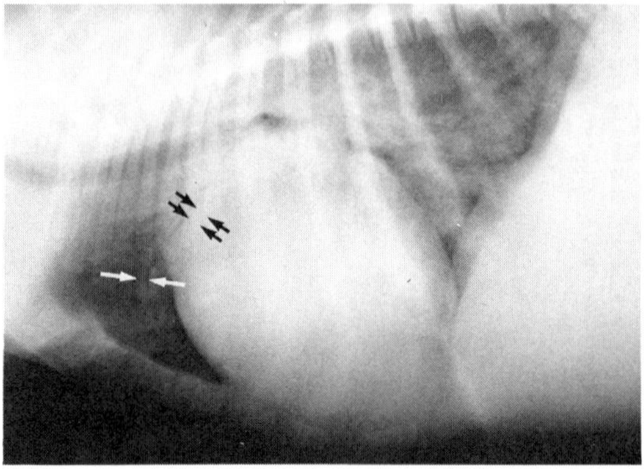

Fig. 10-1. Patent ductus arteriosus (lateral projection). Three-month-old Poodle. There is generalized heart enlargement, engorgement of the right cranial lobar artery (white arrows) and the right cranial lobar vein (black arrows). Vascular engorgement, perivascular congestion and alveolar edema is seen in the caudal lung lobes. (Courtesy of Dr. Ronald Burk, Animal Medical Center, New York, New York.)

1. Miniature Poodle
2. German Shepherd
3. Collie
4. Pomeranian
5. Shetland Sheep Dog
6. Toy breeds (e.g., Yorkshire Terrier)

B. The defect has been shown to be hereditary in the Miniature Poodle, transmitted as a polygenic trait.

II. History

A. The cat or dog with patent ductus arteriosus may be asymptomatic, or it may manifest heart failure.

B. Symptoms of left or right heart failure can occur at any age. Most animals show severe clinical signs of cardiac disease, particularly up to six to eight weeks of age. Beyond six to eight weeks, pups will usually live to adulthood. Congestive heart failure is common in mature dogs.

C. Dogs with a small defect can often survive for a number of years, while cats rarely survive to a few weeks of age.

III. Physical examination

A. Palpation

1. Animals with a patent ductus arteriosus with a large left-to-right shunt characteristically have a bounding (water-hammer) pulse. The volume overload of the left ventricle raises the systolic pressure and the rapid run-off of blood from the aorta to the pulmonary artery lowers the diastolic pressure.
2. Upon palpation of the thorax, the left or right ventricle will be more prominent based on the function of the particular hemodynamic status associated with the defect. If pulmonary vasculature is normal, the left ventricle will be more prominent.

B. Clinical signs

Clinical signs may include a stunting of growth and poor stamina, coughing, dyspnea, anorexia, weight loss and weakness. Cyanosis is an important physical finding in animals with patent ductus arteriosus and right-to-left shunt. Because the site of the ductus is in the descending aorta, cyanosis is characteristically confined to the posterior extremities.

C. Auscultation

1. Auscultation of the chest usually reveals a continuous or nearly continuous machinery murmur, which is present during systole and diastole and may be auscultated best over the left cranial–dorsal thoracic wall (the aortic–pulmonic region). The murmur will often radiate to other regions of the thoracic cavity.
2. As pulmonary hypertension develops, the pulmonary diastolic pressure approaches systemic levels so that the diastolic portion of the murmur disappears. Eventually, as the pulmonary hypertension increases, the systolic murmur will shorten and eventually disappear.

IV. Electrocardiogram

The electrocardiographic changes in patent ductus arteriosus occur because of the diastolic overload of the left ventricle and accompanying left ventricular enlargement.

A. The R waves are tall in leads II, III, and aVF with amplitudes > 3.0 mV in lead II.

B. Deep Q waves are often present in leads II, III, and aVF.

C. The QRS complexes are increased in duration.

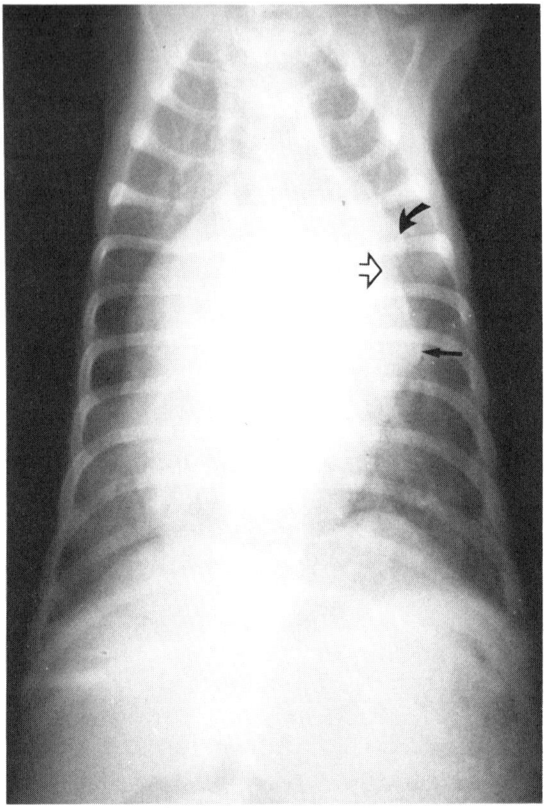

Fig. 10-2. Patent ductus arteriosus (dorsoventral projection). Three-month-old Poodle. There is generalized heart enlargement, an aneurysmal-like bulge of the descending aorta (open arrow), a bulge of the main pulmonary artery (curved arrow) and enlargement of the left auricle (straight arrow). Alveolar infiltrate due to pulmonary edema is present in the caudal lung lobes. (Courtesy of Dr. Ronald Burk, Animal Medical Center, New York, New York.)

D. P mitrale is often present.
E. The mean electrical axis is usually +90 degrees.
F. Animals with pulmonary hypertension may show evidence of right ventricular hypertrophy. Large S waves are present in leads I, II, III, and aVF.
G. Atrial fibrillation and ectopic ventricular arrhythmias may occur in association with congestive heart failure.

H. As will be seen with some of the other congenital heart defects, the ECG can be normal, depending on the hemodynamic characteristics related to the size of the shunt.

V. Thoracic radiographs

The radiographic signs of patent ductus arteriosus (Figs. 10-1 and 10-2) vary considerably with the volume of blood being shunted, the duration of the problem, and the degree of cardiac decompensation.

A. Dorsoventral radiographs often reveal three prominences along the left cardiac silhouette:
   1. The aneurysmal bulge of the aortic arch
   2. The enlarged pulmonary outflow tract
   3. The enlarged left atrium

B. Mild to moderate left ventricular and left atrial enlargement is usually present.

C. Overcirculation of the lung field can often be visualized.

D. Severe cardiomegaly, pulmonary congestion, and pulmonary edema will be present when there is congestive heart failure.

E. Right ventricular enlargement develops in animals with severe pulmonary hypertension.

VI. Other diagnostic techniques

Cardiac catheterization and angiocardiography may be needed to confirm and document the diagnosis of patent ductus arteriosus.

A. Selective angiocardiography

The diagnosis can be made by injecting contrast medium into the ascending aorta. The simultaneous filling of the main pulmonary artery and the aorta is diagnostic for patent ductus arteriosus.

B. Nonselective angiocardiography

Nonselective procedures may be performed by injecting contrast material through a large diameter venous catheter and taking radiographs at approximately one, five and ten seconds. A nonselective angiocardiogram is not always diagnostic.

VII. Differential diagnosis

Angiocardiographic studies are used to differentiate patent ductus arteriosus from other congenital cardiac defects. Two cardiac defects that can resemble patent ductus arteriosus are as follows:

A. Aorticopulmonary window

A round or oval communication is formed between the aorta and

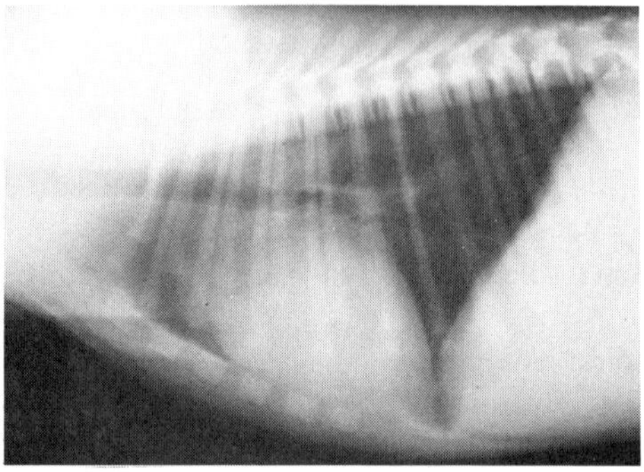

Fig. 10-3. Pulmonic stenosis (lateral projection). Two-month-old mixed breed. There is increased sternal contact of the right heart, due to right heart enlargement, and normal to slightly diminished pulmonary vasculature.

the main pulmonary artery. This rare defect usually results in severe pulmonary hypertension.

B. Aortic stenosis and insufficiency
The systolic murmur of the stenosis and the diastolic murmur of aortic insufficiency almost appear to be continuous. Angiocardiography and echocardiography are often needed to confirm the diagnosis.

Therapy and Prognosis

I. Surgery
   A. As soon as possible after diagnosis, surgery should be performed to occlude the patent vessel. The reader is referred to veterinary surgical textbooks for a detailed description of the procedure.
   B. After the surgery has been successfully performed, the animal without symptoms usually has a normal life expectancy.
   C. If the patent ductus arteriosus is not occluded, serious pathologic consequences are almost sure to follow with aging. Surgery should be strongly advocated before cardiac decompensation occurs. When the procedure is performed on the young asymptomatic patient, the risk is small and the outcome very rewarding. If heart failure is present, the postoperative mortality rate is greater. If the patient is older (over 2 years), the surgical technique is

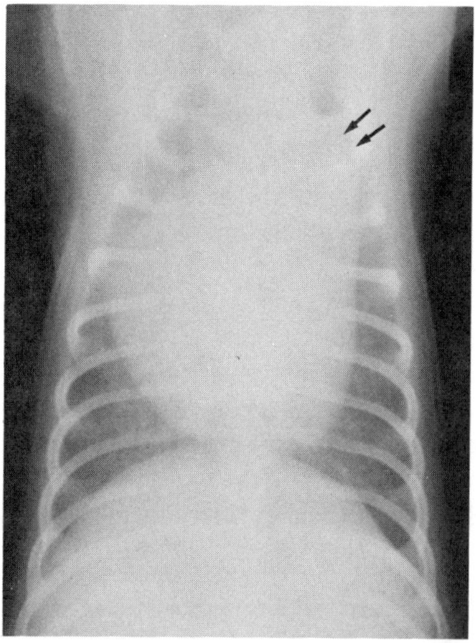

Fig. 10-4. Pulmonic stenosis (dorsoventral projection). Two-month-old mixed breed. There is marked right heart enlargement and prominence of the main pulmonary artery (arrows).

more complicated and existing mitral regurgitation may lead to atrial fibrillation.

D. Correction of patent ductus arteriosus is contraindicated when right-to-left shunting is present. Acute right heart failure and death can occur, since the ductus functions as a relief valve.

II. Medical management

A. When signs of heart failure are present, stabilization of the animal should be attempted with cage rest and drugs for heart failure prior to the operation.

B. Left ventricular failure is treated with digitalis, diuretics, and, if necessary, afterload reduction (e.g., arterial vasodilators).

PULMONIC STENOSIS

INTRODUCTION

I. Anatomy

Obstruction to the outflow of blood from the right ventricle may occur at the following levels:

A. Valvular
B. Subvalvular
C. Supravalvular (Supravalvular type of pulmonic stenosis is rare.)

II. Pathophysiology

A. The consequences of the lesion are in direct proportion to the severity of the obstruction. The major clinical manifestation is right ventricular failure resulting from pressure overload in that chamber.
B. Hemodynamically, valvular pulmonic stenosis results in a pressure gradient across the stenotic valve owing to resistance to right ventricular outflow. Right ventricular hypertrophy is almost always present, the degree varying with the amount of resistance.
C. Turbulence associated with the increase in velocity of blood across the stenotic valve is the probable cause of the poststenotic bulge in the main pulmonary artery segment.

Diagnosis

I. Etiology and breed predisposition

Pulmonic stenosis occurs in both the dog and cat.

A. The defect is more common in the following breeds:
 1. English Bulldog
 2. Fox Terrier
 3. Miniature Schnauzer
 4. Chihuahua
 5. Samoyed
 6. Beagle
B. A polygenic inheritance has been identified in the Beagle.

II. History

A. Animals with mild or moderate pulmonic stenosis are usually asymptomatic. Many animals may live apparently normal lives with mild degrees of pulmonic stenosis.
B. Symptomatic animals with pulmonic stenosis have clinical signs of dyspnea and fatigue secondary to low cardiac output. Exercise-induced syncope may occur, because of the limitation in cardiac output imposed by the stenotic valve.

C. Decompensation and signs of right heart failure occur when right ventricular output is decreased because of a fall in the contractile state of the right ventricular myocardium.

III. Physical examination

A. Palpation

Animals with moderate to severe pulmonic stenosis have easily palpable right-ventricular impulses. A thrill very often can be palpated at the left lower third or fourth intercostal space.

B. Clinical signs

Signs of dyspnea, fatigability and right heart failure may occur as the condition progresses. Cyanosis may be seen with severe pulmonic stenosis commonly due to low cardiac output.

C. Auscultation

A systolic crescendo–decrescendo murmur can be heard best at the left lower third or fourth intercostal space. If the murmur is severe, it may radiate over the cranial thorax and be audible at the thoracic inlet. A split second heart sound due to delayed closure of the pulmonic valve may also be present.

IV. Electrocardiogram

A. Signs of right ventricular hypertrophy predominant, with S waves present in leads I, II, and III and a right shift of the mean electrical axis in the frontal plane to greater than +120 degrees.

B. Arrhythmias are uncommon.

V. Thoracic radiographs

The primary radiographic features (Figs. 10-3 and 10-4) include the following:

A. Right ventricular enlargement and right atrial enlargement

B. Enlargement of the main pulmonary segment

C. Normal to some decreased pulmonary vascularity

VI. Other diagnostic techniques

A. Special studies including phonocardiography, selective or nonselective angiocardiography, and cardiac catheterization may be needed for a definitive diagnosis and to determine whether surgical correction may be indicated.

B. Elevated right ventricular pressures and usually normal or lowered pulmonary artery pressure result in a systolic pressure gradient across the valve. If the gradient exceeds 70 mm Hg, most cardiologists would recommend surgery.

VII. Differential diagnosis

The diagnosis of pulmonic stenosis can usually be made on the basis of history, physical examination, electrocardiogram, and thoracic radiograph. Differential diagnosis should consider the following:

A. Atrial septal defect
B. Ventricular septal defect
C. Innocent or physiological murmurs

THERAPY AND PROGNOSIS

I. Surgery

A. Surgical correction of pulmonic stenosis depends on the type of stenosis present and its severity. Valvular pulmonic stenosis is surgically easier to correct. Animals with significant pulmonic stenosis will have at least a grade IV systolic murmur and right ventricular enlargement on the electrocardiogram. If these are absent, the gradient across the pulmonic valve is usually not significant and the animals will not require surgery.
B. If there is a question, the animal should be catheterized and if the pressure gradient is >70 mm Hg, surgery should be performed.
C. The surgical approach can be done either blindly or through an open right ventriculotomy or pulmonary arteriotomy utilizing venous inflow occlusion. The reader is referred to the veterinary surgical textbooks for a detailed description of the procedure.

II. Medical management

The treatment of right ventricular failure should include digitalis and diuretics.

AORTIC STENOSIS

INTRODUCTION

I. Anatomy

A. Aortic stenosis is a narrowing or reduction of the left ventricular outflow tract dimensions at the subvalvular (fibrous ring or muscular), valvular, or supravalvular level.

B. The subvalvular form is the most common form in the dog in which a fibrous band or ring is located just below the aortic semilunar valves.

C. The supravalvular type is the most common form in the cat.

II. Pathophysiology

A. Aortic stenosis results in a reduction in left ventricular outflow associated with increased resistance at the level of the stenosis. Secondary left ventricular hypertrophy results in increased left ventricular pressure.

B. The velocity of blood flow through the stenotic area is then increased, resulting in turbulence which is evident clinically as a systolic murmur. The turbulence and blood flow is associated with poststenotic bulging of the ascending aorta.

C. The compensatory hypertrophy and aortic stenosis result in an increase in myocardial oxygen consumption. The myocardial hypoxia is partially responsible for the development of left ventricular failure, arrhythmias, and sudden death observed in some cases.

Diagnosis

I. Etiology and breed predisposition

A. A polygenic inheritance has been identified in the Newfoundland Retriever.

B. Other common breeds include the following:

1. Boxer
2. German Shepherd
3. Golden Retriever
4. German Shorthair Pointer

II. History

A. Most immature animals with aortic stenosis are asymptomatic on initial physical examination. Clinical signs of congestive heart failure, exercise intolerance, and lethargy are usually observed in dogs aged 6 to 18 months. Dogs surviving beyond 3 years of age usually

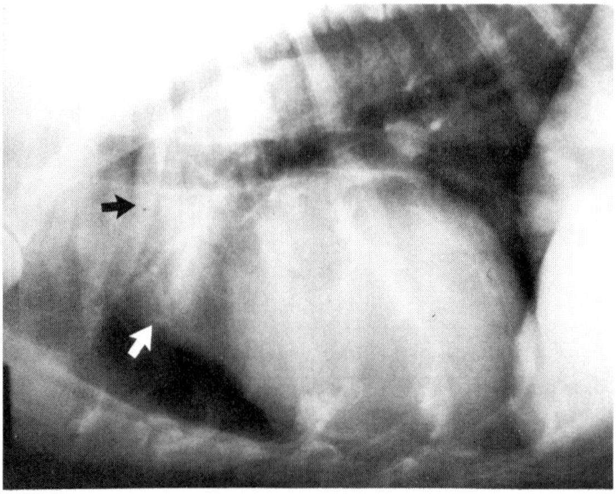

Fig. 10-5. Aortic stenosis (lateral projection). There is marked enlargement of the aortic arch cranial to the heart base (arrows).

do not have a severe enough stenosis to produce a marked effect in left ventricular performance.

B. Sudden death is most likely due to ventricular arrhythmias associated with myocardial hypoxia and can occur at any age.

III. Physical examination

A. Palpation

The femoral pulse may be normal, or if the stenosis is severe, the pulse may be weak. Animals with severe aortic stenosis have easily palpable left ventricular impulses.

B. Clinical signs

Syncope, dyspnea, weakness and sudden death may occur at any age.

C. Auscultation

Aortic stenosis is manifested by a systolic ejection-type murmur heard best over the lower left fourth intercostal space. Frequently, the murmur radiates up the carotid artery and can be auscultated in the mid-cervical area. Occasionally, the murmur may be loudest in the right third or fourth intercostal space midway up the thorax.

IV. Electrocardiogram

A. The ECG may be normal.

B. The ECG may show signs of left ventricular hypertrophy, ventric-

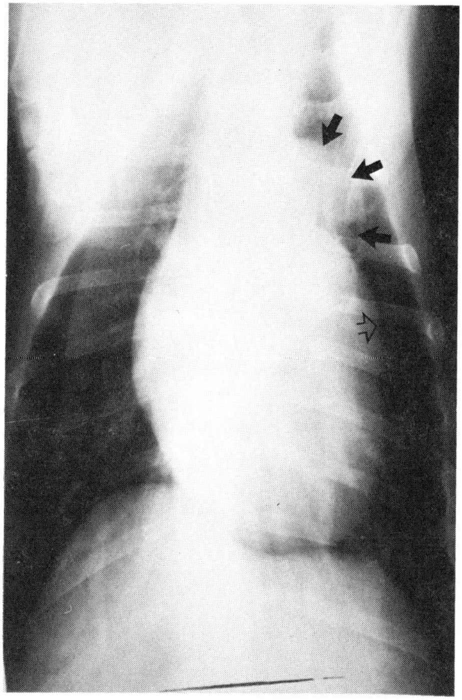

Fig. 10-6. Aortic stenosis (dorsoventral projection). The enlarged aortic arch extends craniolateral to the heart base (arrows). The left auricle (open arrow) extends beyond the cardiac border, and there is slight left ventricular enlargement.

ular or supraventricular arrhythmias, and S-T segment depression.

C. Atrial fibrillation is a common arrhythmia resulting from associated mitral valve disease and secondary left atrial enlargement.

V. Thoracic radiographs

A. Enlarged aortic arch, with poststenotic dilation of the aorta (Figs. 10-5 and 10-6)

B. Both left ventricular and left atrial enlargement occur in those advanced cases with concomitant mitral insufficiency.

C. Survey radiographs may be normal.

VI. Other diagnostic techniques

A. Special studies including phonocardiography, selective or nonselective angiocardiography, and cardiac catheterization are often necessary to substantiate the diagnosis and aid in making an accurate prognosis with and without therapy.

B. Measurement of the left ventricular aortic systolic pressure gradient can provide useful diagnostic and prognostic information.
   1. Between 10 and 40 mm Hg is considered mild stenosis.
   2. 40–80 mm Hg is moderate stenosis.
   3. More than 80 mm Hg is considered severe stenosis.

VII. Differential diagnosis

A. Aortic valvular insufficiency secondary to thickening of the aortic valve leaflets can be associated with subaortic stenosis. The result is a systolic and diastolic murmur that closely resembles the continuous murmur of patent ductus arteriosus.

B. The breed involved, point of maximum intensity of the murmur, as well as other diagnostic tests are, in most cases, useful in differentiating the two congenital defects.

Therapy and Prognosis

I. Surgery

A. Surgical correction of aortic stenosis is probably the method of choice, but surgery requires cardiac bypass, hypothermia, or both; the procedure is not routinely performed.

B. Animals with low pressure gradients may not require surgical correction. Animals with severe pressure gradients may have already developed irreversible compensatory changes making surgical removal of the obstructing fibrous ring ineffective.

II. Medical management

A. Treatment with various cardiac drugs, diuretics, low-salt diets, and rest is usually of minimal benefit in those severe cases that have developed congestive heart failure.

B. β-adrenergic agents (e.g., propranolol) may have some beneficial effects in the long-term management of increased intraventricular pressures and hypertrophy.

VENTRICULAR SEPTAL DEFECT

INTRODUCTION

I. Anatomy
   A. The lower region of the interventricular septum is called the muscular portion, and the upper region is called the membranous portion. In most animals with a ventricular septal defect, the lesion is in the membranous portion.
   B. The opening of the defect in the right ventricle is frequently found under the septal leaflet of the tricuspid valve and in the left ventricle outflow tract just below the aortic valve.

II. Pathophysiology
   A. The obstruction and magnitude of the shunt in an animal with ventricular septal defect is a function of the size of the defect and the relative resistances of the systemic and pulmonary arterial systems. If the defect is small, blood is shunted from left to right. With large defects, the ventricles are in free communication.
   B. If the pulmonary vascular resistance becomes elevated, the shunt will decrease in magnitude and may reverse and become a right-to-left shunt. Right-to-left shunting is due to narrowing of the pulmonary arteries and pulmonary hypertension.
   C. It is possible that the size of the ventricular septal defect could decrease significantly and may even spontaneously close.
   D. Right ventricular hypertrophy can result in narrowing of the right ventricular outflow tract, causing an infundibular pulmonic stenosis.

DIAGNOSIS

I. Etiology and breed predisposition
   A. Ventricular septal defect may occur as an isolated defect or may be seen in conjunction with many other defects including atrial septal defect, patent ductus arteriosus, aortic stenosis, and pulmonic stenosis.

B. The English Bulldog appears to have a higher incidence than other breeds, but the defect is seen in many purebred and mixed breed dogs.
C. Breed incidence in the cat has not been determined.
D. Breed studies in the Keeshond have shown the defect to be polygenic.

II. History
A. The clinical course of animals with ventricular septal defect is largely determined by the size of the defect.
B. Small defects may cause little or no functional disturbances since the shunt volume is small and right ventricular pressures are normal.
C. Animals with a large ventricular septal defect are often stunted because of retarded growth.

III. Physical examination
A. Palpation: With a left-to-right shunt, the left ventricular impulse is pronounced on palpation of the thorax. As pulmonary hypertension develops, and the shunt reverses, a right ventricular impulse becomes prominent. A precordial thrill can often be detected in the right third to fourth intercostal spaces just above the costochondral junction.
B. Auscultation
1. The murmur associated with a ventricular septal defect tends to be maximal in the second to fourth intercostal spaces, just to the right of the sternum. Its characteristics depend on the size of the defect and the height of the right ventricular pressure.
2. The murmur of a small ventricular septal defect may occur only early in systole, while with a large ventricular septal defect, the murmur may be holosystolic.
3. With a larger defect, the murmur is louder and harsher as well as being holosystolic.
4. As the right ventricular pressure rises and the left to right shunt decreases, the murmur occurs in systole then disappears as a shunt becomes balanced.
5. Splitting of the second heart sound may occur due to delayed closure of the pulmonic valve.

C. Clinical signs
1. Congestive heart failure is usually right sided; clinical signs can

include ascites, hepatomegaly, dyspnea, weakness, and weight loss.

2. The signs of left ventricular failure as a result of ventricular septal defect usually occur in the first few weeks to few months after birth.
3. A right to left flow across the defect with resultant cyanosis will occur if pulmonary pressures exceed systemic pressures.

IV. Electrocardiogram

A. The electrocardiogram of an animal with a ventricular septal defect depends on the hemodynamic status.
B. The ECG may be normal in a small defect.
C. The ECG may show evidence of left, right, or biventricular enlargement.
D. Right bundle branch block may also be observed.

V. Thoracic radiographs

A. The appearance of the chest radiographs depends on the size of the defect and the direction and magnitude of the shunt.
B. Small defects are generally associated with a normal survey radiograph.
C. Enlargement of the left atrium, left and right ventricles, and engorged pulmonary vasculature may occur with larger defects.

VI. Other diagnostic techniques

A. Selective angiocardiography can document the location of the ventricular septal defect.
B. Echocardiography may be useful by identifying echodense dye bubbles traversing the defect.

VII. Differential diagnosis

A. Mitral regurgitation
   1. The pathophysiology of mitral regurgitation secondary to congenital mitral valvular dysplasia or acquired mitral valvular fibrosis can be very similar to ventricular septal defect.
   2. Mitral valvular dysplasia is one of the most common defects in cats.
   3. Both ventricular septal defect and mitral regurgitation have harsh, regurgitant holosystolic murmurs. However, the murmur of ventricular septal defect is loudest in the right third to fourth intercostal spaces, while the murmur of mitral regurgitation is heard loudest in the mitral area at the left apex.

4. Angiocardiography is often needed to confirm the diagnosis.

B. Tricuspid valve dysplasia
The harsh, regurgitant holosystolic murmur produced by tricuspid regurgitation may resemble that seen with ventricular septal defect. However, with significant tricuspid regurgitation, a jugular distention and pulse may be present.

Therapy and Prognosis

No treatment is necessary in asymptomatic individuals. Spontaneous closure is quite possible during the first years of life.

I. Surgery
Surgery should only be considered for those animals showing signs of heart failure. Management of the condition may include total surgical correction utilizing heart-lung bypass. Pulmonary artery banding has also been used effectively to increase right ventricular pressure and reduce the amount of blood shunting across the ventricular septal defect.

II. Medical management
When signs of failure develop and surgical correction cannot be considered, medical management with diuretics, low-salt intake, restriction of exercise, digitalis, and the use of vasodilators should be attempted.

III. Prognosis
The prognosis is directly related to the size of the septal defect.

TETRALOGY OF FALLOT

Introduction

I. Anatomy

A. Tetralogy of Fallot is a combination of pulmonic stenosis, high ventricular septal defect, right ventricular hypertrophy, and varying degrees of dextroposition and overriding of the aorta.

B. The right ventricular hypertrophy is secondary to the obstruction to right ventricular outflow. The pulmonic stenosis component may be valvular, infundibular, or both.

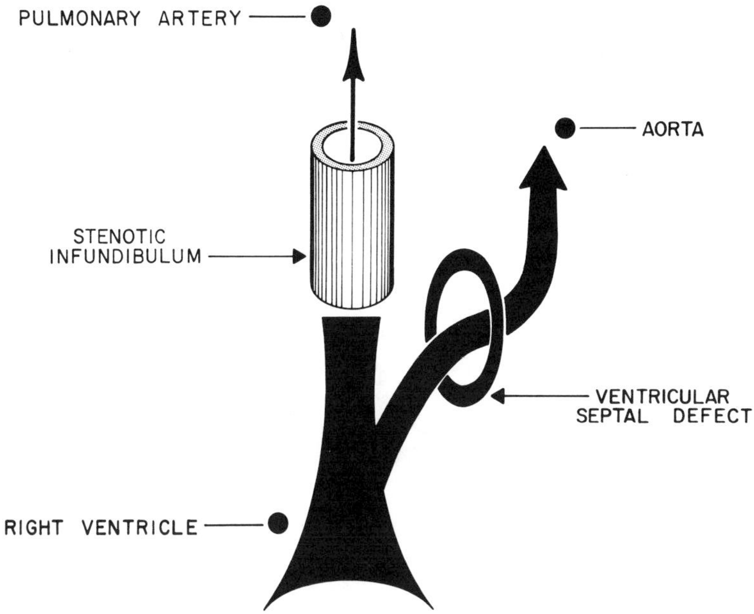

Fig. 10-7. Tetralogy of Fallot. Note diminished blood flow to the lungs and increased blood flow to the body. The small arrow entering the pulmonary artery represents diminished blood flow through the stenotic infundibulum. The heavier arrow represents flow of venous bood through the ventricular septal defect into the aorta. The thick black area identified as the right ventricle indicates the increased pressure in that chamber. (From Fink BW: Congenital Heart Disease: A Deductive Approach to Diagnosis. Year Book Medical Publishers, Chicago, 1975.)

II. Pathophysiology (Fig. 10-7)

A. The hemodynamic consequences of tetralogy of Fallot depend primarily on the severity of the pulmonic stenosis and the ventricular septal defect. Compensatory right ventricular hypertrophy and increased right ventricular pressures are seen with severe pulmonic stenosis.

B. If the pulmonic stenosis is less severe and right ventricular pressures are only moderately elevated, the direction of the intraventricular shunt is from left to right with only a small portion of the venous return entering the overriding aorta. This results in little or no detectable cyanosis.

C. However, if the ventricular septal defect is large, and the pulmonic stenosis severe, the patient will be cyanotic.

D. Secondary polycythemia almost always accompanies those animals with significant right-to-left shunts. The relative hypoxemia tends to stimulate red cell production through increased release of erythropoietin by the kidney.

Diagnosis

I. Etiology and breed predisposition

A. Tetralogy of Fallot occurs in the Keeshond with greater frequency than other breeds but also has been recognized in many other breeds, including cats.

B. In the Keeshond, a polygenic trait has been found.

II. History

Cyanosis usually develops by 3 to 6 months after birth. The animal is usually stunted because of retarded growth.

III. Physical examination

A. Palpation

A thrill may be felt in the third left interspace, near the costochondral junction.

B. Auscultation

A systolic ejection murmur of pulmonic stenosis, loudest in the pulmonic area is sometimes present.

C. Clinical signs

The animal is small, and there is cyanosis, which increases with exercise. Dyspnea is usually present.

IV. Electrocardiogram

A. The electrocardiogram usually displays right axis deviation.

B. Bundle branch block can occur with a bizarre axis shift if bundle branches are interrupted by the ventricular septal defect.

C. Arrhythmias are unusual.

V. Thoracic radiographs

A. The right ventricle is moderately to severely enlarged; on the lateral view, the cardiac apex is often elevated away from the sternum.

B. The lungs will appear undercirculated in right to left shunts and the main pulmonary artery is small.

C. The aorta may also be malpositioned, although usually no aortic displacement is detected.

VI. Other diagnostic techniques

A. Selective angiocardiography may be diagnostic. Using right ventricular injection, simultaneous filling of the aorta and pulmonary artery occurs when a right-to-left shunt is present.

B. Nonselective angiocardiography may support a diagnosis of tetralogy of Fallot.

C. The echocardiogram may show overriding of the aorta and will also show right ventricular enlargement.

D. Secondary polycythemia along with cyanosis may be present.

VII. Differential diagnosis

Atrial and ventricular septal defect as well as patent ductus arteriosus may also develop cyanosis late in the course when pulmonary hypertension leads to shunt reversal.

Therapy and Prognosis

I. Surgery

A. Surgical correction of the pulmonic stenosis and ventricular septal defect is the treatment of choice that requires extensive and complex procedures not generally available.

B. An alternate surgical approach is to create a shunt between the aorta or subclavian artery and pulmonary artery. This surgical procedure increases pulmonary blood flow and improves systemic oxygenation.

II. Medical management

β-adrenergic blockade may be of some value in the management of tetralogy of Fallot by inhibiting sympathetic tone on the hypertrophied right ventricular outflow tract. This medical approach has the possibility of decreasing contractility and allowing the ventricular outflow to stay relatively open during systole, even though its efficacy has not been well documented in the veterinary field.

SUGGESTED READINGS

Alpert JS, Rippe JM: Manual of Cardiovascular Diagnosis and Therapy. Little, Brown, Boston, 1980

Bolton GR, Liu S–K: Congenital heart disease of the cat. Vet Clin North Am [Small Anim Pract] 7:341, 1977

Cohen JS, Tilley LP, Liu S–K, et al: Patent ductus arteriosus in five cats. J Am Anim Hosp Assoc 11:95, 1975

Edwards NJ, Tilley LP: Congenital heart defects, p. 155. In Bojrab MJ (ed): Pathophysiology in Small Animal Surgery. Lea & Febiger, Philadelphia, 1981

Ettinger SJ, Suter PF: Canine Cardiology. WB Saunders, Philadelphia, 1970

Liska WD, Tilley LP: Patent ductus arteriosus. Vet Clin North Am [Small Anim Pract] 9:195, 1979

Liu S–K, Tilley LP: Dysplasia of the tricuspid valve in the dog and cat. J Am Vet Med Assoc 169:623, 1976

Liu S–K, Tilley LP: Malformation of the canine mitral valve complex. J Am Vet Med Assoc 167:465, 1975

Patterson DF: Congenital defects of the cardiovascular system of dogs: Studies in comparative cardiology. Adv Vet Sci Comp Med 20:1, 1976

Perloff JK: The Clinical Recognition of Congenital Heart Disease. ed 2. WB Saunders, Philadelphia, 1978

Pyle RL: Congenital heart disease. p. 933. In Ettinger SJ (ed): Textbook of Veterinary Internal Medicine. ed 2. WB Saunders, Philadelphia, 1983

Thomas WP: The differential diagnosis of congenital heart disease in the dog. Small Anim Vet Med Update Ser 2: No.12, 1979

Thomas WP: Congenital heart disease. p. 301. In Kirk RW (ed): Current Veterinary Therapy—Small Animal Practice. Vol. 8. WB Saunders, Philadelphia, 1983

Tilley LP: Essentials of Canine and Feline Cardiology—Interpretation and Treatment. ed 2. Lea & Febiger, Philadelphia, 1985

11

Cardiovascular Disorders in Systemic Diseases

Philip R. Fox

Many systemic diseases produce associated disorders of cardiovascular structure and function (Table 11-1). The veterinarian may detect cardiovascular abnormalities as the predominant clinical sign, or systemic disease manifestations may overshadow cardiac abnormalities. While cardiovascular disease may sometimes be of no clinical significance, at other times it may constitute the major medical concern. Detection of cardiovascular involvement may be based on clinical signs, radiographic changes, electrocardiographic abnormalities, and laboratory findings.

THE HEART AND ENDOCRINE DISEASE

HYPERTHYROIDISM (THYROTOXICOSIS)

Introduction

I. General features
  A. Thyrotoxic heart disease is common in older cats (range, 6 to 20 years; mean, 13 years).
  B. Thyroid hormone profoundly affects many tissues.
  C. Cardiovascular manifestations (tachycardia, bounding pulses, and heart failure) may be dramatic.

TABLE 11-1. CLASSIFICATION OF IMPORTANT SYSTEMIC DISORDERS AFFECTING THE HEART

Endocrine
Thyroid gland
Thyrotoxicosis
Hypothyroidism
Adrenal gland
Hyperadrenocorticism
Hypoadrenocorticism
Pheochromocytoma
Pancreas
Metabolic
Hypercalcemia
Hypocalcemia
Hyperkalemia
Uremia
Hematologic disorders
Anemia
Neoplastic and infiltrative heart diseases
Physical and chemical agents
Hyperpyrexia
Hypothermia
Arsenic
Lead
Carbon monoxide
Toad poisoning
Oleander toxicity
Cyclophosphamide cardiotoxicity
Doxorubricin cardiomyopathy
Infective inflammatory myocardial diseases
Bacterial
Viral
Mycotic
Protozoal

D. Clinical evidence of thyrotoxic heart disease is unusual before the age of 7 years.

II. Pathophysiology

A. Two biologically active hormones are secreted by the thyroid: Thyroxine (T4) and triiodothyronine (T3). Functional thyroid adenomas (adenomatous hyperplasia) involving one or both lobes is the most common cause of excessive circulatory concentrations of thyroid hormones.

B. Cardiovascular alterations from excess thyroid hormone appear to be due to both direct effects of thyroid hormone on the heart and indirect consequences of augmented sympathetic activity.

C. The thyrotoxic heart usually displays left ventricular hypertrophy. It is physiologically hyperactive with increased heart rate, cardiac output, contractility, left ventricular work, myocardial oxygen consumption, and left ventricular circumferential fiber shortening. Peripheral vascular resistance is decreased, and peripheral arteriovenous shunting increases.

D. The combination of tachycardia, ventricular hypertrophy and increased cardiac output may produce congestive heart failure. Preexisting heart disease, circulatory abnormalities, or anemia may predispose to congestive heart failure.

Diagnosis

I. History and physical examination
  A. Noncardiac manifestations include weight loss, polyphagia, polyuria, polydipsia, vomiting, diarrhea, and hyperactivity or anorexia.
  B. Cardiac manifestations include hyperdynamic circulation, resting tachycardia, loud heart sounds (especially S_1), prominent apex beat, flow murmurs, and arrhythmias.

II. Radiography
  A. Roentgenographic evidence of mild to moderate (occasionally severe) heart enlargement is present in approximately one-half of clinically affected cats.
  B. Pulmonary edema or pleural effusion may occur in about 20 percent of thyrotoxic animals.

III. Electrocardiogram
  A. Sinus tachycardia ($>$240 beats/min) is a distinctive feature. Increased R-wave amplitude in lead II ($\geqslant$0.9 mV) is also common. Supraventricular and ventricular arrhythmias and conduction abnormalities may occur less frequently.
  B. Tachycardia, increased R-wave amplitude, and some arrhythmias may resolve after successful therapy.

IV. Echocardiography
  A. Left atrial enlargement, left ventricular hypertrophy, and elevated

indices of contractility (fractional shortening and velocity of circumferential fiber shortening) are readily confirmed with M-mode echocardiography.

V. Clinical pathology
   A. Elevated serum values for alkaline phosphatease, lactate dehydrogenase, aspartate transaminase, and alanine transaminase can be recorded (one or more of these enzymes is usually increased).
   B. Mild azotemia is present in approximately 25 percent of cases.
   C. Packed cell volume and mean corpuscular volume are increased in almost one-half of affected cats.
   D. Baseline serum thyroid hormone concentrations are elevated (T4, 4 to 54 μg/dl; T3, 54 to 1000 mg/dl).

VI. Thyroid imaging
   A. Thyroid scans show enlargement and increased radionuclide accumulation of affected thyroid lobes.
   B. Occasionally, an affected thyroid lobe will be present in the caudoventral cervical region or in the cranial mediastinum.

Therapy

A. Current therapy involves using β-adrenergic blockade (i.e., propranolol, 2.5 to 5 mg BID-TID) to control the sinus tachycardia, temporary use of antithyroid drugs (propylthiouracil 50 mg TID or methylamazole, 5 mg TID) to convert the hyperthyroid state to euthyroidism, followed by surgical removal of affected thyroid lobes.

B. Antithyroid drug therapy without surgery is used when surgical intervention is contraindicated. A lupuslike response may occur with prolonged antithyroid drug therapy resulting in antinuclear antibody-positive Coombs' positive anemia and thrombocytopenia.

C. Radioactive iodine therapy is possible but requires special and stringent measures regarding radiation safety.

Prognosis

The prognosis for remission of sinus tachycardia, voltage changes, arrhythmias, and congestive heart failure is favorable when the hypermetabolic state is controlled through the medical or surgical techniques discussed.

HYPOTHYROIDISM

Introduction

I. General features
   A. The clinical status of the heart in the hypothyroid state is not clear.
   B. Primary hypothyroidism usually occurs in dogs middle-aged and older without sex predilection.
   C. Its occurrence in cats has been limited to postoperative cases following surgical removal of unilateral or bilateral functional thyroid tumor.

II. Pathophysiology
   A. In primary hypothyroidism, thyroid atrophy occurs by chronic lymphocytic thyroiditis or idiopathic thyroid atrophy.
   B. In hypothyroid humans, resting cardiac output is significantly reduced.
   C. Heart muscle from experimentally produced hypothyroidism in cats exhibits reduced contractility.
   D. There is little evidence that congestive heart failure is common in hypothyroid states in the absence of underlying cardiac pathology.
   E. Large breed dogs with hypothyroidism and dilated cardiomyopathy have a worse clinical course.
   F. Atherosclerosis has been recorded with hypothyroid large-breed dogs, especially Doberman Pinschers. Experimental support for this association has come from cholesterol-fed animals in which atherosclerosis, enhanced by hypothyroidism, is reduced when euthyroidism is established.

Diagnosis

I. History and physical examination
   A. In hypothyroid dogs, signs suggestive of but not necessarily due to impaired cardiac function develop (i.e., fatigue and exercise intolerance).

B. Pulse rate may be slowed. Apex beat and femoral pulse may be weakened.
C. Onset of signs is very gradual.
D. Noncardiovascular signs are often profound and include alopecia, hyperpigmentation, follicular hyperkeratosis, and dry hair coat.

II. Electrocardiography
A. Low-voltage QRS–T complexes may be seen. The T waves may be inverted.
B. Atrial fibrillation in giant-breed dogs occasionally accompanies hypothyroidism. Supplementation of thyroid hormone does not cause conversion to sinus rhythm.

III. Clinical pathology
A. Measurement of plasma T4 concentration is the most useful screening procedure.
B. Measurement of plasma T4 to thyroid-stimulating hormone (TSH) stimulation is suggested for diagnostic confirmation or when T4 is reduced by nonthyroidal factors.

Therapy

I. Canine hypothyroidism is treated by once-daily oral administration of L-thyroxine dosed at 20 μg/kg.

II. In treating hypothyroid dogs with underlying organic heart disease, a slow L-thyroxine replacement program over a 3- to 4-week period is initiated. The animal's response to cardiac glycosides may be altered in hypothyroid states.

Prognosis

There are few complications in the treatment of hypothyroidism.

HYPERADRENOCORTICISM (CUSHING'S SYNDROME)

Introduction

I. General features
A. Causes of canine Cushing's syndrome include adrenocortical hyperplasia from excess pituitary adrenocorticotropic hormone

(ACTH) or excess ACTH from ectopic nonendocrine tumors, adrenocortical adenoma or carcinoma, and iatrogenic response to excessive glucocorticoid administration.

B. Pituitary-dependent hyperadrenocorticism is a disease of middle-aged and older dogs (usually older than 6 years of age), with no sex predilection.

C. Dogs with functional adrenocortical tumors tend to be older. Females have been reported to be affected more frequently.

II. Pathophysiology

A. Excess cortisol leads to protein wasting, increased gluconeogenesis, increased hematopoiesis, increased enzyme activity, increased renal free-water clearance, and sodium retention (due to the weak mineralocorticoid activity of cortisol).

B. Systemic hypertension occurs in more than 85 percent of humans who have Cushing's syndrome. The presence of hypertension in canines with hyperadrenocorticism has been reported but its true incidence is unknown.

C. Morphologic changes reflect end-organ injury resulting from systemic hypertension (i.e., cardiac hypertrophy or changes secondary to heart failure).

D. Many affected dogs have coexisting atrioventricular valvular insufficiency with associated cardiac changes and, occasionally, heart failure.

E. Altered ventilatory mechanics are often present due to weakness of muscles of respiration, increased thoracic fat deposition (decreasing chest wall compliance), and increased diaphragmatic abdominal pressure from adipose tissue and hepatomegaly. Mild respiratory distress or rapid respiratory rate at rest often results. Also, many dogs have collapsing tracheas or chronic obstructive pulmonary disease, which further exacerbates respiratory distress with excitement.

F. The triad of mitral/tricuspid insufficiency, respiratory disease, and Cushing's syndrome may create intractable dyspnea due to cardiopulmonary failure.

Diagnosis

I. History and physical examination

A. The major clinical features are systemic manifestations of hypercorticism and include polydipsia, polyuria, polyphagia, abdominal enlargement, muscle weakness and lethargy, alopecia, skin atrophy, and obesity.

B. The predominant cardiovascular abnormality is left ventricular hypertrophy. The pathophysiology is unclear, since many of these animals have mitral regurgitation. Note that the incidence of hypertension in canine Cushing's syndrome has not been extensively investigated, although systolic and diastolic blood pressure elevations have been recorded in some dogs.

II. Laboratory findings

A. Excessive production of cortisol may result in neutrophilia, monocytosis, elevated fasting plasma glucose, elevated serum alkaline phosphatase, elevated plasma cholesterol, and lipemia.

B. No particular characteristic changes are consistently observed in thoracic radiographs or electrocardiograms. Cardiomegaly with ECG evidence of left ventricular hypertrophy may be present in dogs with mitral valvular insufficiency.

C. Clinical diagnosis is facilitated by the ACTH stimulation test combined with the dexamethasone suppression test.

Therapy

A. Pituitary-dependent hyperadrenocorticism is most easily treated with chemotherapy using Lysodren (o,p′-DDD).

B. Functional adrenocortical tumor. Surgical removal of the affected adrenal gland is recommended.

C. Management of heart failure, if present is undertaken through standard therapeutic protocols.

Prognosis

A. Excellent prognosis is confirmed with resectable, benign adrenal tumors.

B. Chemotherapy with o,p′-DDD for pituitary dependent hyperadrenocorticism has potential side effects, but most treated dogs respond well to therapy.

Adrenocortical Insufficiency (Addison's Disease)

Introduction

I. General features
  A. Idiopathic adrenocortical atrophy is the most common form of primary adrenal insufficiency, thought to be due to humoral and/or cell-mediated autoimmune adrenocortical destruction.
  B. Secondary adrenal insufficiency may occur following acute withdrawal of long-term, high-dose glucocorticoid therapy owing to suppression of the hypothalmic–pituitary–adrenal axis.
  C. Hypoadrenocorticism can be produced iatrogenically with the adrenocorticolytic drug, o,p′-DDD.
  D. Canine Addison's disease is most common in young to middle-aged female dogs (aged 2 to 5 years) but may occur from 6 months to 15 years of age.

II. Pathophysiology
  A. Adrenocortical destruction is generally a chronic process. Clinical manifestations are due to deficiencies of both cortisol and aldosterone.
    1. Initially, "relative" adrenocortical insufficiency causes an inability to respond to stressful situations (e.g., surgery, trauma, infections), although basal hormonal secretion is adequate.
    2. Progressive adrenal destruction causes inadequate basal hormone production and metabolic crisis ensues.
    3. Adrenocortical insufficiency causes hyposensitivity to pressor amines with failure of appropriate vasoconstriction.
  B. Arterial hypotension is the most common cardiovascular finding in adrenocortical insufficiency.
  C. Cortisol insufficiency results in increased pituitary ACTH secretion, increased insulin sensitivity, systemic arterial hypotension, decreased hematopoiesis, and decreased muscle activity.
  D. Aldosterone insufficiency causes renal sodium wasting, potassium retention, hypovolemia, and worsening of hypotension.
  E. Hypovolemia contributes to decreased heart size and hypotension.

Diagnosis

I. History and physical examination
  A. Presenting clinical features include a history of waxing, waning illness with depression, weakness, anorexia, vomiting, or diarrhea. Hemorrhagic vomiting and diarrhea may be the prominent signs in some dogs with anemia secondary to blood loss.
  B. Other signs include weight loss, polyuria, polydipsia, and shivering.
  C. Transient improvement after intravenous fluid therapy or corticosteroid administration with subsequent relapse days or weeks later can occur.
  D. Bradycardia, weak femoral pulses, dehydration, and occasionally hypothermia occur less frequently.
  E. Acute adrenal crisis presents as hypovolemic shock with alteration of consciousness, hyponatremia, and hyperkalemia.

II. Radiography
  A. Heart size may be normal or significantly reduced in dogs presenting with adrenal crisis.
  B. Decreased pulmonary perfusion is usually evident in hypovolemic states.

III. Electrocardiography
  A. The ECG is abnormal in most dogs with significant adrenocorticoid insufficiency, although changes are nonspecific (e.g., bradycardia, ST segment and T-wave alterations, P-R and Q-T interval prolongation).
  B. ECG changes with experimentally induced hyperkalemia have been recorded:
    1. Peaking of the T wave with a narrow base is the earliest ECG abnormality and may be observed when serum K^+ exceeds 5.7 to 6.0 mEq/liter.
    2. P-wave morphology is altered, its amplitude reduced, intra-atrial conduction delayed, and P-R interval prolonged when serum K^+ exceeds 7.0 mEq/liter.
    3. P waves become unrecognizable at plasma K^+ levels > 8.5 mEq/liter.
    4. The QRS widens uniformly at plasma K^+ levels > 9 mEq/liter.

5. Sinoatrial exit block or junctional rhythms with and without escape complexes may be present.
6. Ventricular fibrillation and ventricular asystole may occur at plasma K^+ levels of >10 mEq/liter.

C. Correlation between serum K^+ levels and ECG changes during addisonian crisis may not be as reliable as in experimentally induced hyperkalemia.
1. Other acid–base and electrolyte abnormalities (metabolic acidosis, hyponatremia, hypochloremia) occur in states of clinical addisonian crisis.
2. These abnormalities may influence the ECG features of hyperkalemia.

IV. Clinical pathology
A. Mild to severe anemia (normocytic, normochromic) with minimal reticulocyte response may be present with eosinophilia and lymphocytosis.
B. Prerenal azotemia is common.
C. Metabolic acidosis is often present.
D. Classic electrolyte abnormalities include hyperkalemia, hyponatremia, and hypochloremia. Normal concentrations of sodium, chloride, and potassium do not exclude a diagnosis of hypoadrenocorticism early in the disease or after recent parenteral fluid therapy.
E. Hypercalcemia develops in approximately 25 percent of affected dogs.
F. It is unusual for dogs with untreated Addison's disease to have urine specific gravities of >1.030.
G. Determination of plasma cortisol levels before and after ACTH injection is the best test for diagnosis and confirmation of adrenal insufficiency. Low to normal baseline cortisol with no increase after ACTH stimulation is diagnostic of hypoadrenocorticism.

Therapy

I. Acute crisis
A. Rapid intravenous administration of 0.9 percent normal saline (20 to 80 ml/kg of body weight per hour) for 1 to 2 hours, followed by isotonic saline thereafter (60 ml/kg-day) is initiated.

B. Intravenous administration of a soluble glucocorticoid (i.e., dexamethasone, 5 to 10 mg, or prednisolone, 50 to 200 mg) is initiated.

C. Mineralocorticoid replacement with desoxycorticosterone acetate (DOCA) should be given intramuscularly (1 to 5 mg, proportional to the size of the dog).

D. If life-threatening hyperkalemia is present, intravenous regular crystalline insulin (0.5 unit/kg of body weight) with 2 gm dextrose/unit insulin can be given. Frequent ECG monitoring is advised.

II. Maintenance therapy

A. Intravenous saline administration may be discontinued once oral alimentation is possible.

B. Parenteral glucocorticoid therapy can be changed to oral maintenance prednisone (0.2 to 0.4 mg/kg-day) or cortisone (1 to 2 mg/kg-day) by the third or fourth day.

C. Oral replacement therapy with 9-fluorohydrocortisone acetate or subcutaneous implantation of desoxycorticosterone acetate pellets can be instituted after discontinuing daily intramuscular DOCA injections.

Prognosis

I. Excellent prognosis with therapy is possible for normal life with few if any restrictions.

II. Many dogs appear to do better with a small daily maintenance dose of prednisone or cortisone. During illness or other stressful periods, however, larger doses of glucocorticoids are necessary to avoid relapse into acute adrenal crisis.

Pheochromocytoma

Introduction

I. General features

A. These tumors of adrenal medullary origin are uncommonly detected in dogs.

B. Pheochromocytomas are catecholamine-producing tumors derived from chromaffin cells.
C. In addition to important effects on the cardiovascular system, catecholamines have significant metabolic effects, stimulating glycogenolysis and gluconeogenesis.

II. Pathophysiology
A. Myocardial injury may result from catecholamine excess (i.e., myonecrosis with subsequent fibrosis and interstitial inflammation).
B. Major hemodynamic effects include fixed or paroxysmal hypertension due to excessive catecholamine secretion. Blood pressure and pulses of affected dogs may be variable, depending on the predominant catecholamine secreted and its pattern of release.
C. Cardiac arrhythmias are common.

Diagnosis

I. History and physical examination
A. Hypertension is difficult to assess clinically; its characterization has not been thoroughly investigated in dogs.
B. Arrhythmias may be the most commonly detected clinical abnormality, especially those of ventricular origin.

II. Radiography
Cardiomegaly may be present.

III. Electrocardiography
A. Nonspecific ST-segment and T-wave changes may be noted.
B. Arrhythmias, especially ventricular premature complexes or paroxysmal ventricular tachycardia, can occur.

IV. Clinical pathology
A. Diagnosis of pheochromocytoma is difficult.
B. Demonstration of elevated 24-hour urinary excretion of vanillylmandelic acid, total metanephrines, fractionated catecholamines, and plasma catecholamines is diagnostic in humans.
C. Abdominal ultrasound may constitute a localizing procedure.
D. Angiography can be used in some situations to evaluate adrenal masses invading the caudal vena cava.

Therapy

I. Adrenergic α- and β-blocking drugs may help control arrhythmias and hypertension.
II. Surgical tumor removal is the only definitive treatment.

Prognosis

Dogs with inoperable lesions have a poor prognosis. Long-term α- and β-adrenergic blockers may be used in these instances.

HYPOGLYCEMIA

Introduction

I. General features
   A. Hypoglycemia may be caused by hyperinsulinism due to a functional β-cell pancreatic carcinoma or from endogenously administered insulin for treatment of diabetes mellitus.
   B. Other clinical entities associated with hypoglycemia include nonpancreatic tumors, glycogen storage diseases, juvenile hypoglycemia, neonatal hypoglycemia, septic shock, and hepatic disease.
II. Pathophysiology
   Irrespective of the etiology, hypoglycemia triggers catecholamine release, which causes tachycardia, increases in myocardial oxygen demand, and potentially arrhythmias.

Diagnosis

I. History and physical examination
   Clinical manifestations of hypoglycemia range from lethargy to episodic weakness and seizures.
II. Laboratory findings
   A. Acute, severe hypoglycemia may cause ST depression, T-wave flattening, QT prolongation, and arrhythmias.

B. A low blood glucose (<60 mg/dl) is usually present; elevated immunoreactive insulin (IRI) levels or IRI/glucose ratio abnormalities may be demonstrated with insulinomas.

Therapy

I. Hypoglycemic crisis, regardless of cause, is managed by slow, intravenous administration of 50 percent dextrose to effect.
  A. Resolution of neurologic signs due to hypoglycemia is usually abrupt and virtually complete.
  B. Prolonged, untreated hypoglycemia may result in cerebrocortical hypoxic damage.
  C. Lack of symptom amelioration after therapy may indicate cerebral hypoxia and edema.
  D. ECG changes usually return to normal.
II. Regulation of the decompensated diabetic, reeducation of the client regarding insulin administration, or treatment of the underlying β-cell carcinoma is required to prevent future hypoglycemia episodes.

THE HEART AND METABOLIC DISORDERS

Disorders Associated with Hypercalcemia

Introduction

I. General features
  A. Hypercalcemia occurs when serum calcium concentration consistently exceeds 12 mg/dl in mature dogs and 11 mg/dl in cats. Young, actively growing dogs may normally have calcium values of >12.0 mg/dl.
  B. Many different disorders may cause hypercalcemia. Increased

calcium bone reabsorption, increased gastrointestinal calcium absorption, increased serum protein binding of calcium, increased calcium binding to anions, and decreased renal and intestinal calcium removal from serum comprise possible pathogenic mechanisms of hypercalcemia.

C. The following conditions are associated with hypercalcemia (in decreasing order of occurrence):
   1. Young growing puppy (normal)
   2. Paraneoplastic syndromes (lymphosarcoma, anal sac apocrine gland adenocarcinoma, other nonbony-involving neoplasia, primary and metastatic bony tumors)
   3. Hypoadrenocorticism
   4. Primary renal failure
   5. Septic osteomyelitis
   6. Hypervitaminosis D
   7. Hemoconcentration (hyperproteinemia)
   8. Primary hyperparathyroidism
   9. Disuse osteoporosis
   10. Severe hypothermia
   11. Laboratory error

II. Pathophysiology
   A. Cardiovascular effects of experimentally induced acute hypercalcemia raises systolic and diastolic blood pressure, especially with renal failure.
   B. Clinically, elevated calcium levels have little if any direct adverse effect on cardiac function. In hypercalcemic crisis (>16 mg/dl serum calcium), cardiac arrhythmias or arrest may occur.
   C. Animals with hypercalcemia may be more predisposed to complications of digitalis intoxication.
   D. Long-standing hypercalcemia may predispose to calcification of myocardium, blood vessels, and other soft tissues. These deposits are of little clinical significance.

Diagnosis

I. History and physical examination

Regardless of its cause, hypercalcemia affects the kidney (renal dysfunction, polyuria, polydipsia, nocturia, nephrocalcinosis, renal failure, uremia), gastrointestinal system (anorexia, constipation, and vomiting from decreased gastrointestinal smooth muscle excitability), and nervous system (generalized skeletal muscle weakness from decreased neuromuscular activity).

II. Radiography
  A. Thoracic radiographs may indicate mediastinal mass(es), metastasis, abnormal bony densities or osteolysis.
  B. Abdominal radiographs may show organomegaly, abnormal bone density, sublumbar masses, or sublumbar lymphadenopathy.
  C. Osteopenia, metastatic calcification, or focal bony lesions may be present.

III. Electrocardiography
  A. The characteristic ECG finding is a short QT interval. In extreme cases, the ST segment may fuse with the upstroke of the T wave.
  B. Hypercalcemia may predispose to arrhythmias of digitalis intoxication.
  C. ECG changes resolve after correction of the serum calcium.

IV. Clinical pathology
  A. Hypercalcemia often causes diminished urinary concentrating ability, and the urine is usually hyposthenuric (1.002 to 1.008 specific gravity) or isosthenuric (1.008 to 1.012 specific gravity).
  B. Early in the course, normal renal function is maintained, but primary renal failure (increased BUN and serum creatinine) may develop from progressive structural and functional alterations in the kidney.
  C. Hypophosphatemia or hyperphosphatemia may be recorded depending on the presence or absence of renal failure and the underlying etiology of hypercalcemia.
  D. Serum alkaline phosphatase may be elevated if severe bone disease or concomitant hepatic disease is present.
  E. A hemogram may be normal, display hemoconcentration or anemia, or occasionally show evidence for leukemia (when this disease is associated with the underlying etiology).
  F. Bone marrow evaluation may be unremarkable or disclose evidence of lymphosarcoma, leukemia, or multiple myeloma.
  G. Skeletal survey radiographs may exhibit isolated bony lesions that could account for hypercalcemia.

Therapy

I. Initial treatment is directed at reducing the systemic effects of hypercalcemia.
  A. Preexisting dehydration should be corrected and hydration maintained.
  B. Administration of 0.9 percent NaCl should be used to enhance renal excretion of calcium.
  C. Diuretic therapy (furosemide, 5 mg/kg initially and 5 mg/kg-hr thereafter) may also help in lowering serum calcium.
  D. Glucocorticosteroids may limit bone resorption, decrease intestinal calcium absorption, increase renal calcium excretion, and be cytolytic in certain neoplasms.

II. Definitive treatment is directed at the underlying etiology.

Prognosis

I. Prognosis depends on early detection, ability to establish a definitive diagnosis, and success of treatment. The prognosis of many causes of hypercalcemia is guarded to poor.

Disorders Associated with Hypocalcemia

Introduction

I. General features
  A. Hypocalcemia, although infrequently encountered, can cause profound clinical signs. It occurs when serum calcium concentration is <7 mg/dl in the dog and <6 mg/dl in the cat.
  B. The following conditions may be associated with hypocalcemia:
    1. Canine chronic polyuric renal failure
    2. Feline chronic polyuric renal failure
    3. Eclampsia (puerperal tetany)
    4. Canine acute pancreatitis
    5. Hypoparathyroidism
      a) Idiopathic
      b) Postoperative (during bilateral thyroid surgery)

6. Pseudohypoparathyroidism
7. Hyperphosphatemia
8. Hypocalcemia due to hypoalbuminemia where calcium values are not adjusted for serum protein concentration.

II. Pathophysiology
 A. Hypocalcemia causes an excitatory effect on nerve and muscle cells. Neuromuscular irritability, tetany, and seizures may result. Handling or stress may precipitate tetany.
 B. The major cardiovascular manifestation involves ECG abnormalities.
 C. Animals with coexisting congestive heart failure may experience decreased cardiac function that improves with restoration of calcium levels (due to the augmenting effects of calcium on myocardial contractility).
 D. Acutely induced hypocalcemia (i.e., treatment with chelating agents) can potentially cause sharp reductions in blood pressure and shock.

Diagnosis

I. Physical examination
 A. Tetany, seizures, anorexia, vomiting, and abdominal discomfort are the predominant signs in affected animals.
 B. Cataracts can develop.

II. Laboratory findings: Clinical pathology will reflect abnormalities associated with the underlying disease process. Hypocalcemia is usually diagnosed when low serum calcium levels are detected during clinical investigation of tetany, seizures, renal failure, pancreatitis, or other disorders by analysis of a serum biochemical profile.

III. Electrocardiography: The typical ECG manifestation of hypocalcemia consists of QT prolongation.

Therapy

I. Severe hypocalcemia (<6 mg/dl) is a life-threatening emergency.
 A. Ten percent calcium gluconate is administered intravenously (0.5 to 1.5 mg/kg body weight) slowly over a 15- to 30-minute interval.

B. Electrocardiographic monitoring should accompany administration:
   1. Calcium infusion should be temporarily interrupted if ST-segment elevation or bradycardia occur—to be reinstated at a slower rate when these changes have abated.
   2. Gradual QT interval shortening from its prolonged state may accompany calcium infusion.
   3. Calcium is cardiotoxic if replaced too quickly; even a normal concentration of serum calcium may be toxic if replenished to that level too rapidly.

C. Subsequent intravenous calcium administration may be repeated every 6 to 12 hours, or as needed.

II. Clinical signs of hypocalcemia may abate slowly despite calcium infusion. Resolution of clinical signs may not provide a reliable guide as an end point of adequate calcium administration. Some hypocalcemic signs may persist (i.e., weakness, anorexia) when cardiotoxic effects of calcium infusion occur.

III. Hypocalcemia may not respond to treatment when low-serum magnesium is present and uncorrected.

IV. Vitamin D therapy may be required in some disorders to maintain eventual control of hypocalcemia. In treatment of postoperative parathyroid insufficiency, care must be taken to detect recovery of parathyroid function in order to avoid vitamin D-associated hypercalcemia.

Prognosis

For most causes of hypocalcemia that are carefully managed, the prognosis is good to excellent.

Disorders Associated with Hyperkalemia

Introduction

I. General features

A. Ninety-five percent or more of body potassium is intracellular with only 2 to 5 percent extracellular. Therefore, serum potassium values are not always reliable indicators of total body potassium stores.

B. Clinical causes of hyperkalemia include the following:
   1. Increased administration
      a) High doses of intravenous potassium Pennicillin-G
      b) Excessively rapid intravenous administration of potassium or potassium supplemented fluids
   2. Decreased renal elimination (renal failure, i.e., acute oliguric renal failure or end-stage oliguric chronic renal failure)
   3. Hypoadrenocorticism (Addison's disease)
   4. Ruptured urinary bladder, ureter, or kidney
   5. Potassium-sparing diuretics (i.e., spironolactone)
   6. Intracellular to extracellular transfer
      a. Metabolic acidosis
      b. Rapid release from tissue during severe injury

Diagnosis, Therapy, and Prognosis

Identification and treatment of the underlying cause of hyperkalemia are essential. See section on hypoadrenocorticism (Addison's disease).

Disorders Associated with Hypokalemia

Introduction

I. General features

A. When potassium loss has been severe and the animal is symptomatic for hypokalemia, severe muscle weakness or paralysis may develop.

B. Clinical causes of hypokalemia include the following:
   1. Decreased intake: Anorexia, especially when combined with potassium deficient fluid administration
   2. Excessive gastrointestinal loss
      a) Chronic vomiting

b) Severe diarrhea
c) Overuse of enemas, laxatives, or exchange resins
3. Excessive urinary loss
a) Renal (renal tubular acidosis, postobstructive diuresis, chronic pyelonephritis)
b) Drugs (diuretics, amphotericin B)
c) Secondary hyperaldosteronism (liver failure, congestive heart failure, nephrotic syndrome)
4. Extracellular to intracellular transfer
a) Metabolic alkalosis
b) Insulin and glucose administration
c) Hyperinsulinism (insulinoma)
d) Ketoacidotic diabetes mellitus

II. Pathophysiology
A. Severe hypokalemia causes hyperpolarization of nerve and muscle fiber membranes.
B. Electrocardiographic changes are manifested in delayed and abnormal repolarization.

III. Clinical signs
A. Muscle weakness may be mild or manifest as profound weakness and depression.

Diagnosis

I. History and physical examination
Clinical pathology may be reflective of the underlying disease process contributing to hypokalemia.

II. Electrocardiography
A. Earliest changes consist of a U-wave being taller than the T-wave.
B. As serum potassium falls, the ST segment becomes more depressed and there is a gradual blending of T-waves with what appears to be a tall U-wave.

Therapy

I. Correction of the primary disease process should be accomplished.
II. Parenteral potassium replacement may be given subcutaneously or intravenously.

TABLE 11-2. GUIDELINES FOR POTASSIUM SUPPLEMENTATION

Serum Potassium (mEq/liter)	mEq KCl to Add to 250 ml Fluid	Maximum Fluid Rate (ml/kg-hr)
2.0	20	6
2.1–2.5	15	8
2.6–3.0	10	12
3.1–3.5	7	16

III. Prolonged oral maintenance therapy is rarely indicated.
IV. Intravenous replacement is recommended when potassium loss is severe and the animal is symptomatic for hypokalemia. Guidelines for supplementation are given in Table 11-2.
V. Return to alimentation and treatment of the primary disease responsible for hypokalemia will replace potassium deficits.
VI. Hypokalemia markedly increases the likelihood of toxicity when digitalis is being administered. Serum potassium should be promptly checked and corrected when digitalis toxicity is suspected.

Prognosis

The prognosis is good if the underlying condition can be corrected or managed.

Uremia

Introduction

I. General features
   Cardiovascular manifestations can include ventricular and supraventricular arrhythmias.
II. Pathophysiology
   A. Hypertensive cardiovascular disease, electrolyte imbalance, fluid overload, and anemia can contribute to the production of disturbances.
   B. Oliguric or anuric animals may have potassium retention with associated changes registered on the ECG.

C. Hypertension is a sequela of experimentally produced renal ischemia in dogs and may occur in clinical situations.

Diagnosis

I. Nonspecific signs may accompany uremia, including depression, anorexia, lethargy, and weight loss.
II. Varying degrees of anorexia, vomiting, and diarrhea may occur.
III. Clinical pathology may reveal abnormalities in the hemogram, urinalysis, and biochemistry profile consistent with uremia.
IV. Electrocardiography
   A. Nonspecific ECG abnormalities may be attributed to hypertension, anemia, electrolyte abnormalities, and pericarditis.
   B. Conduction defects or arrhythmias may occur.

Therapy

Treatment is directed at managing uremia and its underlying causes.

Prognosis

Resolution of the uremic state may improve ECG abnormalities, although arrhythmias may persist.

HEMATOLOGIC DISORDERS AND THE HEART

Anemia

Introduction

I. General features
   A. Anemia is a sign of a disease, not a disease entity.
   B. Evaluation should emphasize history (drug or toxin exposure),

clinical signs related to other disorders complicated by anemia (fever, lethargy, bleeding, weight loss), physical examination (petechiae, lymphadenopathy), and clinical pathology.

C. Symptoms of reduced cardiac reserve associated with anemia depend on the severity of anemia and on the presence and extent of underlying cardiac disease.

II. Pathophysiology

A. The combination of tissue hypoxia and reduced blood viscosity leads to decreased systemic vascular resistance and is associated with increased cardiac ouput.

B. When anemia is associated with increased viscosity (multiple myeloma or macroglobulinemia) cardiac output may fail to rise.

C. Lowered blood viscosity, although important, is not the sole cause of increased cardiac output. The precise mechanism of increased cardiac output in chronic anemia is not clear.

D. Physiologic consequences depend on the developmental rate of anemia.

1. With acute blood loss (i.e., hemorrrhage), hypovolemic shock may predominate.
   a) In normal dogs, left ventricular function can become depressed when the hematocrit is reduced below 24 percent in acute anemia.
   b) When heart failure occurs it usually suggests the presence of underlying heart disease that had been compensated until the burden of augmented cardiac output was added.
2. With chronic anemia where blood volume is maintained, cardiac output may rise due to tachycardia with little change in stroke volume.
3. In severe, chronic anemia, heart rate may be normal or only minimally elevated, and cardiac output is increased principally due to augmented stroke volume. This augmented stroke volume is associated with cardiac dilation and hypertrophy.
4. Chronic anemia is usually well tolerated because of compensatory mechanisms which include increased cardiac output, redistribution of blood flow and decreased oxygen affinity of red blood cells. As in thyrotoxicosis, most animals in which congestive heart failure with anemia develops have underlying heart disease aggravated by increased cardiac work caused by anemia.

Diagnosis

I. History and physical examination
  A. Chronic anemia produces few symptoms, which may include fatigue and mild exertional dyspnea.
  B. The precordium may be hyperactive, with arterial pulses bounding or pistol shot, mucous membrane color pale (or icteric), and capillary refill time prolonged.
  C. A medium-pitched, mid-systolic murmur at the left apex, generally grade 1/6 to 3/6, is common with severe anemia.
  D. Heart sounds may be accentuated.

II. Radiology
Thoracic radiographs may display mild cardiac enlargement, but this will vary depending on the presence and extent of previously existing heart disease.

III. Electrocardiography
The electrocardiogram usually does not show specific changes.

IV. Clinical pathology
Abnormalities occur in red cell morphology and may be referable to the severity of anemia and its underlying causes.

Therapy

I. Treatment of anemia depends on the underlying cause.

II. In animals with anemia associated with congestive heart failure, correction of the anemia may be necessary before optimal response of the heart failure to pharmacotherapy can occur. Rapid infusion of whole blood to a severely anemic animal with severe underlying cardiac disease may precipitate heart failure.

Prognosis

Successful management of anemia and underlying causes confer a good prognosis.

NEOPLASTIC AND INFILTRATIVE HEART DISEASES

Introduction

I. General features
  A. Tumors of the heart are uncommon and present in clinically obscure ways.
  B. Primary tumors of the heart and pericardium are uncommon.
    1. Hemangiosarcoma may originate in the right auricle, right atrium, especially in German Shepherd dogs.
  C. Metastatic tumors invade the heart, pericardium or both.
    1. Cardiac metastasis may occur with most types of primary tumors.
    2. Hemangiosarcoma frequently metastasizes to the heart.
    3. Lymphosarcoma is the most common tumor that metastasizes to the heart in cats.
  D. Infiltrative myocardial disease involving nonneoplastic cells is rare in the dog and uncommon in the cat.

II. Pathophysiology
  A. Tumors from other tissues gain direct access to the heart by invasive growth from adjacent structures or spread by hematogenous or lymphatic vessels.
  B. The relative infrequency of cardiac metastasis has been attributed to metabolic peculiarities of striated muscle, rapid coronary blood flow, efferent lymphatic drainage from the heart and the vigorous kneading action of the myocardium.

Diagnosis

I. History and physical examination
  A. Secondary cardiac involvement may not display clinical manifestations.
  B. More commonly, involvement of the heart involves clinical signs which depend on the site and extent of metastasis.

C. Pericardial involvement may cause pericardial effusion.
   1. Pericardial effusion may be detected by auscultating muffled heart sounds, ECG evidence of depressed QRS voltages, electrical alternans, echocardiographic detection, progressive radiographic cardiac enlargement or clinical signs of pericardial tamponade.
   2. Pericardiocentesis may detect cytologic evidence of neoplasia.

II. Radiography
   A. Radiographic evidence of progressive cardiac enlargement may be observed.
   B. Pneumopericardiography or angiocardiography may assess thickness and irregularities of the pericardium, epicardium and endocardium.

III. Electrocardiography
   A. Reduced QRS voltage on the ECG, electrical alternans and pericardial tamponade may be recorded.
   B. Atrial or ventricular arrhythmias, conduction disturbances, and complete heart block can occur.
   C. Arrhythmias, conduction abnormalities, or complete heart block may be present without accompanying heart failure and are often refractory to antiarrhythmic drug therapy.
   D. Infiltrative myocardial neoplasia may cause congestive heart failure due to diastolic dysfunction or arrhythmias.

IV. Echocardiography
   A. Echocardiographic evidence of pericardial effusion may be demonstrated.
   B. Two-dimensional echocardiography may facilitate identification of intracavitary and pericardial masses.

Therapy

I. Pericardiocentesis may offer temporary relief from cardiac tamponade.

II. Animals with myocardial infiltration of tumors sensitive to chemotherapy or radiotherapy may respond favorably.

III. Congestive heart failure may respond to appropriate pharmacotherapy.

Prognosis

In most cases, antemortem diagnosis is not appreciated, etiology cannot be defined or therapy is not effective.

PHYSICAL AND CHEMICAL AGENTS AFFECTING THE CARDIOVASCULAR SYSTEM

Many noninfectious stimuli may cause myocardial injury. Damage may be acute and transient or chronic and lead to permanent myocardial change. Effects are usually related to the severity, dose, and rate of exposure.

Hyperpyrexia (Heat Stroke)

Introduction

I. General features
   A. Hyperpyrexia is usually associated with heart stroke when rectal temperature rises to 41° to 44°C (106° to 111°F).
   B. High ambient temperature is usually present in an animal confined in an enclosed environment with poor ventilation.
   C. High humidity reduces evaporation of water from oral and nasal cavities and reduces the ability of small animals to regulate their temperatures.
   D. Lack of available water as well as obesity, puppyhood, old age, and brachiocephalic conformation are contributing factors to heat stroke.
   E. Malignant hyperthermia is a rare but potentially fatal abnormal response to anesthetic agents, characterized by an acute, rapid rise in body temperature and severe biochemical changes accompanied by muscle rigidity.

II. Pathophysiology
   A. With heat stroke, panting is the initial compensatory mechanism in response to increased ambient temperature.

B. Potentially significant alterations can follow hyperpyrexia:
   1. Respiratory alkalosis may result.
   2. Mild hyperkalemia and hypophosphatemia may occur.
   3. Hemoconcentration may occur.
   4. Disseminated intravascular coagulation may result.
   5. Cerebral edema is a common complication.
   6. Subendocardial and subepicardial hemorrhage is common.
   7. Right heart dilation may occur.
   8. Mechanisms suggested for myocardial injury include direct thermal effects, circulatory collapse with secondary myocardial hypoxia, decreased coronary blood flow and secondary metabolic injury.

Diagnosis

I. History and physical examination
   A. Depending on the duration and severity of the heat stroke, clinical signs may include panting, sinus tachycardia, bright red oral mucous membranes, and hyperthermia.
   B. Extremities become hot to the touch.
   C. Red mucous membranes may turn pale because of diminished circulation or vasoconstriction.
   D. Watery diarrhea may occur, which can progress to bloody diarrhea.
   E. Stupor and coma with respiratory arrest can follow.
   F. With malignant hyperthermia, an acute, profound temperature elevation may be the first noticable sign to the surgeon.
      1. If the heart rate is monitored, tachycardia may be the earliest indication.
      2. Skeletal muscle hypertonus may occur.
   G. ST-segment and T-wave abnormalities may be seen on the ECG; atrial or ventricular arrhythmias are usually absent.
   H. Clinical pathologic alterations relate to the stage and severity of the hyperpyrexia.

Therapy

I. Lowering the body temperature is the first objective of therapy.
   A. Cold water enemas, submergence in cold water, or wetting the extremities with rubbing alcohol are useful techniques.

B. Rectal temperature should be recorded every 5 to 10 minutes and cooling ceased when the rectal temperature reaches 39.5°C (103°F) to prevent hypothermia.

II. When malignant hyperthermia is anesthetic related, all inhalation agents and relaxants should be discontinued, and help should be immediately summoned. Hyperventilation with 100 percent oxygen should be started and an intravenous line inserted.

III. Prevention of cerebral edema should be treated by administering steroids (dexamethasone, 2 mg/kg IV) and later, mannitol (2.0 g/kg of a 20 percent solution over 10 to 15 minutes) if stupor or coma develops.

IV. Balanced intravenous fluids are administered to prevent or treat shock and maintain adequate circulation.

V. Blood gas analysis should be performed if available.

VI. If bleeding tendencies are noted, DIC should be assumed to be present and therapy for DIC initiated.

Prognosis

I. Prognosis for heat stroke is guarded to good if detected and treated early.

II. Malignant hyperthermia is rare but seems to offer a worse prognosis.

III. Coagulopathy and renal failure may be expected after correction of hyperthermia and confers a worse prognosis.

Hypothermia

Introduction

I. General features

A. Lowering of body temperature may occur accidently, due to deep cooling from external cold, drugs, or interference with thermoregulatory centers during anesthesia.

B. Physiologic lesions of hypothermia depend on the extent and duration of exposure.

II. Pathophysiology

A. Cardiac dilation with epicardial and subendocardial hemorrhage can result from severe hypothermia.

B. Microinfarcts can occur in myocardial tissue.
C. Lesions may result from circulatory collapse, hemoconcentration, capillary sludging, or decreased cellular metabolism.

Therapy

I. Treatment initially involves rewarming the patient.
   A. External warming produces temperature changes initially in the body surface or shell.
   B. Vasodilation of skin vessels may initially transfer cooled blood to the body core, further decreasing internal temperature. However, this is rarely a significant clinical complication.
   C. Internal (core) rewarming can be accomplished by peritoneal dialysis.
II. Appropriate supportive care (e.g., intravenous fluids, ventilation) must be administered.
III. Cardiac output and ECG abnormalities improve after warming.
IV. Evaluation of the patient for underlying systemic disorders which could have predisposed the animal to hypothermia should be made once normothermia has been achieved.

Arsenic Toxicity

Introduction

I. General features
   Used in pesticides, arsenic is toxic to the gastrointestinal system, central nervous system, kidneys, and hematopoietic sytems.
II. Pathophysiology
   A. Myocardial involvement may occur with acute and chronic exposure.
   B. Arsenic interferes with sulfhydryl enzyme systems and can cause myocardial hypoxia.
   C. Subepicardial and subpericardial hemorrhage can result in interstitial myocarditis.

Diagnosis

I. History and physical examination
  A. Onset of clinical signs varies from 30 minutes to several hours.
  B. Initial signs include restlessness, vomiting, abdominal pain, and diarrhea.
  C. Tachycardia results and the pulse becomes weak as shock develops.
II. Electrocardiography
  A. ST-segment depression, QT-interval prolongation and T-wave inversion may be recorded on the ECG.
  B. ECG changes may revert to normal after successful therapy.

Lead Poisoning

Introduction

I. General features
  Lead toxicity is very common in small animals; sources include lead-containing paint, linoleum, plumbing supplies, batteries, putty, solder, golf balls, roofing materials, lubricants, toys, rug pads, and miscellaneous objects.
II. Pathophysiology
  A. Once absorbed from the gastrointestinal system, lead is carried by the red blood cells and is deposited in major organs, eventually to be redistributed to bone.
  B. Myofibrillar swelling with interstitial fibrosis may occur.

Diagnosis

I. History and physical examination
  Prominant features usually are exhibited as gastrointestinal and central nervous system dysfunction.
II. Laboratory findings
  Nucleated erythrocytes (5 to 40 per 100 white blood cells) without

evidence of severe anemia and basophilic stippling in red blood cells are common features.

III. Electrocardiography
ECG changes can include nonspecific ST- and T-wave changes, sinus bradycardia, and occasionally arrhythmias.

IV. Radiography
Radiographic changes may include the presence of radiopaque material in the gastrointestinal tract.

Therapy

I. Enemas are used to remove lead from the gastrointestinal tract.
II. Therapy with calcium ethylenediaminetetraacetate (EDTA) is usually associated with resolution of clinical signs.
III. Supportive treatment may be required for neurologic complications.

Prognosis

Treatment is often successful.

Carbon Monoxide Poisoning

Introduction

I. General features and pathophysiology
   A. Myocardial infarction or injury may be due to hypoxia (carbon monoxide diminishes oxygen transport capacity) and to direct effects causing mitochondrial toxicity.
   B. Tissue oxyhemoglobin dissociation is decreased, and oxygen in oxyhemoglobin is replaced by carbon monoxide.
   C. Myocardial hemorrhage and necrosis may occur.

Diagnosis

I. History and physical examination
   A. Sinus tachycardia, pulmonary edema, or cardiovascular collapse may occur.
   B. ECG abnormalities may include ST-segment changes, conduction abnormalities, or arrhythmias.

Therapy

I. Administration of 100 percent oxygen is given to relieve tissue hypoxia.
II. General supportive care should be administered.

Prognosis

Clinical recovery usually occurs if the situation is detected and treated early.

Toad Poisoning

Introduction

I. General features
   Animals biting toads of the species *Bufo alvarious* or *Bufo marinus* may encounter a potent toxin that has a digitalislike action.
II. Pathophysiology
   Bufagins, a component of the toxic chemical complex secreted by the toad, has a digitalislike action.

Diagnosis

I. History and physical examination
   A. Signs develop in affected animals within minutes and may include salivation, pulmonary edema, convulsions, and ultimately death.

II. Laboratory findings
   A. Arrhythmias can occur with gradual worsening to ventricular fibrillation.
   B. Increase in packed cell volume, blood urea nitrogen, and SGOT can be recorded.

Therapy

I. Treatment involves flushing out the animal's mouth with water, atropinization to reduce salivation, barbiturate administration to control convulsions, and use of β-adrenergic blocking drugs (i.e., propranolol) for its cardioprotective effects.
II. Supportive measures should be instituted.

Prognosis

If treatment is delayed, prognosis is poor.

Oleander Toxicity

I. General features
   The common oleander (*Nerium oleander*) is a common ornamental plant and can be consumed by small animals.
II. Pathophysiology
   Toxic principles include cardiac glycosides.
III. Clinical signs
   Nausea, depression, increased pulse rate, mydriasis, bloody diarrhea, arrhythmias, and ultimately death can occur.
IV. Therapy
   There is no effective treatment. Supportive measures should be implemented.

Cyclophosphamide Cardiotoxicity

Introduction

I. General features
   Cyclophosphamide is an alkylating agent that inhibits cell division by causing irreversible crosslinkages of DNA chains.

II. Pathophysiology
   A. High doses in humans have been associated with ECG changes and congestive heart failure.
   B. The heart can become dilated with subepicardial and subendocardial ecchymoses.
   C. Myocardial injury results from direct endothelial damage and resultant fibrin microthrombi in capillaries.
   D. Myopericarditis has been reported with low-output heart failure.

Therapy

I. Congestive heart failure should be treated with appropriate therapy and cyclophosphamide should be discontinued.
II. Myelosuppression is usually a principal side effect, first detected by leukopenia.

Doxorubricin Cardiomyopathy

Introduction

I. General features
   The anthracycline drugs (adriamycin, daunorubicin) are antitumor drugs that inhibit nucleic acid synthesis.
II. Pathophysiology
   A. A dose-related incidence of dilated cardiomyopathy can be demonstrated with cumulative dosage of as little as 150 mg/m^2.
   B. Dilated cardiomyopathy and congestive heart failure are cardiotoxic sequelae of these drugs.

Diagnosis

I. History and physical examination
   A. Congestive heart failure usually develops acutely.
   B. Clinical manifestations include sinus tachycardia, tachypnea, car-

diomegaly, pulmonary edema, ascites or pleural effusion, and hepatomegaly.

II. Radiography
Generalized cardiomegaly may be coupled with radiographic signs of pulmonary edema and/or pleural effusion.

III. Electrocardiography
   A. Electrocardiographic abnormalities include ST-segment and T-wave changes, left ventricular enlargement patterns, intraventricular conduction abnormalities, and atrial and ventricular arrhythmias.
   B. ECG changes may be acute.

IV. Clinical pathology: Myelosuppression seen as leukopenia is also a significant side effect.

Therapy

I. Congestive heart failure is usually poorly responsive to therapy.
II. Anthracycline administration should be discontinued.
III. Sequential chest radiographs, ECGs and echocardiograms may be of value in detecting this complication of cardiotoxicity.

INFECTIOUS INFLAMMATORY MYOCARDIAL DISEASES

Introduction

I. General features
   A. The heart may be involved in an inflammatory process due to many infective agents.
   B. Myocardial cells, interstitium, or vessels may be affected.

II. Pathophysiology
   A. Myocardial injury may occur from direct myocardial invasion of an infectious agent, from a myocardial toxin produced by the agent or by a resultant immune-mediated reaction.
   B. Important causes of myocardial injury in small animals include the following:

1. Bacterial myocarditis
   a) Pyogenic bacteria originate in septicemic states or from other septic foci.
   b) Clinical signs range from subclinical to nonspecific (weight loss, lethargy) to specific (arrhythmias, congestive heart failure).
2. Viral myocarditis has been associated with canine parovovirus and distemper virus in dogs and with suspected but not yet identified viral pathogens in felines. Clinical abnormalities include cardiomegaly, arrhythmias, nonspecific ECG abnormalities and congestive heart failure (with canine parvovirus) to subclinical myocarditis (with canine distemper virus).
3. Fungus and algae may infect the heart secondary to a disseminated disease process, often in conjunction with reduced host defense.
4. Protozoal myocarditis may occur in dogs with canine trypanosomiasis (*Trypanosoma cruzi*) or in dogs and cats with toxoplasmosis (*Toxoplasma gondii*).
   a) Clinical abnormalities with trypanosomiasis include lethargy, depression, diarrhea, lymphadenopathy, tachyarrhythmias, congestive heart failure, or sudden death.
   b) Toxoplasmosis may produce signs dominated by the extent and severity of multiorgan system involvement.

Therapy

Treatment is often supportive and usually focused on the most prominent systemic manifestation of the disease process.

SUGGESTED READINGS

Case AA: Poisoning and injury by plants. p. 145. In Kirk RW (ed): Current Veterinary Therapy VIII. WB Saunders, Philadelphia 1983

Chew DJ, Meuten DJ: Primary hyperparathyroidism. p. 880. In Kirk RW (ed): Current Veterinary Therapy. VIII. WB Saunders, Philadelphia, 1983

Christy JH, Clements SD: The heart and endocrine disease. p. 1547. In JW Hurst (ed): The Heart. ed 5. McGraw-Hill, New York, 1982

Feldman EC: The adrenal cortex. p. 1650. In Ettinger SJ (ed): Textbook of Veterinary Internal Medicine. ed 2. WB Saunders, Philadelphia, 1983

Fisch C: Electrolytes and the heart. p. 1599. In Hurst JW (ed): The Heart. ed 5. McGraw-Hill, New York, 1982

Fox PR: Feline myocardial diseases. p. 337. In Kirk RW (ed): Current Veterinary Therapy. VIII. WB Saunders, Philadelphia, 1983

Fox PR, Tilley LP, Liu S–K: The cardiovascular system. p. 249. In Pratt PW (ed): Feline Medicine. American Veterinary Publications, Santa Barbara, Calif, 1983

Goodwin JF, Roberts WC, Wenger NK: Cardiomyopathy. p. 1299. In Hurst JW (ed): The Heart. ed 5. McGraw-Hill, New York, 1982

Grossman W, Braunwald E: High cardiac output states. p. 818. In Braunwald E (ed): Heart Disease. Vol 1. WB Saunders, Philadelphia, 1980

Lees GE: Hypoparathyroidism. p. 876. In Kirk RW (ed): Current Veterinary Therapy. VIII. WB Saunders, Philadelphia, 1983

Mandell WJ (ed): Cardiac Arrhythmias. JB Lippincott, Philadelphia, 1980

Palumbo NE, Petti S: Toad poisoning. p. 760. In Kirk RW (ed): Current Veterinary Therapy. VIII. WB Saunders, Philadelphia, 1983

Peterson ME: Hyperadrenocorticism. p. 863. In Kirk RW (ed): Current Veterinary Therapy. VIII. WB Saunders, Philadelphia, 1983

Peterson ME, Kintzer PP, Cavanagh PG, et al: Feline hyperthyroidism: Pretreatment clinical and laboratory evaluation of 131 cases. J Am Vet Med Assoc 183:103, 1983

Rosenthal DS, Braunwald E: Hematologic–oncologic disorders and heart disease. p. 1801. In Braunwald E (ed): Heart Disease. Vol. 2. WB Saunders, Philadelphia, 1980

Tilley LP, Bond BR, Patnaik AK, Liu S–K: Cardiovascular tumors in the cat. JAAHA 17:1009, 1981

Tilley LP, Liu SK, Fox RP: Myocardial disease. p. 1029. In Ettinger SJ (ed): Textbook of Veterinary Internal Medicine. ed 2. WB Saunders, Philadelphia, 1983

Wenger NK: Cardiovascular disorders in systemic diseases. p. 374. In Chung EK (ed): Quick Reference to Cardiovascular Diseases. ed. 2. JB Lippincott, Philadelphia, 1982

Williams GH, Braunwald E: Endocrine and nutritional disorders and heart disease. p. 1825. In Braunwald E (ed): Heart Disease. Vol 2. WB Saunders, Philadelphia, 1980

Wynne J, Braunwald E: The cardiomyopathies and myocardities. p. 1438. In Braunwald E (ed): Heart Disease. Vol. 2. WB Saunders, Philadelphia, 1980

Section III
TREATMENT OF CARDIAC FAILURE AND DISTURBANCES OF CARDIAC RHYTHM

12

Pathophysiology and Treatment of Heart Failure

Mark D. Kittleson

INTRODUCTION

DEFINITION

Heart failure is a clinical syndrome caused by a cardiac disease that results in systolic and/or diastolic dysfunction severe enough to produce clinical signs of edema and/or inadequate perfusion.

PATHOPHYSIOLOGY

I. Systolic function (the ability of the heart to contract and pump blood into an arterial system) is determined by myocardial contractility, preload, afterload (systolic myocardial wall stress), heart rate, and the presence or absence of leaks (shunts or regurgitant leaks) in the system.
  A. Systolic dysfunction most commonly is caused by a decrease in myocardial contractility (myocardial failure) or a regurgitant leak or left-to-right shunt. Less commonly, it can occur because of a decrease in venous return (mitral stenosis), an increase in afterload (aortic stenosis), or a decrease in heart rate (e.g., third-degree atrioventricular block).
  B. The initial net result of systolic dysfunction is a decrease in car-

diac output. The decreased cardiac output may cause clinical signs of weakness, fatigue, and exercise intolerance.

C. The body elicits a neurohumoral response to compensate for the decreased cardiac output. Blood and intraventricular volumes are increased by renal salt and water retention and increased thirst. Heart rate is increased. Myocardial hypertrophy ensues to offset changes in systolic myocardial wall stress (afterload). Contractility may increase in early stages if myocardial failure is not present.

II. Diastolic dysfunction

Primary diastolic dysfunction can result from diseases that cause massive myocardial hypertrophy (e.g., hypertrophic cardiomyopathy), that result in endocardial or myocardial fibrosis (e.g., restrictive cardiomyopathy) or that result from pericardial diseases (e.g., constrictive pericarditis, pericardial tamponade). All result in abnormal filling of the ventricles during diastole. These disease processes generally produce chambers that are stiffer than normal so that diastolic pressures are increased resulting in congestion and edema. If filling is impeded to the point of decreased end-diastolic volume of the ventricle, stroke volume may be decreased.

III. The cardiovascular system works within a system of priorities:

A. *The first priority* is to maintain systemic arterial blood pressure to ensure flow and oxygen delivery to the critical vascular beds (brain, heart, kidneys). The high pressure is needed because these organs have high innate vascular resistance. Without adequate flow to these organs, death will occur within a short period.

B. *The second priority* is to maintain cardiac output high enough to supply the entire body with an adequate amount of oxygen. If cardiac output becomes inadequate, death can occur in hours to days.

C. *The third priority* is to maintain normal venous blood pressures. Death can occur in hours to weeks with high venous pressures.

D. In heart failure, these cardiovascular functions are lost sequentially, with the lesser priority functions being lost first.

1. When an acute disease results in systolic dysfunction, cardiac output initially decreases. This causes a decrease in systemic arterial blood pressure. The immediate response is peripheral vasoconstriction in an effort to increase systemic blood pressure back toward normal. However, this is done at the expense of cardiac

output, since increasing blood pressure increases afterload and will serve to decrease cardiac output further.

2. To compensate for an inadequate cardiac output, the body increases intracardiac diastolic volumes by increasing blood volume and by constricting systemic veins. The increase in blood volume is brought about by renal salt and water retention and increased thirst. The increased intracardiac volumes increase cardiac output but also, if severe enough, cause increased diastolic and venous pressures, resulting in pulmonary congestion and edema. The increased blood volume compensates for the systolic dysfunction in order to maintain cardiac output, which helps maintain systemic blood pressure.
3. When overwhelming systolic dysfunction is present, increased blood volume can no longer compensate and cardiac output becomes inadequate at rest. If the decrease in cardiac output is marked, systemic arterial blood pressure can decrease as well.

Classifications of Heart Failure

Backward versus Forward Heart Failure

I. Backward heart failure is tissue congestion and edema due to increased capillary hydrostatic pressures resulting from increased diastolic intraventricular pressures or increased atrial pressures. It can be due to primary diastolic dysfunction or to an increased blood volume occurring secondary to a disease that causes a primary loss of systolic function.

II. Forward heart failure is clinical or laboratory evidence of inadequate tissue oxygen delivery due to a poor cardiac output. It is usually seen in later stages of diseases that cause primary systolic dysfunction. It can be provoked in earlier stages with exercise.

Right-versus Left-Sided Heart Failure

I. Right-sided backward failure may result in hepatic congestion, ascites, and hydrothorax. Right-sided forward failure is a decreased right ventricular cardiac output. It can result in a decreased amount of blood flow to the left ventricle, resulting in inadequate systemic blood flow.

II. Left-sided backward failure is due to increased left ventricular diastolic and/or left atrial blood pressures causing pulmonary congestion and edema. Left-sided forward failure is poor left ventricular cardiac output, resulting in inadequate tissue blood flow.

High-Output versus Low-Output Heart Failure

Some diseases result either in poor tissue oxygen delivery by means other than a low cardiac output (e.g., arteriovenous fistula, anemia) or in increased tissue oxygen demand (e.g. hyperthyroidism). In either situation, a normal or even a high cardiac output may be unable to carry enough oxygen to peripheral tissues. As a result, signs of heart failure can occur despite normal or even high cardiac output. In the more common diseases, cardiac output is low when signs of forward failure are present.

Types of Heart Failure

Myocardial Failure

I. This is the result of a disease that causes a decrease in myocardial contractility. It can be due to a primary myocardial disease (myocarditis) or secondary to prolonged increases in myocardial workload (e.g. aortic stenosis, mitral regurgitation). The most frequently diagnosed disease that results in myocardial failure is dilated cardiomyopathy. When myocardial failure is present, systolic function is poor, resulting in a low cardiac output and secondary fluid retention.

II. The myocardial disease can result in a loss of myocardial compliance and altered diastolic ventricular function. Mitral regurgitation is frequently present because of mitral valve annular dilation, which occurs secondary to left ventricular dilation.

Heart Failure Due to Volume Overloads

I. Mitral and tricuspid regurgitation result in a loss of forward stroke volume back into the left and right atria, respectively. The increased systolic atrial blood flow results in increased atrial pressures, which can cause congestion and edema. To compensate for the forward stroke volume loss, fluid retention occurs, producing dilated (larger end-diastolic volume) ventricular and atrial chambers on the affected side. This increases diastolic intraventricular and atrial pressures, which can cause congestion and edema. When this mechanism can no longer compensate for the loss in forward stroke volume, cardiac output becomes inadequate and signs of forward heart failure become evident. Myocardial failure may develop very late in the course of the disease in dogs with mitral regurgitation. In those dogs that have signs of heart failure, regurgitant fractions (the percentage of the stroke volume flowing into the left atrium) are usually greater than 80 percent.

II. Congenital left-to-right shunts share many characteristics with regurgitant lesions, such as a loss of forward stroke volume (i.e., that stroke volume that travels to the tissues), which is compensated for by fluid retention and increased blood volumes in the affected chamber(s) and blood vessels. Myocardial failure may develop, exacerbating the heart failure.

Heart Failure Due to Pressure Overload

Congenital stenotic lesions of the pulmonic or aortic valves cause increased intraventricular pressures. If severe, these lesions can produce signs of heart failure. If mild, heart failure usually does not develop. Heart failure is most commonly seen in animals with moderate to severe disease that develop myocardial failure as adults. Concentric hypertrophy associated with stenotic lesions produces a ventricle that is stiffer than normal. This effect can contribute to increased intraventricular diastolic pressures and congestion or edema. The stenotic lesion increases ventricular afterload, thereby contributing to the poor systolic function.

Heart Failure Due to Decreased Ventricular Compliance

Hypertrophic cardiomyopathy (HCM) results in decreased ventricular compliance (increased stiffness) because of concentric hypertrophy. Restrictive cardiomyopathy is caused by fibrosis of ventricular endocardium or myocardium, which increases ventricular stiffness. Both diseases result in high diastolic intraventricular pressures, whether the diastolic volume is normal or even decreased. The high diastolic intraventricular pressures result in pulmonary congestion and edema (left-sided backward failure). In HCM, systolic function is usually exaggerated because of a decreased afterload resulting from the left ventricular hypertrophy. By contrast, systolic function is generally normal in restrictive cardiomyopathy.

Heart Failure Due to Pericardial Disease

I. Constrictive pericarditis is caused by diseases that result in pericardial and epicardial scarring. The scarring results in cardiac constriction. The pathophysiology is the same as for restrictive cardiomyopathy. Pericardial effusion can result in cardiac tamponade.

II. Cardiac tamponade (compression of the heart due to fluid in the pericardial sac causing signs of right heart failure) can be acute or chronic.
   A. Acute tamponade is usually due to hemorrhage into the pericardial space (e.g., traumatic heart rupture). The acute impediment to ventricular filling causes a decreased stroke volume, which will result in a decreased cardiac output, hypotension, shock, and death if untreated. Diastolic intraventricular and venous pressures are increased, especially on the right side, resulting in jugular venous distention and an elevated central venous pressure.
   B. Chronic tamponade is seen with chronic pericardial effusions. The effusions increase intrapericardial pressure, as in acute tamponade, but here the body has time to compensate. Cardiac output is frequently normal, but systemic venous pressures are increased so signs of right-sided backward failure predominate.

Diagnosis

History

A thorough history should be obtained from a client whose animal is being examined for heart disease. Clinical signs not evident on physical examinations, previous medications and responses, and previous histories of cardiovascular diseases may then be recorded. In this manner, an assessment of the progression of disease and the presence of any preexisting complicating disease can be made.

I. Cough

Cough is often the presenting complaint in a dog with left-sided backward failure. It is unusual in the cat. The clinician must remember that cough is not specific for heart failure, so that other diseases capable of producing a cough must be ruled out or pulmonary edema as the cause must be ruled in before therapy is initiated. Older small dogs with mitral regurgitation commonly have tracheal collapse, chronic pulmonary disease, compression of the left mainstem bronchus by an enlarged left atrium, or pulmonary edema. Such problems singularly or collectively could cause a cough.

II. Dyspnea

By the time dyspnea is usually seen by an owner, severe pulmonary edema or severe hydrothorax is frequently present. It may therefore be a late sign of heart failure in the dog and cat. Dyspnea is frequently observed with exercise, however. By contrast, in humans, dyspnea is an early clinical sign of heart failure, as it is experienced by the patient as difficulty in breathing.

III. Orthopnea

Orthopnea is difficult breathing when recumbent. An owner may notice that the animal is reluctant to lie down (because lying down causes discomfort) or that the animal breathes heavily when lying down. Orthopnea may be present before dyspnea.

IV. Paroxysmal nocturnal dyspnea

This occurs after an animal has been sleeping for a period of time. Generally it occurs in dogs at night; the owner complains that the dog wakes up coughing or dyspneic and that it then has to walk around before becoming comfortable again and going back to sleep.

This sign is caused by a shift in blood volume from systemic veins to the heart and pulmonary circulation, resulting in pulmonary edema when the animal is recumbent.

V. Ascites, hydrothorax, and peripheral edema

Ascites is a common finding in dogs with right-sided heart failure. When severe, it can be detected readily by visualization and/or ballottement. Small amounts of ascites may be detected with abdominal radiographs. Hydrothorax and peripheral edema are other clinical signs of right-sided heart failure. Systemic venous congestion may be evident. Central venous pressure is increased to >10 cm H_2O.

VI. Exercise intolerance

Exercise intolerance can be one of the first signs of heart failure. However, since many pets do not exercise, this clinical sign is often not observed. Exercise intolerance occurs because cardiac output is inadequate for the increased tissue oxygen demand created by exercise. This results in tissue hypoxia and muscle fatigue. Dyspnea is also present and is probably related either to the poor cardiac output or to elevated pulmonary capillary pressures.

Physical Examination: Cardiovascular Findings in Heart Failure

Dysrhythmias

I. Atrial fibrillation is a common finding in dogs with dilated cardiomyopathy but may also be present in dogs with chronic mitral regurgitation or long-standing patent ductus arteriosus. It is rare in the cat.

II. Atrial arrhythmias, other than atrial fibrillation, are also common in many different cardiovascular diseases that can lead to or are associated with heart failure.

III. Ventricular arrhythmias are common in Boxers and Doberman Pinschers with cardiomyopathy but can be detected in many different cardiac diseases.

Gallop Sounds

Gallop sounds are common in patients with severe left ventricular volume overload and/or decreased myocardial compliance. Especially prevalent in cats with congestive or hypertrophic cardiomyopathy, they are caused by low-frequency vibrations and appear to originate from the left ventricle. They occur during early diastole with rapid ventricular filling (S_3) and late diastole during atrial systole (S_4).

Signs of Backward Failure

I. Pulmonary edema may occasionally be detected by auscultation, but auscultation is neither a sensitive nor a specific diagnostic test for this condition. If pulmonary edema is suspected because of cough, dyspnea, or hyperpnea, chest radiographs should be evaluated.
II. Systemic veins may be distended with right-sided heart failure. Manual compression of the cranial abdomen may demonstrate exaggerated jugular venous distention (hepatojugular reflux). In addition, ascites, hydrothorax, or peripheral edema may be present.

Signs of Forward Failure

I. *Mild or moderate heart failure:* Signs of forward failure are usually only present when the animal exercises. Clinical signs are those of fatigue and dyspnea.
II. *Severe heart failure:* Cardiac output may be low at rest causing pale mucous membranes, a prolonged capillary refill time, or a low venous oxygen tension.

Laboratory Tests

If cardiac output is unable to supply oxygen to meet the demand for oxygen by the resting peripheral tissues, the mixed venous oxygen tension ($P\bar{v}O_2$) will be decreased. Mixed venous samples are difficult to obtain clinically, so free-flowing jugular samples are usually substituted. If the cardiac output is only inadequate with exercise, resting venous oxygen tensions will be normal, but samples taken during exercise will be low. If arterial hypoxemia is present, the $A-VO_2$ difference should be calculated. Normal jugular venous PO_2 is 35 to 45 mm Hg. Noncritical animals with inadequate cardiac outputs have venous PO_2 values of 25 to 35 mm Hg at rest. Animals with venous PO_2 values of <25 mm Hg at rest are usually in the very late stages of heart failure and may be critically ill.

Electrocardiogram

The electrocardiogram may indicate atrial and/or ventricular arrhythmias. Determination of a mean electrical axis and heart chamber enlargement will provide baseline data. The ECG does not provide any definitive criteria for heart failure.

Thoracic Radiographs

I. Signs of heart failure on thoracic radiographs are limited to those of left-sided or right-sided backward failure.
   A. The earliest sign of left-sided failure is pulmonary venous congestion.
   B. As pulmonary venous and capillary pressures increase, interstitial and then alveolar edema appear. The edema may be centrally located around the base of the heart (perihilar) but can also be generalized.
   C. The cardiovascular silhouette is usually enlarged in heart failure.
      1. The enlargement can be due to chamber dilation (volume overload), chamber dilation and eccentric myocardial hypertrophy, concentric hypertrophy, or pericardial effusion.
      2. Cardiac enlargement is not a sign of heart failure per se and may be absent in diseases such as constrictive pericarditis and restrictive cardiomyopathy.

II. Pleural effusion, hepatomegaly, and ascites may be present with right-sided backward failure.

ECHOCARDIOGRAPHY

Echocardiography is extremely helpful in differentiating cardiac diseases that cause heart failure and in identifying types of heart failure, such as myocardial failure, heart failure due to a volume overload, and heart failure due to decreased ventricular compliance.

CARDIAC CATHETERIZATION

I. This diagnostic tool can be used to elucidate the underlying heart disease, to confirm the presence of heart failure, and to assess the severity of heart failure.

II. Since most animals with heart failure are anesthetic risks, it is desirable to either avoid cardiac catheterization, do the procedure with sedation and local anesthesia or do it with light anesthesia and keep the procedure as short as possible.

III. In dogs that require invasive testing to assess the severity of cardiac disease, catheterization of the right side of the heart with a balloon-tipped thermodilution catheter is preferred. This type of catheter can be placed with the dog sedated, the catheter can then be maintained in place, if desired, to monitor the disease or response to therapy. The catheter is usually used to evaluate cardiac output and filling pressures of the right ventricle.

IV. Diagnosis of underlying disease in a dog or cat usually requires general anesthesia and catheterization of the specific chambers involved. Angiography may be required, but its use should be minimized to prevent further volume overload.

PROTOCOL FOR THE DIAGNOSIS OF HEART FAILURE

I. Confirmatory tests
   A. Left-sided backward failure is absolutely confirmed by measuring pulmonary capillary pressures but is usually more loosely confirmed by identifying pulmonary edema on a chest radiograph in association with left heart disease and/or left heart enlargement.

B. Right-sided backward failure is confirmed by identifying ascites, hydrothorax, or peripheral edema and either ruling out other causes or ruling in increased systemic venous pressure, usually by identifying an increased central venous pressure.
C. Forward failure may be difficult to confirm. If heart failure is mild to moderate, cardiac output may only be inadequate when the animal exercises. Exercise testing is rarely done in veterinary medicine. If forward failure is present at rest, it can be documented by determining that a low cardiac output is responsible for decreasing tissue oxygen delivery below the amount required by tissue oxygen consumption. This can be done by first assessing the adequacy of tissue oxygen delivery by measuring the difference in oxygen content between arterial and mixed venous blood or by measuring mixed venous oxygen tension. Then a low cardiac output as the cause for the decreased tissue oxygen delivery can either be ruled in by measuring cardiac output or other causes can be ruled out by determining hemoglobin concentration and arterial oxygen saturation. Such determinations are clinically difficult. The author generally substitutes a jugular venous sample or a mixed venous sample for determination of the venous oxygen tension and then rules out arterial hypoxemia and anemia as causes of poor tissue oxygen delivery.

II. Differential diagnoses
A. Noncardiac pulmonary disease frequently mimics heart failure. Both can cause coughing and dyspnea. It is not unusual for heart disease and pulmonary disease to be present in the same patient. One or both may be responsible for clinical signs. Thoracic radiographs are usually the best diagnostic test to differentiate the causes of cough and dyspnea, but false-negative and false-positive results do occur for all diseases assessed in this manner. Although measurements of left ventricular end-diastolic or pulmonary capillary wedge pressure are the ideal means of confirming pulmonary edema due to left-sided heart failure, they cannot be done on a practical basis.
B. Ascites, peripheral edema, and hydrothorax can be caused by diseases other than right-sided backward failure. Usually the measurement of central venous pressure will confirm whether or not right heart failure is the cause.

THERAPY

MEDICAL THERAPY

Medical management is directed at treating and improving the clinical signs associated with heart failure. Signs of congestion and edema can be treated with diuretics, low-salt diet, positive inotropic agents, venodilators, and arteriolar dilators. Signs of inadequate cardiac output may be treated with positive inotropic agents and arteriolar dilators. The appropriate treatment regimen for a given dog or cat depends on the clinical signs present, the severity of the clinical signs, and the underlying disease.

THERAPY FOR DECREASING CONGESTION AND EDEMA

Low-Sodium Diets

I. Low-sodium diets can effectively decrease blood volume and reduce congestion and edema, especially in mild and moderate heart failure.
   A. Unfortunately, many low-salt diets are not very palatable. As a result, owner and patient compliance with this form of therapy can be poor. Salt substitutes containing KCl can be added to improve flavor.
   B. Commercial low-salt diets have a very low sodium content (30 to 50 mg/100 g dry weight) and probably are most appropriate as the sole caloric source in dogs with severe heart failure. In dogs with mild to moderate heart failure, dog food with sodium content on the lower end of the range (350 to 400 mg/100 mg dry weight) can be mixed 50 : 50 with a commercial low-sodium diet for the pet.
   C. Booklets can be obtained from the American Heart Association, its local chapters, or the USDA, detailing the sodium content of various foods or listing those foods recommended for the patient on a low-salt diet.

Diuretics

I. Diuretics used in heart failure increase urinary sodium excretion by decreasing sodium retention within renal tubules. By doing so they decrease blood volume and so decrease diastolic pressures within the heart. The choice and dose of diuretic depend on the severity of clinical signs. Oral doses for the most frequently used diuretics are listed in Table 12-1.

A. If only congestion or mild edema is present, a thiazide diuretic or low-dose furosemide can be used.
B. Moderate to severe edema is usually treated with furosemide. The dose and frequency depend on the severity of the edema. If a patient is refractory to furosemide, it can be combined with triamterene or a thiazide diuretic to promote additional diuresis. It is unusual for a dog or cat to become hypokalemic because of chronic diuretic administration, but if it does occur, concurrent triamterene administration may alleviate the problem.
C. Life-threatening pulmonary edema must be treated aggressively with intravenous furosemide. Doses up to 8 mg/kg may be given to dogs as frequently as every hour until diuresis is evident. Intravenous doses in cats should not exceed 2 mg/kg. Although hyponatremia and hypokalemia are common with this intensive therapy, they result in death far less frequently than does severe pulmonary edema that is not treated aggressively.

Therapy for Increasing Myocardial Contractility

Such therapy should ideally be used only to treat heart failure when myocardial failure (decreased myocardial contractility) is present. As myocardial function is usually difficult to assess in a clinical situation, clinical decisions are generally made on the basis of population characteristics. For example, dogs and cats with dilated cardiomyopathy have poor myocardial contractility and should always be treated with positive inotropic drugs. Small dogs with mitral regurgitation usually have normal or relatively normal myocardial function for at least 6 months to 1 year after they start showing signs of heart failure severe enough to require diuretic therapy and may not require digitalis during this period. In some diseases, such as hypertrophic cardiomyopathy, the use of positive inotropes is contraindicated.

TABLE 12-1. DIURETIC THERAPY IN DOGS WITH HEART FAILURE

Generic Name	Trade Name	Route of Administration	Dosage
Hydrochlorothiazide	Hydrodiuril	PO	2–4 mg/kg bid
Chlorothiazide	Diuril	PO	20–40 mg/kg bid to tid
Bendroflumethiazide		PO	0.2–0.4 mg/kg bid
Furosemide	Lasix	PO	2–4 mg/kg bid to tid if needed
		IV	2–8 mg/kg up to every hour (see text)
Spironolactone	Aldactone	PO	2–4 mg/kg-day
Triamterene	Dyrenium	PO	2–4 mg/kg-day

Digitalis Glycosides

I. The digitalis glycosides are the only positive inotropic agents available for long-term oral use. Newer positive inotropic agents will soon become available for clinical use that will replace digitalis in some situations and augment the use of digitalis in others.

  A. The use of digitalis glycosides is indicated in dogs and cats with signs of forward or backward heart failure due to myocardial failure. The myocardial failure may be primary (e.g., dilated cardiomyopathy) or secondary to increased cardiac workloads (e.g., aortic stenosis). Digitalis is also indicated as an antiarrhythmic agent in supraventricular arrhythmias and to slow the ventricular response to atrial flutter and fibrillation.

  B. Digoxin and digitoxin are the two most commonly used cardiac glycosides. Digoxin has a half-life of 24 to 36 hours in the dog and approximately 33 to 58 hours in the cat. The half-life of digitoxin is 8 to 12 hours in the dog and is extremely long in the cat. Digoxin is poorly protein bound and is excreted via glomerular filtration. Digitoxin is highly protein bound and metabolized by the liver. About 60 percent of the digoxin in tablets is absorbed from the gastrointestinal tract and 75 percent of the elixir is absorbed (doses of digoxin should be reduced by 20 percent when the elixir is used). Approximately 95 to 100 percent of digitoxin is absorbed.

C. Digoxin and digitoxin should usually be administered as chronic oral maintenance doses. Parenteral administration and loading doses result in toxicity in many patients with myocardial failure. Parenteral administration or loading doses may be used in patients without myocardial failure (dogs with mitral regurgitation) when the glycoside is being used to abolish or control a supraventricular dysrhythmia.

D. The dosage of digoxin is 0.22 mg/m^2 of body surface area bid in dogs. Body surface area can either be calculated (BSA $=$ kg$^{2/3}$ $\times$ 0.112) or the conversion from body weight can be found in standard veterinary texts (Kirk RW: Current Veterinary Therapy VIII. W.B. Saunders, Philadelphia, 1983 or Ettinger SJ: Textbook of Veterinary Internal Medicine. W.B. Saunders, Philadelphia, 1975). Dosage for tincture of digitoxin (Foxalin) is 0.03 to 0.04 mg/kg tid in dogs.

E. Because of digitoxin's long half-life it is not used in cats. Digoxin dosage in cats is 0.005 to 0.01 mg/kg given once a day or divided bid for tablets (1⁄4 of 0.125 mg digoxin tablet every other day for cats weighing 2 to 3 kg; 1⁄4 tablet daily for cats weighing 4 to 6 kg; 1⁄4 tablet bid for cats weighing 7 or more kg). Cats dislike the taste of the elixir.

F. Another method of dosing digoxin in the dog is oral maintenance (0.01 to 0.02 mg/kg divided bid). These dosages need to be adjusted downward depending on numerous factors; discussed in the next section. Rapid oral digitalization is 0.02 to 0.06 mg/kg divided bid for the first day and then a maintenance level should be established.

G. Numerous factors alter digitalis dosages.
   1. Dogs or cats with hypernatremia, hypokalemia, or hypercalcemia require less digitalis.
   2. Both hyper- and hypothyroid animals need less digitalis.
   3. Animals with myocardial failure can be extremely sensitive to digitalis, so their doses must be titrated carefully.
   4. Dogs or cats with renal failure excrete less digoxin, resulting in high serum concentrations and toxicity. Digitoxin is preferred in dogs with renal failure.

5. Digoxin is preferred in cats with renal failure, but doses must be reduced and signs of toxicity must be watched for carefully.
6. Digoxin does not diffuse into fat, so estimates of lean body weight should be used to calculate body surface area.
7. Quinidine, verapamil, and drugs that inhibit hepatic microsomal enzymes (chloramphenicol, tetracycline) should not be administered concurrently with digoxin.

H. Patients that are adequately digitalized and that respond with an increase in myocardial contractility show improvement in clinical signs. Perfusion and exercise tolerance improve, and congestion and edema decrease. The heart rate usually decreases in animals treated for supraventricular tachyarrhythmias. ECG changes are insensitive and nonspecific indicators of adequate serum digitalis concentrations. About 40 to 50 percent of dogs with dilated cardiomyopathy do not respond to digoxin administration. Dogs that do not respond have an average survival time of 6 weeks as compared with 6 months for those that do respond.

I. Animals that become toxic on digitalis or that do not respond to its administration may benefit from measuring serum concentrations of digoxin or digitoxin.
1. Therapeutic digoxin serum concentrations range from 1.0 to 2.5 ng/ml. Moderately toxic serum concentrations are 2.5 to 6.0 ng/ml; very toxic concentrations are >6.0 ng/ml. Serum should be collected 8 hours after the last dose for analysis.
2. Therapeutic concentrations of digitoxin are 15 to 35 ng/ml; toxicity occurs at concentrations >40 ng/ml. Dogs that do not respond clinically to digitalis but that have serum concentrations in the therapeutic range are refractory to the cardiac glycoside. Low serum concentrations suggest poor owner compliance, inadequate absorption from the gastrointestinal tract, or inadequate dosing.

J. Treatment of digitalis toxicity.
1. Mild intoxication produces anorexia and vomiting and can be treated by drug withdrawal.
2. Severe toxicity may produce many different cardiac arrhythmias. Ventricular tachyarrhythmias are the most serious, as they frequently cause death. Lidocaine and phenytoin are the antiarrhythmics of choice in this situation.

3. Phenytoin can be used prophylactically in dogs that may be more sensitive to the effects of the digitalis glycosides (dogs with severe myocardial failure).
4. Propranolol may be beneficial in digitalis-induced tachyarrhythmias. Procainamide is less effective and quinidine is contraindicated.
5. Cholestryamine may be administered orally in digitoxin intoxication to bind the glycoside. It may also be useful if administered early after the ingestion of a large amount of digoxin.

Milrinone

I. Milrinone* is a new orally active agent that has positive inotropic and mild arteriolar dilating properties. Its mode of action is unknown but is not the same as that of the digitalis glycosides or the sympathomimetics. Milrinone is much safer than digitalis.
   A. When administered orally, the effects of milrinone can be observed within 30 minutes. Drug effect lasts at least 12 hours, but the positive inotropic effect is less than half the initial effect at 12 hours. Dogs with milder signs of heart failure may require dosing only every 12 hours. Dogs with severe heart failure may require dosing every 6 to 8 hours. The oral dose ranges from 0.5 to 1.0 mg/kg.
   B. The positive inotropic properties of milrinone along with its arteriolar dilating properties make it a very attractive drug for treating myocardial failure. In studies to date, milrinone appears to be effective in almost 100 percent of dogs with myocardial failure and milder signs of heart failure and 70 to 80 percent effective in patients with more severe signs. The drug may also be beneficial in treating dogs with mitral valve fibrosis because of the arteriolar dilation produced. Caution must be exercised, however, since the increase in force generated by the left ventricle may rupture chordae tendineae.
   C. Milrinone has exacerbated ventricular arrhythmias in a small number of dogs with myocardial failure. Electrocardiographic monitoring is advised when the drug is first administered. If a

*Milrinone is an experimental drug not yet approved for use in dogs or cats.

ventricular arrhythmia is present before milrinone administration, it should be treated appropriately (see Chapter 13). If it develops after milrinone administration, the drug should be discontinued or the arrhythmia treated.

Dobutamine–Dopamine

I. The sympathomimetics are used only to treat acute heart failure. Their short half-life (1 to 2 minutes) and extensive hepatic metabolism make them inappropriate for oral use. This class of drugs stimulates various adrenergic receptors, so that drug effects can vary markedly from one drug to another.
   A. Dobutamine increases myocardial contractility by stimulating β_1 receptors. Both β_2 and α_1 receptors are stimulated in peripheral vasculature, so there is no major change in blood pressure. Dobutamine is generally regarded as being less arrhythmogenic than other catecholamines (except dopamine) in heart failure patients.
      1. Dobutamine can be used to treat dogs with acute myocardial failure due to anesthetic overdose, severe metabolic abnormalities, or myocardial depression following cardiac arrest. It can also be used to stabilize patients with chronic heart failure while waiting for other drugs to render support. As an example, a dog with severe heart failure due to dilated cardiomyopathy may benefit from short-term dobutamine administration while maintenance doses of digitalis are given.
      2. Dobutamine, like other sympathomimetics, should be administered as a constant-rate infusion. Usual infusion rates range from 5 to 20 μg/kg-min. Heart rate usually increases at infusion rates of $>$20 μg/kg-min.
   B. Dopamine acts similarly to dobutamine, with three major differences:
      1. Dopamine dilates renal and mesenteric vasculature favoring flow to these vascular beds, while dobutamine favors flow to myocardial and skeletal muscle.
      2. The infusion rate for dopamine is 1 to 10 μg/kg-min, and infusion rates $>$10 μg/kg-min produce vasoconstriction.

3. Dopamine may increase diastolic intraventricular pressures in chronic heart failure patients so dobutamine is favored in this group.

Therapy to Decrease Cardiac Workload

I. Vasodilators can be used to treat acute or chronic heart failure. Vasodilators dilate systemic arterioles, systemic veins, or both. Selected vasodilators may also have effects on the pulmonary vasculature.
   A. Types of vasodilators
      Little is known about the effectiveness, pharmacodynamics, and pharmacokinetics of most of the vasodilators. Dosage recommendations are mostly derived from clinical experience. When using a drug that dilates arterioles, care must be taken not to induce hypotension. Titrating the drug dosage upward from a low dose is the best means of avoiding this complication. Venodilators require less monitoring, since side effects are usually not life threatening.
      1. Arteriolar dilators (e.g., hydralazine) decrease aortic input impedance, usually lower systemic arterial blood pressure, and so decrease systolic myocardial wall stress (afterload). This results in increased myocardial fiber shortening and an increased stroke volume. In mitral regurgitation, the decreased impedance and systolic intraventricular pressure induced by arteriolar dilators results in lesser regurgitant flow and greater aortic blood flow. This results in lowered left atrial pressures along with increased forward stroke volume.
      2. Venodilators (e.g., nitroglycerin, isosorbide dinitrate) decrease diastolic intracardiac volumes by redistributing blood away from the heart and pulmonary circulation into the peripheral veins. These agents are used to treat signs of congestion and edema. They are usually used when diuretics lose their effectiveness.
      3. Combination vasodilators (e.g., nitroprusside, prazosin, captopril) decrease congestion and edema and increase cardiac output.
   B. Hydralazine is the most extensively studied vasodilator in veterinary medicine. Its arteriolar dilating effect lasts 11 to 13 hours. Its dosage ranges from 1 to 3 mg/kg.
      1. Before drug administration, baseline thoracic radiographs should

be taken. Mucous membrane color should be evaluated carefully. Jugular venous oxygen tension should be evaluated, if possible. If systemic arterial blood pressure can be obtained, it should be recorded.

2. An initial dose of 1 mg/kg hydralazine should be administered to dogs per os. To determine whether this dose is effective, blood pressure can be repeated in 1 hour and blood gas in 3 hours, or clinical signs can be reevaluated anywhere from 5 hours to 1 day later.
3. If mean blood pressure has decreased 15-20 mmHg or is <70 mmHg, the titration is complete and the 1 mg/kg dose should be continued at 12-hour intervals. The same is true if the venous PO_2 was <35 mm Hg and is now >35 mm Hg. If the mucous membrane color has improved dramatically, or if pulmonary edema has decreased, the dosage given was effective.
4. If no improvement has occurred, drug titration should continue and another 1-mg/kg dose (total dose, 2 mg/kg) administered if it has been <8 hours since the last dose. If it has been >12 hours, a 2-mg/kg total dose should be administered. The dog should be reevaluated as appropriate.
5. If there is still no response, a total dose of 3 mg/kg can be administered.
6. The total dose should be administered every 12 hours.
7. Side effects of hydralazine include hypotension and tachycardia. Significant hypotension (i.e., mean systemic arterial blood pressure <60 mm Hg, oliguria, altered consciousness) should be treated with dopamine at infusion rates of >10 μg/kg-min.
8. If heart rate is >180 beats/min, use of a digitalis glycoside and/or propranolol may be considered to decrease the heart rate. Some dogs and cats have gastrointestinal disturbances associated with hydralazine use. This complication may be severe enough to preclude further therapy.
9. Dosage titration for cats should start at a total dose of 2.5 mg and can go as high as 10 mg.

C. Captopril can be very effective in treating selected dogs with dilated cardiomyopathy and mitral regurgitation. The author has noted renal failure in 3 dogs treated with captopril at doses of 3 mg/kg bid or tid. Doses > 2mg/kg tid are strongly discouraged.

D. Suggested doses for other vasodilators are listed in Table 12-2.

With any drug possessing arteriolar dilating properties, a low dose should be administered initially and the dose titrated to an effective end point.

II. *Restriction of physical activity* decreases tissue oxygen consumption, placing less demand on the heart for supplying oxygen delivery. The dog with mild heart failure may need only curtail hunting activity or be confined to the yard. Dogs with severe heart failure may require cage rest. Dogs with life-threatening heart failure should be placed on cage rest and usually cannot tolerate even the slightest amount of physical activity. Even struggling during restraint or fighting oxygen administration given by mask may cause death. Dogs in these situations may benefit from sedation with morphine (≤1 mg/kg SC or IM).

Therapeutic Strategies for Treating Heart Failure

I. Management of dogs with mitral valvular fibrosis (see also Chapter 5)
  A. If only a murmur is present but no signs of heart failure exist (class I), no treatment is needed.
  B. Mild heart failure (class II)
    1. If signs are present only with heavy exercise, this activity should be curtailed.
    2. If exercise cannot be curtailed or if even light exercise causes coughing, dyspnea, or fatigue, recommend a low-salt diet and consider administering a thiazide diuretic or low-dose furosemide.
  C. Moderate heart failure (class III)
    1. If normal activity produces clinical signs, low to moderate doses of furosemide can be given. Use of digitalis is most often indicated.
    2. Attempt to place the animal on a low-salt diet.
  D. Severe heart failure (class IV)
    1. Administer moderate to maximum doses of furosemide when signs of heart failure are present at rest.
    2. Insist that the dog be fed a low-salt diet.

TABLE 12-2. VASODILATER THERAPY IN DOGS WITH HEART FAILURE[a]

Generic Name	Trade Name	Mechanism of Action	Route of Administration	Dosage
Isosorbide dinitrate	Isordil	Venodilation	PO	1–1.5 mg/kg tid to qid
Nitroglycerin ointment	Nitro-BID Nitropaste	Venodilation	Cutaneous	0.25–2 inches tid to qid
Hydralazine	Apresoline	Arteriolar dilation	PO	1–3 mg/kg bid
Prazosin	Minipress	Arteriolar and venodilation	PO	1 mg tid for dogs weighing <15 kg; 2 mg tid for dogs weighing >15 kg
Nitroprusside[b]	Nipride	Arteriolar and venodilation	IV	1–5 μg/kg/min
Captopril	Capoten	Arteriolar and venodilation	PO	0.5 to 2 mg/kg tid (do not exceed 2 mg/kg tid)

[a]Dosages for vasodilators except hydralazine are based only on limited clinical experience or are extrapolated from data generated from normal dogs. In general, dosages should be titrated to an effective end point in each patient.
[b]Nitroprusside should only be used when blood pressure can be monitored.

3. When furosemide is no longer effective or when forward heart failure is present, begin hydralazine therapy. Other vasodilators, such as captopril, should be considered, if the patient does not tolerate hydralazine.
4. If sinus tachycardia, paroxysmal atrial tachycardia, or atrial fibrillation are present, begin a course of digitalis glycoside therapy.
5. Digitalis should also be administered if the dog's condition is refractory to hydralazine.

E. Life-threatening heart failure (class V)
1. Cage rest to avoid stress is of paramount important. Such maneuvers as taking chest radiographs, placing jugular catheters, and administering oxygen by mask often prove fatal, especially when the animal struggles.
2. Oxygen administration via an oxygen cage is recommended.
3. Intravenous furosemide ($\leq$8 mg/kg-hr) can be administered if

a venous catheter is in place or if it can be administered without stress. If not, intramuscular injections can be given. When diuresis is established, furosemide doses should be decreased to maintenance levels.

4. Oral hydralazine (initial dose of 2 mg/kg) can be beneficial. Other arteriolar dilators may also be considered, but should not be administered concurrently with hydralazine.
5. If fluid therapy is needed, half-strength saline with 2.5 percent dextrose or 5 percent dextrose solutions should be used. Slow administration is advised, with careful monitoring, to prevent fluid overload.

II. Management of dogs or cats with dilated cardiomyopathy (see also Chapter 6)

A. Mild heart failure

1. It is unusual to see this stage in the dog and rare in the cat.
2. Exercise restriction and diuretic administration usually are beneficial.

B. Moderate and severe heart failure

1. Administer milrinone or a digitalis glycoside.
2. Furosemide dosage should be adjusted so that edema is controlled but dehydration and poor perfusion are not produced.
3. Keep on a low-salt diet.
4. If the animal is refractory or becomes refractory to milrinone and digitalis, consider using vasodilators.

C. Life-threatening heart failure

1. Administer oral milrinone (1 mg/kg), or start a constant-rate infusion of dobutamine to dogs.
2. Administer intravenous furosemide ($\leq$8 mg/kg every hour until diuresis is established in the dog; 2 mg/kg in the cat).
3. Administer oxygen via an oxygen cage.
4. Intravenous nitroprusside can be given to dogs if blood pressure can be monitored. Oral hydralazine and topical nitroglycerin cream may be beneficial.

III. Management of cats with hypertrophic cardiomyopathy

A. Mild to moderate heart failure

1. Administer propranolol (2.5 to 5.0 mg bid to tid).
2. Low doses of furosemide may be needed to control pulmonary edema.

B. Severe heart failure
   1. Administer furosemide (1 mg/kg per PO or IM bid to tid).
   2. Give propranolol (2.5 to 5.0 mg bid to tid); propranolol is contraindicated when severe heart failure is present.
C. Life-threatening heart failure
   1. Administer furosemide (1 to 2 mg/kg IV or IM).
   2. Place on cage rest and oxygen administration.
   3. Propranolol is administered when clinical signs have improved.

IV. Management of dogs with pressure overloads (see also Chapter 10)
A. Heart failure secondary to aortic stenosis can be managed with milrinone or a digitalis glycoside, diuretics, and a low-salt diet. Surgical relief of the obstruction may be very beneficial.
B. Heart failure secondary to pulmonic stenosis can be treated surgically. Medical management includes diuretics and milrinone or a digitalis glycoside. A drug having venodilating properties, such as captopril, may help control ascites.

V. Management of dogs with heartworm disease and heart failure (see also Chapter 8)
A. Cage rest, diuretics, and arsenical therapy are the mainstays of therapy for this condition. Milrinone may also be beneficial.
B. Dogs should be cage-rested for at least 1 week before arsenical therapy.
C. Heart failure therapy can often be discontinued 4 to 8 weeks after arsenical administration.

SUGGESTED READINGS

Braunwald E: Vasodilator therapy—a physiologic approach to the treatment of heart failure. N Engl J Med 297:331, 1977

Calvert CA, Rawlings CA: Diagnosis and management of canine heartworm disease. p. 348. In Kirk RW (ed): Current Veterinary Therapy. VIII. WB Saunders, Philadelphia, 1982

Clemmer TP: Oxygen transport. Int Anesth Clin 19:21, 1981

Ettinger SJ (ed): Textbook of Veterinary Internal Medicine. WB Saunders, Philadelphia, 1975

Fox PR: Feline myocardial diseases. p. 337. In Kirk RW (ed): Current Veterinary Therapy. VIII. WB Saunders, Philadelphia, 1982

Kirk RW (ed): Current Veterinary Therapy. VIII. WB Saunders, Philadelphia, 1983

Kittleson MD: Concepts and therapeutic strategies in the management of heart failure. p. 279. In Kirk RW (ed): Current Veterinary Therapy. VIII. WB Saunders, Philadelphia, 1983

Kittleson MD: Drugs used in the management of heart failure. p. 285. In Kirk RW (ed): Current Veterinary Therapy. VIII. WB Saunders, Philadelphia, 1982

Kittleson MD: Dobutamine. J Am Vet Med Assoc 177:642, 1980

Kittleson MD, Hamlin RL: Hydralazine pharmacodynamics in the dog. Am J Vet Res 44:1501, 1983

Kittleson MD, Eyster GE, Knowlen GG, et al: Myocardial function in small dogs with chronic mitral regurgitation and severe congestive heart failure. J Am Vet Med Assoc 184:455, 1984

Kittleson MD, Eyster GE, Knowlen GG, et al: The effect of digitalis glycosides on peripheral tissue oxygen delivery and myocardial function in dogs with congestive cardiomyopathy. Scientific Proceedings of the American College of Veterinary Internal Medicine, Salt Lake City, Utah, 1982

Kittleson MD, Eyster GE, Olivier NB, et al: Oral hydralazine therapy for chronic mitral regurgitation in the dog. J Am Vet Med Assoc 182:1205, 1982

Kittleson MD, Pipers FS, Knauer KW, et al: Efficacy of milrinone for the treatment of myocardial failure in dogs. Scientific Proceedings of the American College of Veterinary Medicine, New York, 1983.

Smith TW, Braunwald E: The management of heart failure. p. 509. In Braunwald E (ed): Heart Disease: A Textbook of Cardiovascular Medicine. WB Saunders, Philadelphia, 1980

13

Treatment of Cardiac Arrhythmias and Conduction Disturbances

Michael S. Miller

INTRODUCTION

DEFINITION

Arrhythmias are defined as abnormalities of cardiac impulse formation, conduction, rate, and regularity. Other terms such as dysrhythmia and ectopic rhythm are also used to describe electrophysiologic cardiac disturbances. Many cardiac arrhythmias are benign and clinically insignificant and require no specific therapy. Other arrhythmias may cause severe clinical signs or degenerate into malignant arrhythmias leading to cardiac arrest and sudden death. In the latter case, immediate therapeutic intervention may be life saving.

GENERAL MECHANISMS

The current view on the mechanisms for cardiac arrhythmias includes isolated or concurrent abnormalities in impulse initiation (automaticity), propagation (including reentry), and triggered activity (early and delayed afterdepolarizations). The interested reader should consult the Suggested Readings list at the end of this chapter for further information about the mechanisms of cardiac arrhythmias. Arrhythmias can be classified according to the mechanism underlying the arrhythmias (Table 13-1).

TABLE 13-1. CLASSIFICATION OF CARDIAC ARRHYTHMIAS

Normal sinus impulse formation
Normal sinus rhythm
Sinus arrhythmia
Disturbances of sinus impulse formation
Sinus bradycardia
Sinus tachycardia
Disturbances of supraventricular impulse formation
Atrial premature complexes
Sinus arrest and/or block
Atrial tachycardia
Atrial flutter
Atrial fibrillation
Atrioventricular (AV) junctional rhythm
Disturbances of ventricular impulse formation
Ventricular premature complexes
Ventricular tachycardia
Ventricular asystole
Ventricular fibrillation
Disturbances of impulse conduction
Atrial standstill
First-degree AV block
Second-degree AV block
Complete AV block (third degree)
Disturbances of both impulse formation and impulse conduction
Sick sinus syndrome
Ventricular preexcitation and the Wolff–Parkinson–White (WPW) syndrome

General Etiology

Cardiac arrhythmias may occur in either the presence or absence of specific cardiac disease (Table 13-2). Numerous systemic disorders may be correlated with abnormal cardiac rhythms. Specific arrhythmias are more likely to occur in patients with heart disease (e.g., atrial fibrillation associated with dilated cardiomyopathy in large-breed dogs) and may be useful as clues to the underlying disease. The amount of structural damage to the heart is not always correlated with the type and severity of any arrhythmia.

TABLE 13-2. ETIOLOGIES OF CARDIAC ARRHYTHMIAS

A. Cardiac

1. Dog

a. Heredity (genetics not documented in all cases)
   1) Doberman (His bundle degeneration)
   2) English Springer Spaniel (persistent atrial standstill)
   3) Miniature Schnauzer, Dachshund, Cocker Spaniel (sick sinus syndrome)
   4) Pug and Dalmatian (sinus node disease)
   5) Pug (stenosis and degeneration of the His bundle)
   6) Wolff-Parkinson-White syndrome

b. Atrial and/or ventricular arrhythmias
   1) Atrial enlargement, secondary to congenital defects or acquired disease
   2) Cardiomyopathy
   3) Congenital heart disease
   4) Congestive heart failure
   5) Mitral valve disease (congenital and acquired)
   6) Myocarditis, endocarditis
   7) Neoplasia
   8) Trauma

c. Conduction system disease
   1) Acquired sinus and AV node disease (sick sinus syndrome)
   2) Cardiomyopathy
   3) Neoplasia
   4) Surgical damage to conduction tissue
   5) Trauma
   6) Vascular (e.g., microscopic intramural myocardial infarction)
   7) Ventricular septal defect and other congenital defects

2. Cat

a. Heredity (rare)
   1) Wolff-Parkinson-White Syndrome

b. Atrial and ventricular arrhythmias
   1) Cardiac enlargement secondary to congenital heart defects
   2) Cardiomyopathy
   3) Neoplasia
   4) Trauma

c. Conduction system disease
   1) Cardiomyopathy
   2) Neoplasia

B. Non-cardiac
1. Dog and cat
   a. Acidosis or alkalosis
   b. Autonomic nervous system imbalance (parasympathetic or sympathetic); central nervous system (e.g., pain, excitement, fear); respiratory, gastrointestinal or organic brain disease

(Cont.)

c. Drug toxicity (e.g., digitalis, preoperative sedatives, or anesthetic agents, catecholamines, antiarrhythmic agents, bronchodilators)
d. Electrolyte disorders (e.g., hyperkalemia, hypercalcemia, hypokalemia, hypocalcemia, hypomagnesemia)
e. Endocrinopathies (e.g., hypothyroidism, hyperthyroidism, Addison's disease, pheochromocytoma)
f. Hypothermia
g. Hypovolemia
h. Hypoxia
i. Mechanical stimulation (e.g., cardiac catheterization, intravenous catheter)
j. Neoplasia
k. Shock
l. Toxemia or sepsis
m. Trauma

FUNDAMENTAL APPROACH TO THE INTERPRETATION OF CARDIAC ARRHYTHMIAS

Initial Evaluation

I. Review all pertinent clinical data: age, breed, medical history, physical examination, previous ECG strips, and all laboratory tests.
II. Make a general inspection of the ECG.
  A. Is normal sinus rhythm or a cardiac arrhythmia present?
  B. If an arrhythmia is present, does it occur rarely, frequently, intermittently, or continuously? Is it uniform or multiform?
  C. Is the arrhythmia clinically insignificant or significant? Does it correlate with specific clinical signs?
  D. Are provocative maneuvers (e.g., exercise, ocular or carotid sinus pressure) or pharmacologic intervention (e.g., intravenous lidcoaine) required to further evaluate an arrhythmia?

Systematic Approach to the ECG Strip

I. Sinus rhythm or arrhythmia?
II. Heart rate rapid, slow, or normal?

III. Do the P (atrial) waves occur at regular or irregular intervals? What is the height, width, direction?
IV. Do the QRS (ventricular) complexes occur with regularity, and uniformity? What is their morphology?
V. What is the relationship between the P waves and the QRS complexes? The P-R interval is a measurement of atrioventricular (AV) conduction time. Is the P-R interval of normal duration, regular or irregular, or is there no consistent relationship between the P wave and QRS complex?
VI. In summarizing the above findings, is the predominant rhythm sinus, atrial, AV junctional or ventricular? Is the arrhythmia a disorder of impulse formation, conduction, or both?

QUESTIONS TO BE ANSWERED IN THE FINAL INTERPRETATION OF A CARDIAC ARRHYTHMIA

I. What is the possible mechanism for the arrhythmia?
  A. Is there an abnormal impulse formation?
  B. Is it atrial, AV junctional, or ventricular in origin?
  C. Is there a conduction abnormality?
II. Is the P wave present? Where does it start? Is it related to the QRS complex?
  A. If the P wave is not related to the QRS complex, what is the abnormality causing the AV dissociation?
III. What reason or abnormality explains the absence of the P wave?
  A. Is the P wave superimposed on a portion of the QRS complex, S-T segment, or T wave?
  B. Is the arrhythmia atrial standstill, atrial fibrillation, atrial flutter, AV junctional escape rhythm, or atrial tachycardia?
IV. If AV dissociation is present, where does the QRS complex evolve from?
  A. Is there an AV junctional and/or purkinje or idioventricular foci involved?
V. Is the wide and bizarre QRS complex due to a ventricular arrhythmia or caused by a premature atrial impulse that is aberrantly conducted (refer to atrial premature complexes, P : QRS characteristics)?

A. What are the differential possibilities of the arrhythmia?

VI. What is the clinical significance of the arrhythmia?

A. Is specific therapy required?

B. What is the best immediate therapy?

THERAPEUTIC APPROACH

I. Have a precise diagnosis for the arrhythmia, if possible.

II. Eliminate noncardiac causes (e.g., acid–base and electrolyte abnormalities, hypothermia, hypovolemia, hypoxemia, and other systemic problems) before using an antiarrhythmic drug.

A. Stop other drug therapy if it may be the cause of the arrhythmia (e.g., digitalis, quinidine, procainamide, xylazine, and acetylpromazine).

B. Correct electrolyte disturbances or metabolic abnormalities with appropriate fluid and supportive therapy (e.g., hypokalemia may predispose to an arrhythmia that is refractory to therapy).

III. The purpose of drug therapy for cardiac arrhythmias is to prevent clinical signs such as weakness, syncope, seizures, personality changes, and congestive heart failure. Also drug therapy may decrease electrical instability and the likelihood of progression to a malignant arrhythmia (e.g., ventricular fibrillation).

IV. Select the antiarrhythmic drug best suited to the underlying cause of the arrhythmia (e.g., phenytoin for digitalis-induced tachyarrhythmias, lidocaine to terminate supraventricular arrhythmias, or atrial fibrillation over an anomalous pathway in the Wolff–Parkkinson–White syndrome (WPW) rather than digoxin or propranolol).

V. Be familiar with recommended dose ranges of the various antiarrhythmic drugs (see section on antiarrhythmic therapy).

VI. Be aware of synergistic effects of antiarrhythmic drugs (e.g., digoxin and propranolol may additively delay AV conduction) and antagonistic effects (e.g., quinidine may increase serum digoxin levels, increasing the possibility of digoxin toxicity). Refractory arrhythmias may require a combination of antiarrhythmic agents, although the possibility of drug-related toxicity may increase (e.g., digoxin and propranolol, procainamide and propranolol, quinidine and propranolol, procainamide and diazepam, and quinidine and diazepam).

VII. Be aware that some arrhythmias may rquire antiarrhythmic drugs in addition to other therapeutic modalities (e.g., sick sinus syndrome patients with bradyarrhythmia–tachyarrhythmias may require a permanent cardiac pacemaker for the bradyarrhythmia and an antiarrhythmic drug for the tachyarrhythmia). For ventricular tachycardia due to quinidine or procainamide toxicity, conventional antiarrhythmic drugs may worsen this arrhythmia. Stopping the drug and administering sodium bicarbonate, isoproterenol, or dopamine may prove effective in controlling this toxic arrhythmia.

GENERAL MANAGEMENT OF ARRHYTHMIAS

PREMATURE COMPLEXES

I. Treat the underlying problem (e.g., surgical correction of a pyometra with toxic myocarditis).

II. If premature complexes are frequent (> 20 to 30 per minute) and/or correlated with clinical signs or underlying cardiac disease (e.g., chronic valvular disease, cardiomyopathy), antiarrhythmic agents should be considered.

III. Digitalis may be effective when atrial premature complexes (APCs) or ventricular premature complexes (VPCs) are associated with congestive heart failure (CHF). If digitalis is used for congestive heart failure complicated by frequent VPCs, the ECG should be monitored every few days to determine whether the arrhythmia is worsening or resolving.

MANAGEMENT OF SUPRAVENTRICULAR TACHYARRHYTHMIAS

I. A vagal maneuver (e.g., ocular or carotid sinus pressure) is often effective in terminating paroxysmal atrial or AV junctional tachycardia. The dive reflex (i.e., immersing the head in cool water) may also be an effective maneuver. A vagal maneuver increases parasympathetic stimulation to the sinus and AV nodes.

II. Digitalis is the drug of choice for atrial fibrillation, producing a rapid ventricular response in the dog and cat.

III. If digitalis toxicity is a consideration, the drug should be stopped immediately. Phenytoin may be effective in terminating the arrhythmia in the dog.

IV. Intravenous or oral propranolol may be effective in terminating a supraventricular tachyarrhythmia not complicated by congestive heart failure (beware of hypotension, bradycardia, and AV block).

V. Verapamil, a new antiarrhythmic drug, is effective for the treatment of supraventricular tachyarrhythmias with a reentrant mechanism in the dog. Verapamil is a calcium channel blocker; it is not well established in veterinary medicine.

VI. Direct current (DC) shock (cardioversion, refer to Chapter 14) is reserved for a severe tachyarrhythmia that is refractory to antiarrhythmic therapy in a patient that remains symptomatic. Use of a cardioverter synchronized to the QRS complex of the ECG is mandatory. This method should not be employed by an inexperienced clinician. Electrical shock administered during the electrical vunerable period (Q-T interval on the ECG) will likely result in ventricular fibrillation. Digoxin toxicity is a contraindication for DC shock.

VII. The use of temporary pacemakers and premature electrical stimulation or overdrive suppression of the arrhythmia is another therapeutic modality, although not established in veterinary medicine. Specialized equipment is again required.

Ventricular Arrhythmias

I. Intravenous lidocaine without epinephrine is the drug of choice for the treatment of ventricular tachycardia in the canine patient. Procainamide and quinidine are the next most commonly used drugs.

II. Electrolyte and metabolic abnormalities must be treated with appropriate fluid therapy.

III. Disopyramide and propranolol are less commonly used for the treatment of ventricular tachycardia.

IV. Lidocaine and phenytoin are the drugs of choice for ventricular tachycardia induced by digitalis toxicity.
V. Underlying problems (e.g., congestive heart failure) must also be treated.
VI. DC shock should be reserved for refractory ventricular arrhythmias in patients that are symptomatic and should be administered by clinicians experienced with the specialized equipment.

SPECIFIC CARDIAC ARRHYTHMIAS

Sinus Rhythms

Normal Sinus Rhythm

I. Location
Impulses are generated from the sinus node.
II. Heart rate and rhythm
A. 70 to 160 beats/min (bpm) dog; (up to 180 bpm in toy breeds and 220 bpm in the pup); 160 to 240 bpm in the cat.
B. The rhythm is regular with less than a 10 percent variation in the R-R interval.
III. P : QRS characteristics
There is a normal P wave for each QRS complex, with a constant P-R interval (Fig. 13-1A,B).
IV. Differentials
None.
V. Significance
This is a normal cardiac rhythm in the dog and cat.
VI. Treatment
None.

Sinus Arrhythmia

I. Location
Impulses are generated from the sinus node.

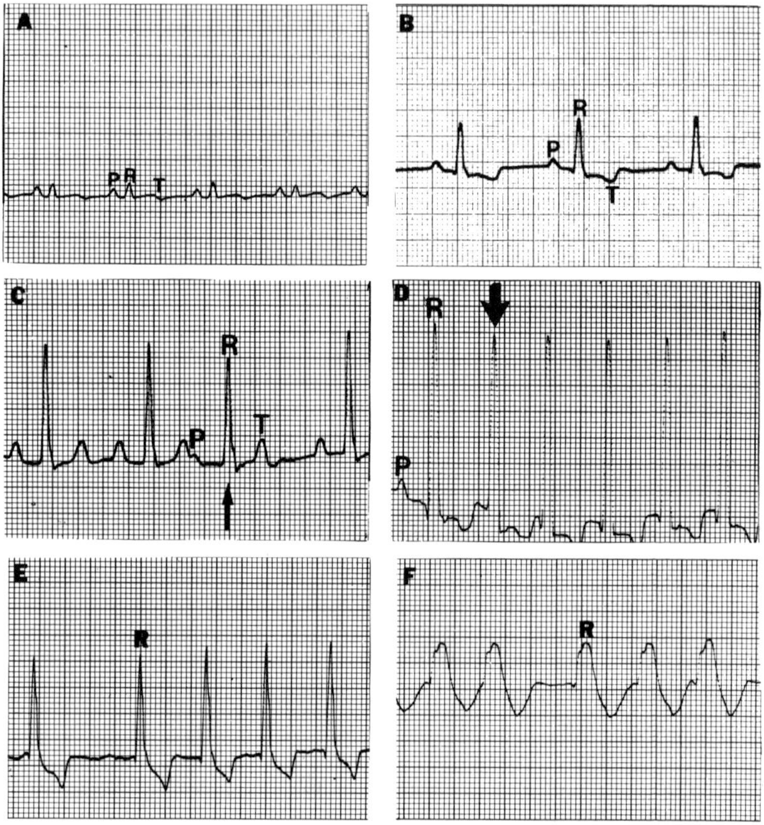

Fig. 13-1. Selected sinus and supraventricular rhythms. Lead II rhythm strips, paper speed = 50 mm/sec; 1 cm = 1 mV. (A) Normal sinus rhythm, cat. (B) Normal sinus rhythm, dog. (C) Atrial premature complex (arrow), dog. (D) Paroxysmal atrial tachycardia (begins at arrow), dog. (E) Atrial fibrillation, dog. (F) Atrial fibrillation with left bundle branch block, dog.

II. Heart rate and rhythm

70 to 160 bpm dog; 160 to 240 bpm in the cat. The rhythm is irregular with greater than a 10 percent variation in the R-R interval.

III. P : QRS characteristics

There is a normal P wave for each QRS complex, with a constant

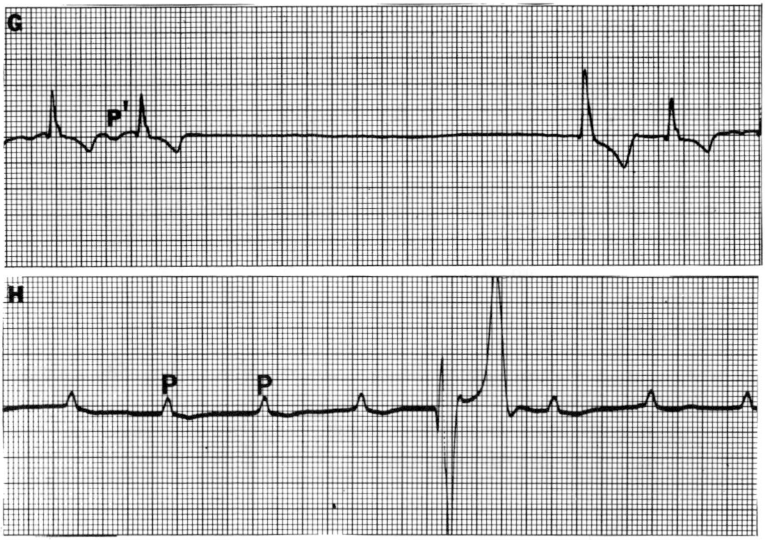

Fig. 13-1(*Cont.*) (G) AV junctional rhythm (negative P′ waves) with a period of sinus block and/or arrest with a low AV junctional or ventricular escape beat, dog. (H) complete AV block, dog.

P-R interval. A wandering pacemaker (P waves vary in shape) is often present.

IV. Differentials

Atrial premature complexes (APCs).

V. Significance

A. Sinus arrhythmia is a normal cardiac rhythm in the dog but is very unusual in the cat.

B. Sinus arrhythmia is correlated with a variation in vagal tone, usually in synchronization with respiration. This rhythm may be coupled with a wandering pacemaker (alteration in P-wave morphology due to a change in site of impulse origination or conduction through the atria).

C. A wandering pacemaker is also of normal variation in the dog.

VI. Treatment

None, unless associated with a symptomatic sinus bradycardia.

Sinus Bradycardia

I. Location

Impulses are generated in the sinus node but at a slower than normal frequency.

II. Heart rate and rhythm

A. Less than 70 bpm in the dog (less than 60 bpm in large breeds) and less than 160 bpm in the cat.

B. The rhythm is regular, with a slight variation in the R-R interval.

III. P : QRS characteristics

A. There is a normal P wave for each QRS complex. The P-R interval is constant.

B. AV junctional or ventricular escape complexes may occur as well as atrial or ventricular premature complexes.

IV. Differentials

Marked sinus arrhythmia.

V. Significance

Sinus bradycardia is associated with:

A. Various clinical abnormalities including hypothermia, endocrinopathies (e.g., hypothyroidism, Addison's disease)

B. Drugs (e.g., acetylpromazine, xylazine, digoxin, propranolol, edrophonium chloride, pilocarpine, general anesthesia)

C. Diseases associated with an increase in vagal stimulation (e.g., neurologic, pharyngeal, gastrointestinal, respiratory)

D. Sick sinus syndrome

VI. Treatment

A. Sinus bradycardia is usually self-limiting and does not require therapy; it is important to correct any underlying disorders.

B. If clinical signs such as weakness or syncope develop, parenteral atropine or glycopyrrolate (intramuscular or subcutaneous route is preferred) is used initially.

C. Sympathomimetic agents such as epinephrine, isoproterenol, or dopamine may be used in emergency (cardiac arrest) situations, although other severe arrhythmias may be triggered by these drugs.

D. Artificial pacing is sometimes necessary with symptomatic bradycardia unresponsive to drug therapy.

Sinus Tachycardia

I. Location
Impulses are generated in the sinus node but at a faster than normal frequency.

II. Heart rate and rhythm
A. The rate is greater than 180 bpm in the dog and 240 bpm in the cat.
B. The rhythm is regular.

III. P : QRS characteristics
A. There is a normal P wave for each QRS complex with a constant P-R interval.
B. The P waves may be partially or completely fused with preceding T waves.

IV. Differentials
A. Paroxysmal atrial tachycardia, atrial flutter with 2 : 1 AV block, and AV junctional tachycardia are included.
B. A vagal maneuver (e.g., ocular or carotid sinus pressure for 5 to 10 seconds) may clarify identification of the arrhythmia.

V. Significance
Sinus tachycardia may occur with stress, anxiety, pain, shock, anemia, fever, congestive heart failure, hyperthyroidism, drugs (e.g., atropine, sympathomimetic agents), functional pheochromocytoma, light anesthesia, and numerous other causes.

VI. Treatment
Depending on the patient's clinical status, the specific cause of the rapid heart rate should be established and treated. Although there are exceptions, antiarrhythmic agents are not required. For congestive heart failure, digitalis and diuretic therapy may improve cardiac output and lessen sympathetic tone to the sinus node. For hyperthyroidism without congestive heart failure, propranolol may be useful in decreasing the cardiac rate.

Supraventricular Rhythms

Atrial Premature Complexes (APCs)

I. Location
Impulses originate from an atrial focus other than the sinus node (ectopic focus).

II. Heart rate and rhythm

The heart rate varies depending on the intrinsic sinus node rate and frequency of the APCs; the rhythm is irregular.

III. P : QRS characteristics

There is usually an abnormal P′ wave (premature P wave) followed by a normal QRS complex; the P′-R interval of the APC may vary from the sinus rhythm P-R interval. The P′ wave may have various morphologies and may be fused with the T wave of the preceding beat. The P′ wave may occur so early in the cardiac cycle that it will find the AV conduction system refractory and the impulse will not be conducted to the ventricles (e.g., APC with physiologic AV block). The pause following the APC is often less than fully compensatory (R wave before and after R wave of APC is equal to two normal R-R intervals) due to premature depolarization and resetting of the sinus node (Figure 13-1C). The QRS complex is usually normal, but an early APC may find the ventricular conduction system in a relative refractory period and result in a bizarre (abnormal shape or direction) QRS complex. This abnormality is termed an APC with aberrant ventricular conduction. This aberrant QRS complex is often confused with a VPC. Aberrant ventricular conduction commonly occurs in humans with a long R wave to R wave interval preceding an APC with a prolonged P-R interval; it is termed *Ashman's phenomenon*. A short coupling interval (duration between previous normal P wave and ectopic P′ wave) to the APC also favors aberrant conduction.

IV. Differentials

A. Marked sinus arrhythmia and VPCs when aberrant ventricular conduction follows an APC.

B. A P′ wave preceding the abnormal QRS complex and a similarity of the initial deflection of the QRS complex with a preceding normal beat would support aberrant conduction.

C. In humans, about 90 percent of aberrantly conducted beats have the pattern of a right bundle branch block.

V. Significance

A. APCs often indicate underlying cardiac disease (e.g., chronic valvular fibrosis, cardiomyopathy, congenital defect, or cor pulmonale).

B. Other causes include electrolyte disturbances, hypoxia, drug toxicity (e.g., digitalis), toxemias, and increased sympathetic tone.

C. APCs may progress to other supraventricular arrhythmias such as paroxysmal atrial tachycardia and atrial fibrillation.

VI. Treatment

A. Infrequent APCs may be a normal variation and do not require treatment.

B. If this arrhythmia is correlated with congestive heart failure, digoxin and diuretic therapy is used initially. If the APCs are correlated with poor hemodynamic status without congestive heart failure, then digoxin, propranolol, quinidine, or procainamide may be considered in the above order of preference.

C. If congestive heart failure is not present, digoxin may increase the frequency of the atrial premature contractions due to its effect of shortening the atrial myocardial cell refractory period as well as by other complex mechanisms.

Sinus Arrest and/or Block

I. Location

A primary disorder in the sinus node resulting in lack of generation of the cardiac impulse or its poor propagation through surrounding tissue may cause sinus arrest and/or sinus block. It is not possible to distinguish between sinus block or arrest in the dog due to the normal variation in the R-R interval (sinus arrhythmia).

II. Heart rate and rhythm

A. The rate is variable and is often correlated with a bradycardia or slow sinus arrhythmia.

B. The rhythm is regularly irregular or irregular with pauses.

III. P : QRS characteristics

There is a normal P wave for each QRS complex with a pause equal to or greater than two times the normal R-R interval (Fig. 13-1G). The P wave may vary in shape if a concurrent wandering pacemaker is present. The P-R interval is constant.

IV. Differentials

Marked sinus arrhythmia and sinus bradycardia are included.

V. Significance

A. Sinus arrest may be consistent with an increase in vagal tone (e.g., ocular pressure, brachycephalic breeds, irritation of the vagus nerve).

B. Pathology of the atria including fibrosis, cardiomyopathy, neoplasia, and drug toxicity (e.g., digitalis, propranolol, quinidine, xylazine, and acetylpromazine) may result in sinus arrest.

C. Sinus arrest is one of the complex arrhythmias in the sick sinus syndrome (SSS) that affects small breed dogs including the Miniature Schnauzer, Dachsund, Pug, and Cocker Spaniel. Often there is concurrent AV nodal disease producing AV block and/or paroxysmal atrial tachycardia.

VI. Treatment

A. Asymptomatic dogs or cats require no specific therapy.

B. When correlated with signs of weakness or syncope, an atropine response test should be performed (0.04 mg/kg IM) followed by a follow-up ECG in 15 to 30 miutes.

C. If there is a decrease in the sinus pauses or an increase in the cardiac rate following atropine, the patient may benefit from oral anticholinergic agents. A poor clinical response suggests the need for a temporary or permanent cardiac pacemaker.

D. Congestive heart failure may also develop, in which case diuretics and vasodilators must be considered as the preferred treatment. Digitalis may exacerbate the sinus arrest in these cases, although it may be warranted if a demand pacemaker is utilized, and/or if the patient is carefully monitored.

Atrial Tachycardia

I. Location

A. Impulses originate from an atrial site other than the sinus node.

B. The atrium and AV junctional areas are also involved (a reentrant circuit that allows the impulse to restimulate the atrium as well as to pass to the ventricles). An abnormal automatic focus in the atrium may also be responsible for this arrhythmia.

II. Heart rate and rhythm

A. The rate is above 160 to 180 in the dog; and above 240 bpm in the cat.

B. The rhythm is usually regular, but may be slightly irregular.

III. P : QRS characteristics

There is a P′ wave for each QRS complex, although the P wave is usually of different morphology than the sinus P wave. The P-R interval is constant. The P wave may not be visualized as it may be fused with the T wave or occur simultaneously with the preceding QRS complex (Fig. 13-1D). The QRS complex may also be of different morphology due to aberrant conduction through the ventricular conduction system. An irregular R wave to R wave interval may be caused by concurrent AV block, or multifocal atrial tachycardia (P′ waves vary in shape; firing of two or more ectopic atrial foci).

IV. Differentials

Sinus tachycardia, AV junctional tachycardia, and atrial flutter.

V. Significance

A. Persistent (nonparoxysmal) atrial tachycardia supports severe myocardial or conduction system disease. This arrhythmia may also be secondary to digitalis toxicity or may occur under general anesthesia.

B. Systemic disease that results in autonomic nervous systemic abnormalities may also be causative.

C. In the cat, this arrhythmia is correlated with feline cardiomyopathy, hyperthyroidism, and other types of systemic disease.

VI. Treatment

A. Sustained (nonparoxysmal atrial tachycardia) is often correlated with weakness, hypotension, and syncope and requires immediate therapy.

B. If acute or chronic congestive heart failure is present, intense therapy including oxygen, cage rest, diuretics and digitalis is required. Intravenous fluid therapy and corticosteroids may be required for hypotension and shock.

C. Vagal maneuver (mild ocular pressure or carotid sinus pressure) may effectively terminate a reentrant atrial tachycardia (Fig. 13-3C). A vagal maneuver may also slow down the sinus rate and reveal sinus tachycardia or cause AV block and unmask atrial flutter (Fig. 13-3D), both differentials of atrial tachycardia.

D. Intravenous digoxin may slow the ventricular response and improve the clinical status. If digoxin is not effective, intravenous propranolol or verapamil (treatment of choice in humans) may convert atrial tachycardia to sinus rhythm or slow down the ventricular rate. The latter two drugs must be used with caution as they may decrease cardiac contractility and exacerbate congestive heart failure. Intramuscular quinidine gluconate has also been used to convert atrial tachycardia to normal sinus rhythm in dogs with refractory atrial tachycardia.

E. Electrophysiologic pacing methods such as overdrive suppression or premature atrial stimulation may also be effective in terminating atrial tachycardia but should only be used by an experienced clinician. DC shock should be reserved for refractory cases and only by a veterinarian experienced with this technique and possessing the proper equipment.

Atrial Fibrillation

I. Location

A high number of disorganized atrial impulses bombarding the AV node is responsible for this arrhythmia. Many of these impulses approach the AV node in a refractory period and are not conducted to the ventricles.

II. Heart rate and rhythm

A. The rate is usually rapid, often above 180 bpm in the dog, and above 240 bpm in the cat.

B. The rhythm is very irregular and is correlated with an arterial pulse deficit.

III. P : QRS characteristics

No P waves are seen and there are normally shaped QRS complexes. Instead of P waves, small or large oscillations (f waves) are present. The interval between successive QRS complexes is very irregular because of intermittent AV block (Fig. 13-1E). There may be some variation and widening of the QRS complexes due to aberrant ventricular conduction or bundle branch block.

IV. Differentials

A. Frequent atrial premature complexes, AV junctional tachycardia with AV block, supraventricular tachycardia with AV block and atrial flutter with AV block are included.

B. Atrial flutter usually shows a regular R-R interval and the atrial oscillations (F waves) are larger than f waves (Fig. 13-3D).

V. Significance
   A. Atrial fibrillation is a severe arrhythmia and commonly occurs in patients with cardiomyopathy, advanced chronic valvular disease, and progressive congenital heart disease.
   B. Other etiologies include severe ischemia or shock (gastric dilatation and after cardiac arrest), atrial tumor (hemangiosarcoma), or electrolyte disturbances (hyperkalemia).
   C. Loss of atrial contraction decreases the stroke volume and cardiac output. The rapid ventricular rate also results in poor cardiac output. Slow atrial fibrillation (below 100 bpm) may signify concurrent AV block.

VI. Treatment
   A. Underlying congestive heart failure must be controlled. Digoxin is used to slow the ventricular response. Diuretics and vasodilator agents may be added as required. After approximately 5 to 7 days, if the ventricular rate is not controlled, propranolol may be added at a low dose. The propranolol dose is increased slowly until the ventricular rate is adequately controlled ($<$ 140 to 160 bpm). The lowest possible dose of propranolol will lessen the negative inotropic effects.
   B. Although it is unusual to convert atrial fibrillation to normal sinus rhythm in dogs, the antiarrhythmic drug quinidine may be useful for this purpose. A normal-size heart and lack of congestive heart failure favors the use of quinidine. In certain cases, digitalis may also convert atrial fibrillation to normal sinus rhythm.
   C. Lidocaine should be avoided, as it may increase AV conduction and lead to an even more rapid ventricular response.
   D. DC shock should be reserved for refractory cases without severe cardiomegaly. Experienced personnel and proper equipment are essential.

Atrioventricular Junctional Rhythm

I. Location

Impulses are generated in the AV junctional tissue and spread backward (retrograde) through the atrium and forward (antegrade) to the ventricles.

II. Heart rate and rhythm
  A. The heart rate is variable (usually > 60 bpm) depending on passive escape rhythm versus enhanced AV junctional rhythm (60 bpm but < 100 bpm in the dog).
  B. The rhythm is usually regular.

III. P : QRS characteristics
The negative P′ wave may occur before, during, or after the normal QRS complex. The P′-R interval is constant, or R-P′ interval may be variable. The P′-wave location depends on the area of impulse generation, and relative speed of retrograde conduction through the atrium compared with antegrade conduction through the AV node, His bundle, and ventricular conduction system.

IV. Differentials
Atrial standstill and slow atrial fibrillation are included.

V. Significance
  A. Digitalis toxicity may cause an AV junctional rhythm. When abnormally rapid, this arrhythmia is difficult to distinguish from atrial tachycardia.
  B. An AV junctional escape rhythm may occur in patients with depressed sinus node function as in the sick sinus syndrome.

VI. Treatment
  A. Usually no treatment is needed and the rhythm reverts spontaneously.
  B. If weakness or syncope is associated with a slow AV junctional rhythm, atropine or isoproterenol may be used in an attempt to accelerate the sinus node in order to help regain function as the primary pacemaker.
  C. Oral anticholinergic agents may also be useful for chronic therapy. If congestive heart failure is present with an enhanced AV junctional rhythm, digitalis, diuretic, and vasodilator therapy may be needed.

Ventricular Arrhythmias

Ventricular Premature Complexes (VPCs)

I. Location
Ectopic impulses are generated from a focus below the AV node and AV junction.

II. Heart rate and rhythm

The rate is variable, depending on the frequency of VPCs; the rhythm is irregular. VPCs are usually related (coupled) to normal beats. If the VPCs are not coupled to a normal beat, the origination site is referred to as a parasystolic focus. There is usually a full compensatory pause (interval between the VPC and following sinus P wave) following a VPC as the ectopic beat does not usually conduct back to the atrium and affect the spontaneous sinus node discharge rate. Interpolated VPCs occur between normal beats and are not usually followed by a full compensatory pause.

III. P : QRS characteristics

P waves that are seen are normal in shape, but are not associated with the QRS complex of the VPCs. The QRS complex is often wide and bizarre. If the major deflection of the QRS complex is negative in lead II, the ectopic focus is in the left ventricle (Fig. 13-2A); if the major deflection is positive in lead II, the ectopic focus is in the right ventricle (Fig. 13-2B).

IV. Differentials

Atrial premature complexes with aberrant ventricular conduction and right or left bundle branch block are included.

V. Significance

A. Frequent VPCs, runs of VPCs, multifocal VPCs, or VPCs occurring during the Q-T interval of the previous beat may be dangerous. The ventricular arrhythmia may be due to cardiac disease (e.g., congestive heart failure, myocarditis, endocarditis).

B. Secondary causes of VPCs include trauma, electrolyte disturbances, autonomic changes, hypoxia, and ischemia. Frequent VPCs may lead to hypotension, shock, or congestive heart failure.

C. Frequent VPCs or VPCs occurring during the preceding Q-T interval may be electrically unstable and may proceed to ventricular tachycardia and/or fibrillation and sudden death.

VI. Treatment

A. VPCs do not always require antiarrhythmic therapy. A medical data base including a thoracic radiograph, CBC and blood chemistry screen, and urinalysis is essential to rule out secondary causes of VPCs, which may require specific supportive therapy. Underlying congestive heart failure should be controlled with digitalis or other inotropic agents, diuretic and vasodilator therapy.

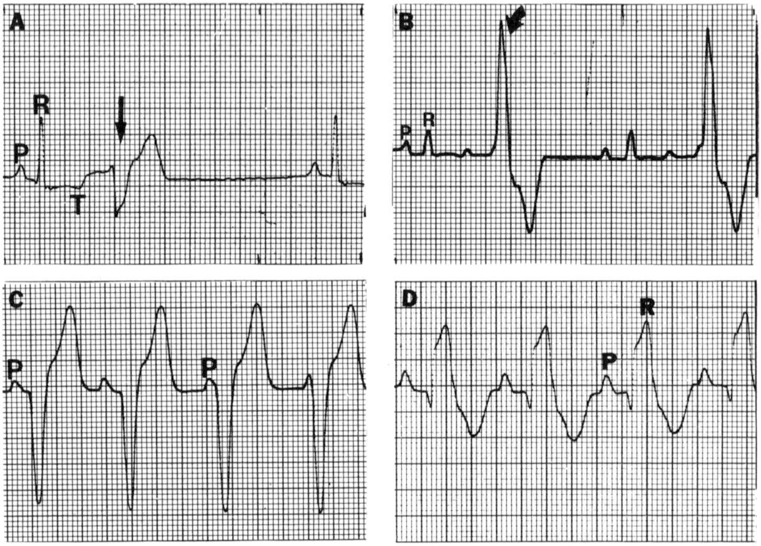

Fig. 13-2. Selected ventricular arrhythmias. Lead II rhythm strips, paper speed = 50 mm/sec; 1 cm = 1 mV. (A) Left ventricular premature complex (arrow), dog. (B) Right ventricular premature complex (arrow), cat. (C) Ventricular tachycardia (P waves not related to QRS complexes), dog. (D) Left bundle branch block (can be confused with ventricular tachycardia, although note the constant P-R interval), dog.

B. Antiarrhythmic therapy is advocated with frequent VPCs (greater than 20 to 30 per minute); repetitive complexes or runs of VPCs; multifocal QRS configurations; R on T phenomena (vulnerable period for development of ventricular fibrillation, Fig. 13-2E), where the VPC occurs during the Q-T interval of the previous complex; and where clinical signs of poor cardiac output (e.g., weakness, dyspnea, and syncope) occur.

C. Ventricular escape complexes (similar to VPC configuration) should not be treated as they represent a safety mechanism for maintaining cardiac output.

D. Antiarrhythmic drugs commonly used to control VPCs include intravenous lidocaine and parenteral or oral procainamide, quinidine, disopyramide, propranolol and phenytoin (digitalis-induced VPCs). New antiarrhythmic agents that are being investigated for VPCs include aprindine, amiodarone, and mexiletine.

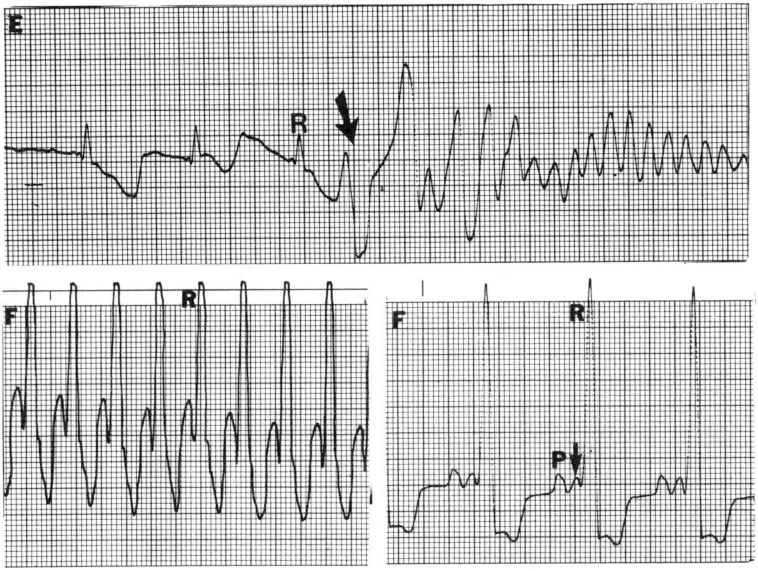

Fig. 13-2(*Cont.*) (E) Ventricular fibrillation initiated by a forceful blow to the chest (during a Q-T interval) in a suspected cardiac arrest, dog. (F) (*left*) Supraventricular or ventricular tachycardia; (*right*) IV lidocaine interrupts the tachycardia and reveals ventricular preexcitation with a short P-R interval and delta wave (arrow) supporting the Wolff–Parkinson–White syndrome.

Ventricular Tachycardia

I. Impulses are repetitively generated (greater than 3 VPCs in a row) from one or more ventricular foci. This arrhythmia may be paroxysmal or sustained.

II. Heart rate and rhythm
   A. The rate is usually above 100 bpm in the dog; and usually above 150 bpm in the cat.
   B. The rhythm is regular unless the arrhythmia is intermittent.

III. P : QRS characteristics
   The P waves that are seen are normal in shape but have no fixed relationship to wide and bizarre QRS complexes. The P waves occur before, during or after the QRS complexes, but have no fixed relationship (Fig. 13-2C).

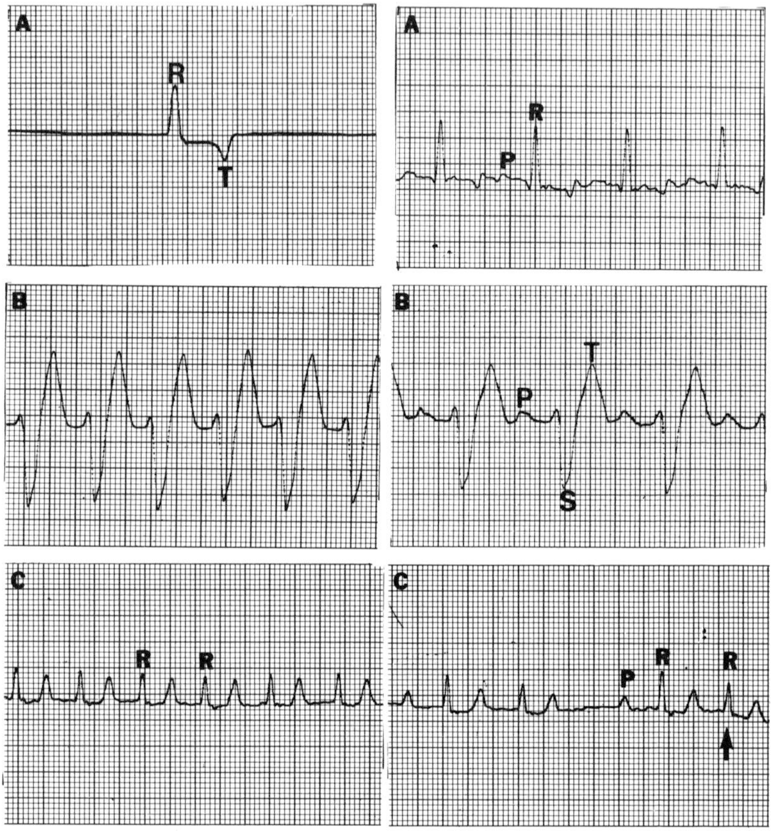

Fig. 13-3. Selected arrhythmias before and after treatment. Lead II rhythm strips, paper speed = 50 mm/sec; 1 cm = 1 mV. (A) (*left*) Atrial standstill; (*right*) Thirty minutes after IV normal saline and sodium bicarbonate, a conversion to normal sinus rhythm, dog. (B) (*left*) Suspected ventricular tachycardia; (*right*) IV lidocaine slows the cardiac rate and reveals right bundle branch block (prelidocaine ECG shows atrial tachycardia with right bundle branch block), dog. (C) (*left*) Supraventricular tachycardia; (*right*) A vagal maneuver breaks the tachycardia abruptly (atrial premature complex, arrow), supporting an atrial tachycardia, dog.

IV. Differentials

A. Sinus tachycardia, atrial tachycardia, or atrial fibrillation with a conduction disturbance (e.g., left or right bundle branch block) (Figs. 13-1F, 13-2D, 13-3B) are included.

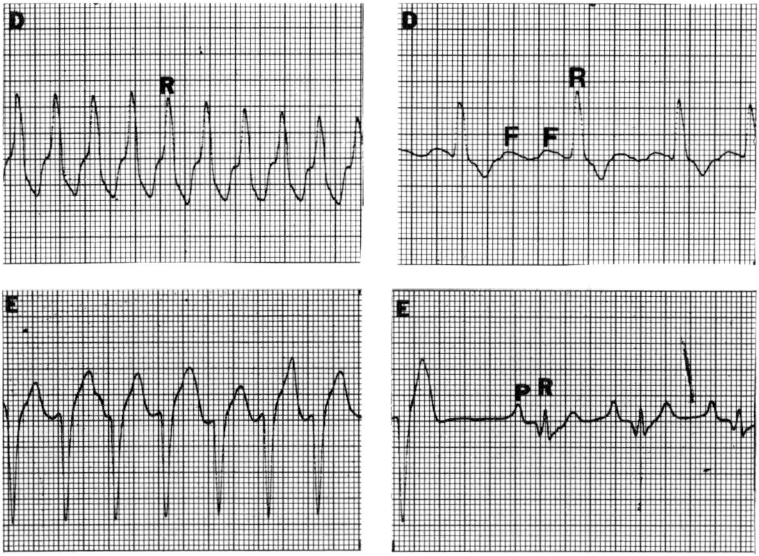

Fig. 13-3(*Cont.*) (D) (*left*) Supraventricular tachycardia; (*right*) a vagal maneuver results in varying degrees of AV block and atrial flutter, with flutter waves (F) and irregular R-R intervals, dog. (E) (*left*) Ventricular tachycardia; (*right*) IV lidocaine converts ventricular tachycardia to normal sinus rhythm, dog.

B. A sustained ventricular rhythm slower than the above rates is termed an idioventricular rhythm.

V. Significance

A. Ventricular tachycardia is a life-threatening arrhythmia that, if sustained, may lead to hypotension, myocardial ischemia, syncope or seizures, and shock.

B. Some patients with ventricular tachycardia may show no clinical signs, especially if there is no underlying primary cardiac disease.

C. This arrhythmia is electrically unstable and may lead to ventricular fibrillation and sudden death.

D. All etiologies of VPCs (e.g., primary and secondary cardiac disease) may lead to a ventricular tachycardia.

VI. Treatment

A. Antiarrhythmic therapy is required in most patients with ventricular tachycardia. Exceptions include patients with complete heart block where the ventricular rhythm may be an escape mechanism, and severe acid–base or electrolyte disturbances, such as hypokalemia or hyperkalemia, which may respond to specific electrolyte or fluid therapy.

B. Lidocaine hydrochloride without epinephrine (2 to 3 mg/kg) via slow intravenous administration is the initial preferred treatment in the dog (Fig. 13-3E). This drug may also be used in the cat (0.5 mg/kg slow IV—beware of seizures). Seizures require intravenous diazepam. Hypotension may also occur if the bolus is administered too rapidly. The lidocaine bolus may have to be repeated several times at 10 minute intervals, although, the higher dosages will increase the incidence of toxicity. A maximum total dose of 8 mg/kg is advised in the dog. Seizures will often occur before this dose is reached in the cat. Seizures may also occur in the dog at toxic doses.

C. The therapeutic effect of lidocaine is short termed and repeat boluses or constant rate infusion may be required for a sustained antiarrhythmic effect (see antiarrhythmic drug section). If the ventricular arrhythmia is stable, intramuscular or oral therapy with procainamide or quinidine may be initiated and the lidocaine infusion slowly reduced over a 24- to 48-hour period. Hypokalemia and acidosis may cause therapeutic failure and must be treated.

D. When treatment with lidocaine is not indicated or practical, intramuscular quinidine or procainamide may be used to provide initial control of ventricular tachycardia. An initial loading dose of 12 to 20 mg/kg followed by repeat doses of four to six hour intervals at 6 to 12 mg/kg. Prolonged therapy may be continued with oral quinidine or procainamide at appropriate doses. Other antiarrhythmic drugs that may be useful include disopyramide, propranolol, phenytoin, and aprindine.

E. DC shock should be reserved for the refractory arrhythmia and requires an experienced clinician and proper equipment.

F. The ECG should be monitored at frequent intervals. If the arrhythmia is poorly controlled, the advantage of increasing the drug dosage versus side effects must be considered. If the arrhythmia worsens, antiarrhythmic drug toxicity must be considered as a cause of this abnormality. Multiform ventricular tachycardia due to procainamide or quinidine toxicity may be a life-threatening complication of antiarrhythmic medication (torsades de pointes).

G. Combinations of drugs such as procainamide and quinidine, procainamide and propranolol, or added diazepam may be beneficial in refractory cases. The disadvantages of toxicity with combination therapy must be weighed against potential benefit.

H. If the arrhythmia is well-controlled, it may be attempted to stop or slowly wean (controversial) the patient off the antiarrhythmic agent after a 2- to 3-week period. Attempting to stop the medication will avoid complications of long-term therapy and the great expense of antiarrhythmic drugs. The ECG must be evaluated before each decrease in dosage, or within one week after stopping the medication.

Ventricular Asystole

I. Location
No impulses are generated from atrial or ventricular pacemakers.

II. Heart rate and rhythm
There is no cardiac rate or ventricular rhythm.

III. P : QRS characteristics
P waves are of normal shape with complete AV block or are not present. No QRS complexes are seen.

IV. Differentials
Artifact (e.g., electrocardiograph is not on a proper lead or is connected improperly).

V. Significance
It is associated with cardiac arrest and has a very grave prognosis.

VI. Treatment

A. Cardiopulmonary resuscitation must be undertaken immediately.

B. Pharmacologic intervention with epinephrine, calcium chloride, sodium bicarbonate, and appropriate fluids is mandatory.

C. An effective approach in human patients is to convert asystole to ventricular fibrillation followed by DC shock.

Ventricular Fibrillation

I. Location

Impulses are generated and propagated in the ventricles in a chaotic, asynchronous manner.

II. Heart rate and rhythm

A. The heart rate is rapid and disorganized.

B. The rhythm is irregular.

III. P : QRS characteristics

None are seen. There are no P waves present and there are no recognizable QRS complexes. There are continuous positive and negative oscillations that are chaotic and bizarre (Fig. 13-2E). The oscillations may be large (coarse) or small (fine).

IV. Differentials

Artifact (e.g., 60-cycle electrical interference or respiratory movement) is included.

V. Significance

A. The most common arrhythmia associated with cardiac arrest is ventricular fibrillation.

B. There is no effective cardiac output.

C. Conditions such as myocardial ischemia, electrolyte imbalance, hypoxia, hypothermia, slow conduction, increased automaticity, drugs, and unstable ventricular arrhythmias trigger ventricular fibrillation.

D. Ventricular fibrillation carries a very grave prognosis.

VI. Treatment

A. Cardiopulmonary resuscitation must be undertaken immediately.

B. Electrical defibrillation requires specialized equipment but is mandatory.

C. Intracardiac lidocaine or propranolol may occasionally be successful in converting ventricular fibrillation to normal sinus rhythm.

D. Open-chest cardiac massage may be effective in converting ventricular fibrillation to normal sinus rhythm if no electrical cardioverter is available. External blows to the chest (thump-version) is less effective.

E. Supportive therapy with IV fluids, and sodium bicarbonate may be useful in reestablishing normal electrolyte and acid–base balance.

Conduction Disturbances

Atrial Standstill

I. Location:
   Impulses are not generated in the sinus node or are poorly conducted through the atrial tissues.
II. Heart rate and rhythm
   A. The rate is less than 60 bpm in the dog; less than 160 bpm in the cat.
   B. The rhythm is regular.
III. P : QRS characteristics
   No P waves are seen (Fig. 13-3A). The QRS complexes are normal or bizarre depending on the intraventricular conduction. The ST segment is elevated or depressed. The T wave may be tall due to shortened repolarization. The rhythm may be regular or irregular.
IV. Differentials
   AV junctional rhythm, idioventricular rhythm, and atrial fibrillation with complete heart block are included.
V. Significance
   A. Atrial standstill is a life-threatening abnormality associated with hyperkalemia (Addison's disease, acute renal failure, urinary obstruction, and diabetic ketoacidosis).
   B. Persistent atrial standstill is a disorder reported in English Springer Spaniels and other breeds and select cats with dilated cardiomyopathy where there is degeneration and fibrosis of the atrial myocardial cells. There is often cardiac enlargement, although the blood electrolytes are normal. This abnormality may be correlated with a fascioscapulohumeral muscular dystrophy as seen in humans.
VI. Treatment
   A. If hyperkalemia is suspected, emergency therapy is undertaken if clinical history supports this possibility. The therapy is designed to

transfer extracellular potassium into the body cells restoring normokalemia.

B. Initially, 2 mEq/kg of sodium bicarbonate is administered slow IV coupled with normal saline, and may restore sinus rhythm within 15 to 30 minutes (beware of paradoxical cerebral acidosis) (Fig. 13-3A).

C. Alternative therapy includes 0.5 unit/kg of regular insulin coupled with 2 g of dextrose per unit of insulin by slow intravenous administration.

D. Calcium gluconate (1 ml of a 10 percent solution/10 kg body weight) by slow intravenous administration.

E. Intravenous normal saline with intravenous corticosteroids (e.g., 20 mg/kg hydrocortisone sodium succinate, 0.5 to 1 mg/kg dexamethasone, or 2 mg/kg of prednisolone).

F. Intravenous 5 percent dextrose in water.

Incomplete AV Block (First- and Second-Degree AV Block)

I. Location

The cardiac impulse is delayed or intermittently blocked in the region of the AV node or AV junction.

II. Heart rate and rhythm

A. The rate is variable, depending on the rate of the sinus node pacemaker.

B. The rate is usually regular in first-degree AV block, unless other arrhythmias are present. The rhythm is usually irregular with second-degree AV block.

III. P : QRS characteristics

A. First-degree AV block shows a prolonged, constant P-R interval (AV conduction) with normal P wave and QRS complexes, at a 1 : 1 ratio.

B. Second-degree AV block has normal P wave and QRS complexes with a constant P-R interval, and with intermittent P waves not followed by QRS complexes. In Mobitz type I (Wenckebach) AV block, the P-R interval gradually prolongs before a dropped ventricular beat occurs. The rhythm is regularly irregular. Mobitz-type II AV block, demonstrates a consistent P–R interval prior to a dropped ventricular beat. The rhythm is often irregular.

IV. Differentials

Complete AV block is included.

V. Significance

A. First-degree AV block and Mobitz type I second-degree AV block are often caused by an increase in vagal tone (e.g., brachycephalic breeds, respiratory, gastrointestinal, or neurologic disease), digitalis, and sedatives (e.g., xylazine, acetylpromazine). Antiarrhythmic drugs (propranolol, quinidine, procainamide and verapamil) and AV nodal disease are also associated with these types of AV block. Physiologic AV block may occur following ectopic beats or atrial tachyarrhythmias that occur during the AV node absolute or relative refractory periods (will slow down or block impulse).

B. Mobitz type II AV block is a more advanced degree of block, occurs in the AV junction, His bundle, or below and may progress to complete heart block. Causes include idiopathic fibrosis (older dogs), hereditary stenosis of the His bundle in the Pug, hypertrophic cardiomyopathy in the dog and the cat, neoplastic infiltration secondary to metastatic neoplasia, and electrolyte disorders.

C. Whether clinical signs develop (e.g., weakness, syncope, or congestive heart failure) may depend on the degree of AV block, ventricular rate, and ventricular function.

VI. Treatment

A. For Mobitz type I AV block, treatment is usually not required. If related to drug toxicity, the drug should be stopped or dosage lowered.

B. For Mobitz type II AV block, therapy depends on the clinical signs. If the cardiac rate is slow and weakness or syncope is evident, then atropine, isoproterenol, or a temporary or permanent cardiac pacemaker is required.

Complete (Third-Degree) AV Block

I. Location

The cardiac impulse is completely blocked in the region of the AV junction and/or His bundle.

II. Heart rate and rhythm

The atrial rate (P-P interval) is within normal limits, and there is a slow idioventricular escape rhythm. The rhythm is usually regular. An idioventricular escape rhythm is below 40 bpm, whereas a low AV junctional (idiojunctional) escape rhythm has a rate of 40 to 60 bpm in the dog. An enhanced AV junctional or idioventricular rhythm (AV dissociation) shows a more rapid rate with the ventricular rate approaching the atrial rate.

III. P : QRS characteristics

A. No relationship; the P wave is completely dissociated from the QRS complex.
B. The P-R interval is variable and there are usually many P waves versus few QRS complexes (Fig. 13-1H).
C. The morphology of the QRS complexes varies depending on the location of the ventricular escape rhythm.

IV. Differentials

Advanced second-degree AV block, atrial standstill, and ventricular tachycardia.

V. Significance

A. Complete AV block is often associated with the clinical signs of weakness, syncope, or congestive heart failure.
B. Underlying conditions resulting in this abnormality include congenital defects (e.g., aortic stenosis, ventricular septal defect, isolated AV block), infiltrative cardiomyopathy (e.g., amyloidosis, neoplasia), idiopathic fibrosis, myocardial infarction, hypertrophic cardiomyopathy, bacterial endocarditis, and idiopathic fibrosis in geriatric dogs (e.g., Cocker Spaniel, German Shepherd). Other reported causes include hypokalemia and hyperkalemia.

VI. Treatment

A. A permanent cardiac pacemaker is the only effective treatment in symptomatic patients.
B. Asymptomatic patients may not require therapy.
C. Drugs used for this abnormality include atropine, isoproterenol, and corticosteroids (anti-inflammatory). An intravenous isoproterenol infusion may be useful in increasing the rate of the ventricular escape rhythm during nonelective surgical procedures.

Arrhythmias and Conduction Disturbances

Sick Sinus Syndrome (SSS)

I. Location

A. The cardiac impulses are generated in the sinus node at a slower than normal rate or are blocked exiting the sinus node.

B. The atria and AV node may also be involved resulting in an atrial tachyarrhythmia (e.g., atrial tachycardia, flutter, or fibrillation).

II. Heart rate and rhythm

The rate is rapid or slow and long pauses (Fig. 13-1G) may be present on the ECG. There may be a bradycardia–tachycardia syndrome with alternating periods of slow and rapid heart rates.

III. P : QRS characteristics

There is a normal P wave for each QRS complex. The P-R interval is constant unless the bradycardia–tachycardia syndrome is present.

IV. Differentials

A. Sinus bradycardia, sinus block and/or arrest, atrial tachycardia; A poor (blunted) response to atropine (e.g., less than 50 percent increase in heart rate may support SSS.

V. Significance

The clinical signs of the sick sinus syndrome are variable.

B. A reduction in cardiac output may result in hypoperfusion of vital organs and show clinical signs of marked weakness and/or syncope.

VI. Treatment

A. If the animal is asymptomatic or has mild clinical signs, no therapy is required.

B. If there are severe clinical signs, injectable atropine or other oral anticholinergic agents (e.g., probantheline) may alleviate these signs.

C. An artificial ventricular-demand pacemaker is required for long-term control of bradyarrhythmias, while digoxin may control the tachyarrhythmia.

Ventricular Preexcitation and the Wolff–Parkinson–White (WPW) Syndrome

I. Location
The cardiac impulses are generated in the sinus node but spread to the ventricle via an anomalous conduction pathway as well as the AV node.

II. Heart rate and rhythm
The cardiac rate and rhythm are normal in ventricular preexcitation. The rate may be very rapid (e.g., 300 bpm) in the WPW syndrome.

III. P : QRS characteristics
The P waves are normal in ventricular preexcitation or are unrecognizable in the WPW syndrome. The QRS complex is widened with notching of the R wave (delta wave) in ventricular preexcitation. The QRS complex may be normal, wide, or bizarre in the WPW syndrome depending on the circuit the atrial tachycardia follows. The P-R interval is short in ventricular preexcitation. In the WPW syndrome, often there is a P wave for every QRS complex (1 : 1 conduction). A short P-R interval may be correlated with a normal QRS complex if the anomalous pathway bypasses the AV node to the area of the His bundle (Lown–Ganong–Levine syndrome, in humans).

IV. Differentials
AV junctional tachycardia, atrial tachycardia, and ventricular tachycardia are included.

V. Significance
Ventricular preexcitation and WPW syndrome may be a congenital problem in the dog or cat occurring with or without other congenital heart defects (e.g., atrial septal defect, valvular dysplasia, or fibrosis).

VI. Treatment
   A. Ventricular preexcitation without tachycardia may not require therapy.
   B. The WPW syndrome requires control and/or conversion of the tachycardia with a vagal maneuver (e.g., ocular or carotid sinus pressure) (Fig. 13-2F) digoxin, lidocaine, propranolol, quinidine, procainamide, verapamil, or DC shock). Digoxin is only indi-

cated in narrow QRS complex WPW syndrome. In wide QRS complex WPW syndrome, digoxin may decrease the refractory period of the anomalous pathway and increase the rate of the tachycardia. Only lidocaine, procainamide, or quinidine should be used in this situation.

ANTIARRHYTHMIC THERAPY

Cardiac arrhythmias and conduction disturbances may have profound effects on cardiac output, coronary artery perfusion, arterial blood pressure, and vital organ perfusion. The clinical signs that result from specific arrhythmias have been previously described. Antiarrhythmic therapy may result in a control or abolishment of the arrhythmia and a return to normal hemodynamic function. It is important to have a thorough knowledge of the properties of the agents available to treat specific rhythm disturbances. Many of the available antiarrhythmic drugs are classified based on their electrophysiologic mechanisms (Table 13-3). The investigative agents are new drugs not available for routine clinical use. Antiarrhythmic drugs may decrease electrical instability (antifibrillatory) and lessen the possibility that an arrhythmia will result in ventricular fibrillation and sudden death. The antifibrillatory activity of an agent does not have to correlate with its antiectopic activity.

Commonly Used Antiarrhythmic Drugs

Atropine Derivatives

I. Indications
   Symptomatic sinus bradycardia, sinus block and/or arrest; incomplete AV block; sick sinus syndrome
II. Pertinent mechanisms
   Parasympatholytic agent; decreases vagal tone to the sinus and AV nodes

TABLE 13-3. CLASSIFICATION OF ANTIARRHYTHMIC AGENTS[a]

Type	Agent	General Mechanism
I	Quinidine Procainamide Lidocaine Disopyramide Phenytoin Aprindine* Encainide* Flecainide* Mexiletine* Tocainide*	Membrane-stabilizing agent (local anesthetic) Decreases the membrane conductance to sodium ions, depresses phase 4 depolarization (automaticity)
II	Propranolol Metoprolol Nadolol* Timolol* Atenolol* Pindolol*	Sympatholytic agent β-adrenergic blockade) Depresses phase 4 depolarization (automaticity)
III	Bretylium* Amiodarone*	Prolongation of action potential duration Depresses phase 4 depolarization (automaticity) Antiadrenergic effects
IV	Verapamil Diltiazem* Nifedipine*	Decreases the slow inward current, primarily the calcium ion Depresses phase 4 depolarization (automaticity) Depresses conduction in fibers with slow current.

[a]Asterisk (*): investigative agents, and/or not established for routine clinical use.

III. How supplied
  A. Atropine sulfate injection 0.4 mg/ml USP, and 0.4-mg tablet (Eli Lilly)
  B. Isopropamide (Darbid 5-mg tablet; Smith, Kline and French)
  C. Probantheline (Pro-Banthine, 7.5, 15mg tablet; Searle and Co.)
  D. Glycopyrrolate (Robinul injection; 0.2mg/ml, Robbins)
IV. Dosage
  A. Dog
    1. Atropine: 0.01 to 0.02 mg/kg IV, IM; 0.02 to 0.04 mg/kg SC q6–8h
    2. Isopropamide: 2.5 to 5.0 mg q8–12h
    3. Probantheline: 7.5 to 15 mg q8–12h
    4. Glycopyrrolate: 0.005 to 0.01 mg/kg IV, IM; 0.01 to 0.02 mg/kg SC q8–12h
  B. Cat
    Atropine: 0.02 to 0.04 mg/kg q4–6h; SC, IM, IV

V. Side effects and toxicity
   A. Sinus tachycardia, ectopic beats, and ocular, gastrointestinal, and pulmonary effects
   B. Initial response may be parasympathomimetic (e.g., bradycardia), especially when administered IV

Digitalis Glycosides

I. Indications
   A. Atrial premature complexes; atrial tachycardia; and atrial flutter or atrial fibrillation
   B. Sinus tachycardia due to congestive heart failure

II. Pertinent mechanisms
   A. Digitalis decreases the velocity of AV conduction by direct and parasympathomimetic effects.
   B. Cardiac contractility and cardiac output improve in congestive heart failure, resulting in diminished sympathetic tone to the sinus and AV nodes.
   C. Parasympathomimetic (vagal) tone is increased and may result in a decreased cardiac rate.
   D. The refractory period of atrial and ventricular cell transmembrane potentials is decreased and may result in ectopia.

III. How supplied
   A. Digitoxin (crystodigin injection 0.2 mg/ml, 0.1- to 0.2-mg tablets; Eli Lilly); (Foxalin 0.1-, 0.25-, 0.5-mg capsule; Halsom).
   B. Digoxin (Lanoxin elixir 0.05 mg/ml; 0.125-, 0.25-, 0.5-mg tablet; Burroughs Wellcome); (Cardoxin elixir, 0.05, 0.15 mg/ml; Evsco).

IV. Dosage
   A. Dog
      1. Digitoxin: oral maintenance: Foxalin, 0.04 to 0.1 mg/kg divided q8h; rapid parenteral: 0.01 to 0.03 mg/kg, one-half of dose IV, wait 30 to 60 minutes and give one-fourth of dose; wait 30 to 60 minutes and give remaining dose if required.
      2. Digoxin: oral maintenance: 0.01 to 0.02 mg/kg divided bid; rapid oral: 0.02 to 0.06 mg/kg divided bid for the first day; then go to

maintenance level; rapid parenteral: 0.01 to 0.02 mg/kg in divided doses as per Digitoxin.

B. Cat
  1. Digitoxin: not routinely administered to cats.
  2. Digoxin: oral maintenance: 0.007 to 0.015 mg/kg SID to every other day (average cat, 1⁄4 of a 0.125-mg tablet every other day; elixir not well tolerated); rapid IV: 0.005 mg/kg lean body weight divided between three doses or to effect; one-half the calculated dose IV, 60 minutes later, one-quarter of the calculated dose, and 60 minutes later the final one-quarter dose if necessary (stop if marked bradycardia, diminished AV conduction, digoxin-related arrhythmias, or clinical signs are evident). Oral maintenance digoxin is started immediately after the last IV dose, in the dog and the cat.

V. Side effects and toxicity
  A. Gastrointestinal (anorexia, vomiting, diarrhea)
  B. Neurologic (lethargy, ataxia)
  C. Cardiac (e.g., AV block, AV junctional rhythm, ectopic beats from atrium or ventricle, ventricular tachycardia, and any other arrhythmia or conduction disturbance)

Epinephrine

I. Indications

Ventricular standstill is the primary indication; high degree or complete AV block, until an artificial or permanent pacemaker is inserted.

II. Pertinent mechanisms

It is a sympathomimetic (α- and β-receptor stimulation) agent. Epinephrine accelerates the atrial and ventricular rate in complete AV block (e.g., enhances automaticity).

III. How supplied

Epinephrine Hydrochloride 1 : 1,000 solution, 1 mg/ml injectable; (Adrenalin, Parke-Davis)

IV. Dosage

Dog and cat; 0.05 to 0.5 mg of 1 : 10,000 dilution IV (15 to 20 mg/kg), 0.5 to 5 μg/kg intracardiac (IC)

V. Side effects and toxicity
Cardiovascular (arterial hypertension, atrial and ventricular ectopia, and atrial or ventricular tachycardia and/or fibrillation

Isoproterenol

I. Indications
Sinus bradycardia; sinus block and/or arrest; complete AV block; and to maintain an escape pacemaker during general anesthesia

II. Pertinent mechanisms
Sympathomimetic effects (e.g., stimulation of the cardiac and respiratory β-adrenergic receptors); cardiac effects are primarily on the sinus and AV nodes

III. How supplied
  A. Isuprel Hydrochloride injection, 0.2 mg/ml, 1 and 5 ml ampule, 10-mg glossets (Breon)
  B. Proterenol 20-, 40-mg tablet (Key Pharm.)

IV. Dosage
  A. Dog
    1. Isuprel: 0.4 mg in 250 ml of 5 percent dextrose/water titrated to effect
    2. Proterenol: 10 to 20 mg q4–6h
    3. Isuprel glossets: 5 to 10 mg per rectum q4–6h
  B. Cat
    Isuprel: 0.4 mg per 250 ml of 5 percent dextrose/water titrated to effect

V. Side effects and toxicity
  A. Gastrointestinal (vomiting)
  B. Neurologic (excitation)
  C. Cardiac (sinus tachycardia, ectopic complexes)

Lidocaine Hydrochloride

I. Indications
Frequent ventricular premature complexes; paroxysmal or persistent ventricular tachycardia; atrial tachyarrhythmias conducted over anomalous pathway in WPW syndrome

II. Pertinent mechanisms
   A. Depresses automaticity in ventricular myocardial cells; has minimal effects on atrial cells
   B. Lidocaine may decrease the refractory period of the AV node causing an increase in the ventricular response in patients with atrial flutter or fibrillation.

III. How supplied:
   Xylocaine (lidocaine), without epinephrine, 2 percent (20 mg/ml), (Astra)

IV. Dosage
   A. Dog
      1. 2 to 4 mg/kg slow IV repeat every 10 minutes to a maximum of 8 mg/kg
      2. Constant-rate infusion (CRI) 25 to 75 μg/kg-min; approximately 2 mg/ml of 5 percent dextrose/water administered in a slow IV drip to effect. CRI equals body weight (kg) $\times$ dose $\times$ 0.36 = total dose in kg slow IV over 6 hours
   B. Cat
      0.5 mg/kg slow IV (cats are sensitive to this drug and may undergo seizures; control with diazepam)

V. Side effects and toxicity
   A. Gastrointestinal (emesis)
   B. Neurologic (tremors, seizures, excitation, control with diazepam)
   C. Cardiovascular (hypotension, increased AV conduction with atrial flutter or fibrillation)

Phenytoin

I. Indications
   Digitalis-induced atrial and ventricular tachyarrhythmias; digitalis-induced AV block; used in place of lidocaine or procainamide with refractory ventricular arrhythmias

II. Pertinent mechanisms
   A. Depresses diastolic depolarization and automaticity, shortens the duration of the action potential and the effect of refractory period
   B. Increases the conduction velocity in the atrium, and counteracts the depressant effect of AV conduction induced by digitalis or procainamide

III. How supplied
  1) 30- and 100-mg capsule, 125 mg/5 ml syrup, 50 mg/ml injectable, (Parke-Davis)

IV. Dosage
  A. Dog: 4 to 8 mg/kg PO divided q6–8h; 4 mg/kg slow IV
  B. Cat: not used; toxic

V. Side effects and toxicity
  A. Skin reactions (dermatoses)
  B. Neurologic (ataxia, tremors, depression)
  C. Cardiac (AV block)

Procainamide

I. Indications
  Ventricular premature complexes; ventricular tachycardia; supraventricular tachycardia in WPW syndrome with wide QRS complexes; supraventricular tachyarrhythmias (not established in the dog).

II. Pertinent mechanisms
  A. Prolongation of refractory period in the atria and the ventricles
  B. Slowing of electrical conduction, depression of automaticity, and prolongation of the refractory period of atrial and ventricular myocardial cells
  C. Indirect vagolytic effects (e.g., AV conduction may improve with low doses and decrease with higher doses)

III. How supplied
  A. Procan sustained-release (SR), 250-, 500-mg tablet (Parke-Davis)
  B. Pronestyl: 200, 500 mg tablet (Squibb)
  C. Pronestyl injection: 100, 500 mg/ml; (Squibb)

IV. Dosage
  A. Dogs
    1. Procan-SR: 8 to 20 mg/kg q6–8h
    2. Pronestyl tablets: 8 to 20 mg/kg q6h
    3. Pronestyl injection: 6 to 12 mg/kg IM q6–8h (the initial dose may be doubled), and 6 to 12 mg/kg IV over 5 minutes; CRI 25 to 40 μg/kg-min
  B. Cats (not routinely administered)

V. Side effects and toxicity
   A. Gastrointestinal (anorexia, vomiting, diarrhea)
   B. Cardiovascular (weakness, hypotension, decreased cardiac contractility; widening of the QRS complex and Q-T interval and AV block; multiform ventricular tachycardia)
   C. Systemic (fever, leukopenia; lupus erythematosus syndrome in humans, not established in the dog)

Propranolol Hydrochloride

I. Indications
   A. Atrial premature complexes and tachyarrhythmias; atrial fibrillation in conjunction with digitalis; and ventricular premature contractions (second choice to quinidine or procainamide)
   B. Propranolol effective with digitalis induced atrial and ventricular tachyarrhythmias.
   C. Atrial tachycardia secondary to Wolff–Parkinson–White syndrome with normal QRS complexes.
   D. Cats with hypertrophic cardiomyopathy.
II. Pertinent mechanisms
   A. Propranolol is a β-adrenergic receptor (B_1 and B_2) blocking agent that inhibits sympathetic stimulation to the heart.
   B. There is also a direct depressant action on the transmembrane potentials of the cardiac cells reducing automaticity and conduction. Propranolol may show antifibrillatory activity.
III. How supplied
   A. Inderal 10-, 20-, 40-, 80-mg tablet; l-ml vial (l mg/ml); (Ayerst)
   B. A selective β_1 blocking drug metoprolol (Lopressor, Geigy) is available in 50- and 100-mg tablets
IV. Dosage
   A. Dog
      1. Propranolol: 0.04 to 0.06 mg/kg IV slowly; 0.2 to 1.0 mg/kg PO q8h
      2. Metoprolol: not accurately evaluated; dosages similar to propranolol
   B. Cat
      1. Propranolol—0.04 mg/kg IV slowly, 2.5 to 5.0 mg q8–12h

V. Side effects and toxicity
   A. Respiratory (bronchoconstriction)
   B. Cardiac (decreased contractility, hypotension, bradycardia, and AV block)
   C. Systemic (hypoglycemia)

Quinidine

I. Indications
   A. Ventricular premature complexes; ventricular tachycardia; acute atrial fibrillation; refractory supraventricular tachycardia; supraventricular arrhythmias with anomalous conduction in the WPW syndrome
II. Pertinent mechanisms
   A. Inhibition of the fast sodium channel of the transmembrane potential
   B. Prolongation of the refractory period in the atria and ventricles
   C. Slows phase 0 of the action potential and depresses spontaneous diastolic depolarization (automaticity)
   D. An indirect vagolytic effect
III. How supplied
   A. Quinidine sulfate USP 200-mg tablet, 300 mg Extentab (Parke-Davis)
   B. Quinidine gluconate USP injection (80 mg/ml, Eli-Lilly); (Quinaglute duratab 324 mg, Cooper)
   C. Quinidine polygalacturonate 275-mg tablet (Cardioquin, Purdue-Frederick)
IV. Dosage
   A. Dog
      1. Quinidine sulfate 6 to 16 mg/kg PO q6h (sulfate), q8h (Extentabs)
      2. Quinidine gluconate 6 to 20 mg/kg IM q6h, 8 to 20 mg/kg PO q6–8h (Quinaglute)
      3. Quinidine polygalacturonate 8 to 20 mg/kg q6–8h (Cardioquin)
   B. Cat
      1. Not routinely administered.

V. Side effects and toxicity
  A. Gastrointestinal (anorexia, vomiting, diarrhea)
  B. Cardiac (weakness, hypotension, decreased cardiac contractility, widening of the QRS complex and Q-T interval, AV block, and syncope due to multiform ventricular tachycardia)
  C. Drug interaction (increases serum digoxin levels)

Less Commonly Used Antiarrhythmic Drugs

Calcium Chloride

I. Indications
  Ventricular asystole (to increase cardiac irritability); electromechanical dissociation (QRS complex is not correlated with effective stroke volume, or arterial pulse)
II. Pertinent mechanisms
  Stimulates excitation–contraction coupling of the myocardial cells.
III. How supplied: 10 percent solution (100 mg/ml), 10-ml vials (Bristol)
IV. Dosage
  A. Dog
    0.05 to 0.10 ml/kg of 10 percent solution IV or IC.
  B. Cat
    0.05 to 0.10 ml/kg of 10 percent solution IV or IC
V. Side effects and toxicity
  A. Neurologic: depression, coma
  B. Systemic: nephropathy.

Disopyramide

I. Indications
  A. The prevention and treatment of ventricular tachyarrhythmias.
  B. Disopyramide has also been reported effective for supraventricu-

lar tachyarrhythmias (atrial fibrillation or flutter) in humans, although it may be less effective for this purpose in the dog.

II. Pertinent mechanisms
  A. Similar to quinidine and procainamide
  B. Decreases the slope of phase IV depolarization (automaticity)
  C. Anticholinergic effects
  D. A potent negative inotropic agent

III. How supplied
  100-mg, 150-mg capsule (Norpace, Searle)

IV. Dosage
  Not well established, due to rapid excretion in the dog; not used in the cat

V. Side effects and toxicity
  A. Should not be administered in patients in congestive heart failure or shock due to its negative inotropic effects
  B. Gastrointestinal (dry mouth, vomiting)
  C. Cardiac (AV block, sinus node depression, multiform ventricular tachycardia)
  D. Systemic (urinary retention, glaucoma, depression)

Diazepam

I. Indications
  A. Refractory supraventricular and ventricular tachyarrhythmias, combined with other antiarrhythmic drugs
  B. Arrhythmias induced by nervous systemic excitation or the autonomic nervous system

II. Pertinent mechanisms
  Sedative effect on the central nervous system that may be indirectly causing a cardiac arrhythmia

III. How supplied
  10-ml vials (5 mg/ml), 2-, 5-, 10-mg tablets (Valium, Roche)

IV. Dosage:
  A. Dog
    2.5 to 20 mg IV, 0.1 to 0.2 mg/kg PO q8–12h
  B. Cat
    2.5 to 5 mg (5 mg/ml) IV, 0.1 to 0.2 mg/kg PO q12h

V. Side effects and toxicity
   Neurologic (marked sedation or coma)

Edrophonium Chloride

I. Indications
   Atrial tachycardia
II. Pertinent mechanisms
   Short-acting parasympathomimetic drug (increases vagal tone)
III. How supplied
   1-ml, 10-ml vials; 10 mg/ml (Tensilon, Roche)
IV. Dosage
   A. Dog
      1 to 2 mg slow IV over 30 seconds; if no response, give 3 to 5 mg additionally (atropine sulfate should be available if marked bradycardia occurs)
   B. Cat
      Not used in the cat
V. Side effects and toxicity
   A. Neurologic (excitation and seizures)
   B. Respiratory (dyspnea)
   C. Gastrointestinal (vomiting, diarrhea)
   D. Cardiac (bradycardia, hypotension)

Potassium Chloride

I. Indications
   Chemical ventricular defibrillator (dog and cat); digitalis-induced ventricular arrhythmias (dog)
II. Pertinent mechanisms
   A. Hyperkalemia decreases automaticity and conduction.
   B. Hypokalemia exacerbates digitalis induced ventricular arrhythmias.
   C. Hypokalemia may result in tachyarrhythmias that are refractory to drug therapy.

III. How supplied
  10-ml ampules (2 mEq/ml), (Abbott)

IV. Dosage
  Monitor serum potassium and ECG.
  A. Dog
    1. 0.5 to 2.0 mEq/kg-day slow IV (40 mEq diluted in 500 ml of 5 percent dextrose/water), not to exceed 0.5 mEq/kg-hour (rate of infusion is critical)
    2. 1.0 mEq of potassium chloride/kg with 6.0 mg of acetylcholine/kg intracardiac (ventricular defibrillation only)
  B. Cat
    1. Should not exceed 0.5 mEq/kg-hr slow IV (e.g., hypokalemia)
    2. 0.25 to 0.75 mEq followed by calcium chloride IC (chemical defibrillation)

V. Side effects and toxicity
  Cardiac arrest

Verapamil

I. Indications
  A. Atrial tachyarrhythmias, particularly those generated by a reentrant mechanism
  B. Reciprocating tachycardia with normal QRS complexes in the WPW syndrome
  C. To decrease the ventricular rate by slowing AV conduction in atrial fibrillation

II. Pertinent mechanisms
  A. Verapamil is a calcium blocking agent, originally developed as an antianginal drug in humans that blocks the influx of calcium and sodium ions at the slow channels of cardiac tissue.
  B. This agent slows the sinus node rate and prolongs the absolute and relative refractory period of AV nodal tissue.

III. How supplied
  A. Verapamil hydrochloride injectable 5 mg/ 2 ml; 80-, 120-mg tablets (Calan, Searle)
  B. 2-ml ampules, 2.5-mg/ml; and 80-, 120-mg tablets (Isoptin, Knoll)

IV. Dosage
  A. Dog
    1. 0.05 to 0.15 mg/kg over 2 minutes, 5 mg total dose
    2. Oral dose not established at this time
  B. Cat
    Dosage not established
V. Side effects and toxicity
  A. Gastrointestinal (constipation)
  B. Systemic problems (urinary retention)
  C. Cardiovascular (hypotension and shock, AV block, sinus bradycardia, and sinus block and/or arrest)
  D. For hypotension and shock, IV fluids, calcium chloride supplementation, and catecholamines (dobutamine, dopamine, or isoproterenol) may reverse these signs
  E. Drug interaction (verapamil may increase serum digoxin levels).

Investigative Antiarrhythmic Agents

Amiodarone

I. Indications
  Acute and chronic atrial and ventricular tachyarrhythmias; atrial tachyarrhythmias correlated with the WPW with narrow or aberrant QRS complexes in humans
II. Pertinent mechanisms
  A. Amiodarone prolongs the duration of the action potential in the atria and the ventricles. This agent shows antifibrillatory effects in humans.
  B. The sympathetic nervous system is inhibited.
  C. The sinus node rate is slowed and the sinus node recovery time is prolonged.
  D. The absolute and relative refractory periods of the AV node and His–Purkinje system are prolonged.
  E. The absolute refractory period of the AV node and anomalous pathway is prolonged in the WPW syndrome.

III. How supplied
Not available for routine clinical usage

IV. Dosage
Not established in small animals

V. Side effects and toxicity (reported in humans)
   A. Gastrointestinal (vomiting)
   B. Systemic (hypothyroidism or hyperthyroidism, pulmonary fibrosis, and corneal deposits)

Aprindine

I. Indications
   A. Supraventricular tachyarrhythmias; ventricular premature contractions and incessant ventricular tachycardia; arrhythmias induced by digoxin toxicity; and supraventricular tachycardias in the WPW syndrome with wide QRS complexes
   B. Ventricular arrhythmias that are refractory to quinidine or procainamide

II. Pertinent mechanisms
Mechanisms are similar to quinidine and procainamide; delays conduction in all levels of the heart; prolongs the effective refractory period of the atria, AV node, and His–Purkinje system

III. Dosage
   A. Dog
      0.5 to 2.0 mg/kg IV or PO, q8h
   B. Cat: Not used

IV. How supplied
100-mg tablets (Eli Lilly)

V. Adverse effects; not well documented in the dog
   A. Neurologic (tremors, ataxia)
   B. Systemic (agranolocytosis and cholestatic jaundice in humans)
   C. Cardiac (decreases contractility)

Bretylium

I. Indications
   A. Life-threatening, drug-resistant ventricular tachycardia, or ventricular fibrillation in humans.

B. Limited clinical experience in the dog does not favor injectable bretylium as an antifibrillatory agent. This drug may actually worsen ventricular tachycardia and promote ventricular fibrillation, although this remains controversial and may depend on the dose administered.

II. Pertinent mechanisms

A. Bretylium has direct membrane effects on the myocardium and indirect effects by blocking the sympathetic nervous system.

B. Bretylium increases the action potential duration and absolute refractory period in isolated tissue.

III. How supplied

Bretylium tosylate injectable, 50 mg/ml (American Critical Care).

IV. Dosage

Not established in small animals.

V. Side effects and toxicity (in man)

A. Gastrointestinal (vomiting)

B. Cardiovascular (hypotension)

Tocanide and Mexiletine

I. Indications

Ventricular arrhythmias that are responsive to IV lidocaine

II. Pertinent mechanisms

Tocanide and mexiletine are synthetic analogs of lidocaine developed in an attempt to find an orally active lidocaine-type preparation. The electrophysiologic mechanisms are similar to those of lidocaine.

III. How supplied

Tocainide HCl (Tonocard, Merck) 400-, 600-mg tablets

IV. Dosage

1 to 2 mg/kg/day divided bid–tid (tocainide and mexiletine); not established in small animals.

V. Side effects and toxicity

Similar to lidocaine in humans; also blood dyscrasias and pulmonary fibrosis

Nonpharmacologic Methods of Treating Cardiac Arrhythmias

Vagal Maneuver (increasing parasympathetic tone to the sinus and AV node via ocular or carotid sinus pressure)

I. Indication
To provide a diagnostic aid in undefined atrial tachyarrhythmias and suspected sick sinus syndrome patients; terminate atrial tachycardia in some patients.

II. Mechanisms

A. In sinus tachycardia, a vagal maneuver usually causes a slight slowing of the heart rate due to the effect on the sinus node.

B. With atrial tachycardia or flutter, physiologic AV block often occurs, and the R-R intervals become irregular, showing an underlying atrial mechanism for the arrhythmia.

C. Supraventricular tachycardia that depends on circus (reentrant) routes through AV junctional tissue may respond to a vagal maneuver by sudden termination of the tachycardia or speeding or slowing of the cardiac rate.

D Although, a tachycardia may be resolved only temporarily, it may aid in establishing the best choice of antiarrhythmic therapy, if needed.

III. Contraindications and complications

A. Sick sinus syndrome (bradycardia–tachycardia syndrome): patients may show a marked symptomatic bradycardia.

B. Breeds that are hypersensitive to a vagal maneuver (brachycephalic breeds) may show a marked symptomatic bradycardia.

Artificial Cardiac Pacing

I. Indications

A. Temporary pacing

1. Symptomatic and drug-resistant second- or third-degree AV block
2. Symptomatic and drug-resistant sinus bradycardia, sinus arrest and/or sinus block, and slow AV junctional rhythm (sick sinus syndrome)
3. Atrial or ventricular tachyarrhythmias unresponsive to drug therapy (use premature stimulation or overdrive suppression)

B. Permanent pacing
1. Symptomatic heart block
2. Symptomatic sinus block and/or arrest, bradycardia, AV block (sick sinus syndrome)
3. Symptomatic chronic second-degree AV block (Mobitz type II)
4. Recurrent drug-resistant tachyarrhythmias benefited by short-term pacing
5. Symptomatic bilateral bundle branch block

II. Mechanisms and types of pacemakers
A. Functions as natural pacemaker by initiating electrical impulses via a battery. The electrical impulse travels through small wires to the heart.
B. An atrial pacemaker is required to suppress atrial arrhythmias.
C. A ventricular pacemaker is satisfactory for complete AV block, although the lack of sequential atrioventricular pumping will result in less than maximal cardiac output.
D. Bifocal pacing (AV sequential pacing) is commonly used in humans.
E. A demand pacemaker (functions only when the heart rate is below a critical level) avoids a major complication of fixed pacemakers, competition between the natural rhythm and pacemaker-induced rhythm.

III. Complications and malfunctions
A. Malfunctioning pacemakers (slowing, irregularity, sensing failure, and loss of capture).
1. Requires replacement of the malfunctioning unit with a new pacemaker.
2. Loss of capture may be due to malposition or fracturing of the electrodes or wires.

B. Ventricular fibrillation

The most common cause is competition of the regular rhythm with a fixed-rate pacemaker and R-on-T phenomenon.

C. Infection at surgical sites or along wire tracts; surgical drainage or removal of the infected sites may be required.

D. Arrhythmias related to underlying heart disease.

Cardioversion and Defibrillation (see Chapter 14)

I. Indications

Electroshock therapy is used as an emergency procedure during ventricular fibrillation and also for the conversion of selected tachyarrhythmias (e.g., atrial fibrillation in which underlying cause has been corrected; atrial tachycardia, atrial flutter, and ventricular tachycardia unresponsive to drugs and correlated with clinical signs).

II. Mechanism

Cardioversion electrically converts arrhythmias to a sinus rhythm by a synchronized discharge of current during the depolarization (QRS complex) part of the electrical cycle. Defibrillation does not require a synchronized delivery of current.

III. Contraindications for cardioversion

A. Digitalis toxicity and/or hypokalemia
B. Severe mitral insufficiency and/or marked left atrial enlargement
C. Chronic atrial fibrillation
D. Atrial fibrillation or atrial flutter with AV block
E. Sick sinus syndrome
F. A cardioverter that is not synchronized to the QRS complex

SUGGESTED READINGS

Anderson JL: Antifibrillatory versus antiectopic therapy. Am J Cardiol 54(2): 7A–12A, 1984

Bolton GR: Handbook of Canine Electrocardiography. WB Saunders, Philadelphia, 1975.

Bonagura J: Therapy of cardiac arrhythmias. p. 360. In Kirk RW (ed): Current Veterinary Therapy. VIII. Small Animal Practice. WB Saunders, Philadelphia, 1983

Bonagura JD: Cardiac dysrhythmias diagnosis and treatment. Scientific Proceedings of the American Animal Hospital Association 87, 1980

Chung EK: Principles of Cardiac Arrhythmias. ed 3. Williams & Wilkins, Baltimore, 1983

Fenster PE: Use of antidysrhythmic drugs. p. 117. In Hurst JW, (ed): Clinical Essays on the Heart. Vol. I. McGraw-Hill, New York, 1983

Jenkins WL, Clark DR: A review of drugs affecting the heart. J Am Vet Med Assoc 171(1):85, 1977

Opie LH (ed): Drugs for the Heart. American Edition. Grune & Stratton, New York, 1984

Mandel WJ: Cardiac Arrhythmias. JB Lippincott, Philadelphia, 1980.

Selzer A: Drug therapy. p. 117. Principles and Practice of Clinical Cardiology. ed 2. WB Saunders, Philadelphia, 1983

Tilley LP: Essentials of Canine and Feline Electrocardiography, Interpretation and Treatment ed 2. Lea & Febiger, Philadelphia, 1985.

14

Cardiopulmonary Arrest and Resuscitation

Wayne E. Wingfield

INTRODUCTION

DEFINITION

The term *cardiac arrest* is used to designate the clinical cessation of myocardial contractility. Since respiratory failure is an important causative factor of cardiac arrest and since it follows circulatory arrest within a matter of 20 to 30 seconds, the more inclusive term *cardiopulmonary arrest* is preferable.

IMPORTANCE

Cardiopulmonary arrest has become a topic of prime importance because of the development of effective resuscitation methods and the experience that prompt recognition and vigorous therapy may avert a fatal outcome. Although cardiopulmonary arrest is frequently the terminal mechanism in severely ill patients, this discussion covers its sudden appearance in apparently healthy subjects or in the presence of minimal overt cardiac abnormalities.

INCIDENCE AND ETIOLOGY

Predisposing Factors

Factors that predispose to cardiopulmonary arrest include:

I. Pathologic states of the heart

II. Hypoxia and/or hypercapnia
III. Electrolyte disturbances, particularly hyperkalemia and hypocalcemia
IV. Acute conditions, such as overwhelming systemic infections or thoracic trauma
V. Drugs and anesthetic agents
VI. Electrical shock
VII. Cardiovascular surgery
VIII. A combination of the above factors

Precipitating Factors

Precipitating factors in cardiopulmonary arrest include:

I. The development of ectopic arrhythmias (e.g., ventricular tachycardia, ventricular fibrillation, sinus arrest)
II. Parasympathetic activity (e.g., ocular or abdominal surgery), especially in the presence of hypoxia, hypercapnia, or hyperkalemia
III. Drug therapy (e.g., digitalis, quinidine, procainamide)
IV. Hypoglycemia; and convulsive seizures
V. Cardiopulmonary arrest may be precipitated during therapeutic procedures:
   A. During angiocardiography
   B. During rapid infusions of antiarrhythmic drugs
   C. Intratracheal intubation
   D. Tracheostomy
   E. Pharyngeal examination

TYPES OF CARDIAC ARREST

Categories

Cardiac arrest in veterinary patients may occur in the following categories:

I. Primary cardiac arrest
II. Cardiac arrest as part of general circulatory failure
III. Cardiac arrest secondary to or coincident with respiratory failure

Electrocardiographic

The cessation of myocardial contractility can usually be correlated electrocardiographically to:

I. Ventricular flutter or fibrillation
II. Electromechanical dissociation of the heart
III. A lack of electrical activity (asystole)

Pathophysiology

I. Asphyxia generalized or localized in a particular tissue such as the myocardium, is either the cause or the inevitable consequence of any form of sudden death.
II. During experimental obstructive asphyxia, four distinct stages may be observed:
   A. Immediately after obstruction of the airway, breath efforts continue; relief of obstruction will result in resuscitation.
   B. Two to 4 minutes after obstruction, breathing efforts stop while circulation remains intact. At this stage, relief of obstruction and ventilation of the lung with air results in resuscitation.
   C. If obstruction continues for 6 to 9 minutes, severe hypotension and bradycardia lead to pulselessness, dilated pupils, and absence of heart sounds. Artificial ventilation, if given quickly, often is life saving.
   D. Within a short period of time, myocardial contractions cease, even though reasonably normal electrocardiographic (ECG) activity usually continues for prolonged periods. Once myocardial contractions stop, artificial ventilation and circulation, usually with drug therapy, are required for resuscitation.
III. Normally, myocardial contraction of the ventricles is excited by the propagation of an action potential throughout the myocardial cells that arises in the sinoatrial node, travels through the atrial fibers to the atrioventricular node, and reaches the ventricular myocardium via the bundle of His and the Purkinje fibers of the ventricular conducting system. This sequence leads to the coordinated contraction that is responsible for the ejection of blood from the ventricles into the pulmonary artery and aorta.

A. Ventricular fibrillation

1. In ventricular fibrillation, the excitatory impulse does not arise at a single focus and spread throughout the ventricle in an orderly manner. Instead, the excitatory impulse wanders continuously along constantly changing pathways.
2. As a result, fully contracted fibers and fully relaxed fibers are present at all times and normal systole and diastole no longer occur.
3. There is no rise in intraventricular pressure, no pumping of blood, and no perfusion of the tissues of the body or the heart itself.
4. Fibrillation of the ventricles can be induced in the normal ventricle if an electrical stimulus of a certain strength and duration is applied to the heart during a critical interval—the "vulnerable period."
   a) The vulnerable period roughly corresponds to the middle third of the T wave.
   b) It occurs at a time when some of the fibers of the ventricle are fully repolarized, some remain in their absolute refractory period, and others, being partially repolarized, are partially refractory and capable of being excited by a strong stimulus.
5. A state of marked incoordination of the spread of electrical activity will arise. Normal action potentials will conduct rapidly into other fully repolarized fibrs but will eventually reach partially depolarized fibers and will conduct slowly or die out. The abnormal action potentials, evoked in partially refractory fibers, may block and die out, or they may gain access to more fully repolarized fibers and begin to conduct more rapidly.
6. Excitation spreads along a number of pathways at a variety of speeds, causing the electrical activity in one group of cells to be out of phase with activity in other groups of cells. This random movement and reentry of excitation constitute the essential abnormality and both initiates and sustains fibrillation (circus movement of excitation).
7. The three mechanisms that may be regarded as the cause of ventricular fibrillation are:
   a) Reentry or circus movement of excitation

b) The appearance of rapid automatic activity in previously normal fibers
c) The triggering of automatic activity in previously quiescent abnormal fibers

B. Electromechanical dissociation
1. Mechanical activity of the myocardium can completely cease, yet electrical impulse generation may continue in a relatively normal manner.
2. The uncoupling of electrical activity from contraction is referred to as electromechanical dissociation or, on the cellular level, excitation–contraction uncoupling.
3. The importance of this phenomenon is that the ECG may seem fairly normal even in the presence of severe inotropic depression.

C. Asystole
1. Cardiac asystole designates a lack of both electrical and contractile activity of the heart.
2. The specialized pacemaker cells of the sinoatrial node fail to initiate excitatory impulses, and the escape mechanisms of the remaining tissues of the cardiac conducting system fail to develop.

DIAGNOSIS

Sudden cardiovascular collapse does not invariably denote a cardiac catastrophe leading to death. Most often it is a benign condition for which a rapid recovery is expected without therapeutic intervention. However, when the collapse is due to inadequate cardiac output, dire consequences ensue. Since cerebral metabolism is aerobic and depends on uninterrupted blood supply, more than four minutes of cardiac arrest may result in brain damage. As little as 2 minutes of elapsed time affects the ease and outcome of resuscitation, a fact probably related to the rapid development of acidosis in the hypoxic heart.

Syncope versus Cardiovascular Collapse

I. Before appropriate action is initiated, it is mandatory to distinguish between simple syncope and cardiovascular collapse. The differential diagnosis for cardiovascular collapse is summarized in Table 14-1.

TABLE 14-1. DIFFERENTIAL DIAGNOSIS OF CARDIOVASCULAR COLLAPSE

I. Cardiovascular causes
  A. Arrhythmias
    1. Tachyarrhythmias
      a. Ventricular
      b. Supraventricular
    2. Bradyarrhythmias
      a. Sinus arrest or block
      b. Atrioventricular blocks
      c. Atrial standstill
    3. Sick-sinus syndrome
    4. Asystole
  B. Low-output states
    1. Congestive heart failure
    2. Cardiomyopathies
    3. Aortic stenosis
    4. Pericardial effusions
    5. Hypotension
      a. Shock
      b. Vasodilator drugs
      c. β-adrenergic blocking drugs
      d. Calcium channel-blocking drugs
    6. Left atrial rupture
    7. Cardiac neoplasia
    8. Pulmonary dirofilariasis
    9. Bacterial endocarditis
    10. Thoracic effusions (air, fluid)

II. Respiratory causes
  A. Pneumonitis
  B. Asphyxia
  C. Bronchial asthma
  D. Collapsing trachea
  E. Chylothorax
  F. Thromboembolism (e.g., dirofilariasis)

III. Central nervous system causes
  A. Thromboembolism
  B. Epilepsy
  C. Infection (meningitis or encephalitis)
  D. Polyradiculoneuritis
  E. Spinal trauma (Shiff–Sherrington syndrome)
  F. Brain trauma
  G. Brain hemorrhage

IV. Metabolic causes
  A. Hypoxia
  B. Hypercarbia
  C. Adrenocortical insufficiency
  D. Hyper- and hypokalemia
  E. Hyper- and hypocalcemia

F. Hyperthyroidism
G. Hypoglycemia

V. Miscellaneous causes
A. Drugs
B. Cirrhosis of the liver
C. Portosystemic shunts
D. Allergic reactions
E. Poisonings
F. Electrical shock
G. Bites and stings
H. Overwhelming infections

II. Syncope is a common clinical sign associated with cardiopulmonary collapse. With syncope, four possible derangements contribute to this transient loss of consciousness:
   A. Diminution or interruption of cerebral circulation
   B. Inadequate cardiac output
   C. Compromise of systemic blood pressure
   D. Inadequate oxygen and/or energy delivery to the brain.

Physical Examination

When encountering a patient in cardiovascular collapse one must first determine whether the problem:

I. Relates to a self-terminating functional derangement or is the result of an organic condition.
   A. A self-terminating dysfunction is benign and resolves with time.
   B. An organic dysfunction is serious, jeopardizes survival, and requires prompt measures.
II. Is noncardiac or cardiac in origin.
   A. Noncardiac causes usually manifest with loss of consciousness but maintenance of respiration, heart sounds, and pulses.
   B. Cardiac causes result in a rapid deepening of cyanosis, absence of heart sounds, and a lack of detectable pulses in the femoral and carotid arteries (Table 14-2). These findings are sufficient to diagnose cardiac arrest.

TABLE 14-2. CLINICAL SIGNS OF CARDIOPULMONARY ARREST

Impending Arrest	Definite Arrest
1. Weak, irregular pulse	1. Unconsciousness
2. Prolonged capillary refill time (>2 seconds)	2. Apnea or agonal gasping
3. Cyanosis	3. Absence of carotid and femoral pulses
4. Darkened, oozing blood	4. Absence of heart sounds
5. Dyspnea	5. Dilated pupils
	6. ECG evidence of arrhythmia of asystole or ventricular flutter/fibrillation

Electrocardiography

Electrocardiography recordings show that the cardiopulmonary arrest may be ventricular flutter/fibrillation, asystole, or electromechanical dissociation.

TREATMENT OF CARDIOPULMONARY ARREST

Following the diagnosis of cardiac arrest, the primary responsibilities are directed to maintenance of an open airway for ventilation, ensuring adequate circulation, and reestablishing normal sinus electrical rhythm. Maintenance of an airway and adequate circulation are discussed under Basic Life Support; reestablishing a normal sinus rhythm is discussed under Advanced Life Support (ALS).

Basic Life Support

Basic life support (BLS) is that phase of emergency treatment that either prevents circulatory or respiratory arrest or insufficiency through prompt recognition and intervention or externally supports the respiration and circulation through cardiopulmonary resuscitation (CPR).

Accomplishing BLS involves the sequential steps listed in Figure 14-1. The ABC's of CPR are as follows:

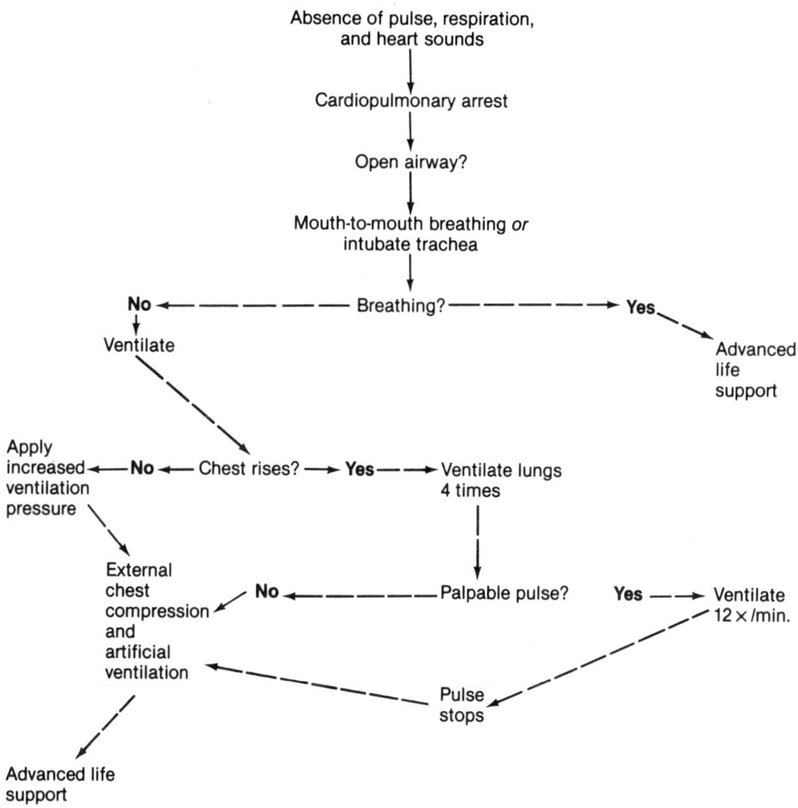

Fig. 14-1. Sequential steps in the performance of basic life support in cardiopulmonary arrest.

Airway

I. Opening the airway
   A. Airway obstruction is infrequently the cause of cardiopulmonary arrest. The most important action for resuscitation is to ensure a patent airway.

B. Opening the mouth and pulling the tongue outward will permit visualization of the mouth and pharynx.
C. Foreign materials or vomitus should be removed as best as possible.
D. Use of an endotracheal tube is preferred in order to maintain an open airway and provide artificial ventilation.

Breathing

If the animal is not making breathing movements, artificial ventilation is instituted.

I. Mouth-to-mouth ventilation may be required in the absence of an endotracheal tube. This is best accomplished by cupping one's hands about the animal's nose and holding the mouth closed. Blow air into the animal's nose with sufficient force to expand the animal's chest. Unless chest expansion occurs, the lungs have not been ventilated.
II. Positive pressure can be applied to the endotracheal tube by any method available, such as mouth-to-tube, a self-inflating resuscitation bag (Ambu bag), or a reservoir bag on an anesthetic machine or nonrebreathing circuit.
III. Four quick respirations are given; then a check is made to detect a femoral and/or carotid pulse. If a pulse is felt, it indicates there is sufficient circulation to permit resuscitation by artificial ventilation alone. If a pulse is not felt, two situations are possible. First, the heart may be in cardiac arrest. Second, the heart may be beating so weakly that a pulse cannot be felt. Skilled observers are usually not able to feel a pulse when the systolic pressure falls below 60 mm Hg.
IV. If a pulse is not felt, give three or four breaths and again check for pulse. In some instances when a weak circulation exists, enough oxygen may be transported to reoxygenate the heart and restore circulation.

Cardiac Compression

If a pulse is not felt after 30 seconds of ventilation, artificial circulation must be started. External cardiac compression consists of a rhythmic application of pressure over the thoracic wall.

I. Positioning
  A. Because of the chest configuration of the dog and cat, an oblique position will provide the best position for application of thoracic pressure.
  B. To maintain this position, large and medium-size animals are supported on the down side with a sandbag or other firm substance to maintain a 30- to 45-degree angle between the table surface and the sternum.
  C. One's doubled-up fist may serve as a thoracic support if necessary.
  D. In small dogs and all cats, application of pressure is achievable by grasping across the sternum and squeezing the thoracic walls toward each other.

II. Blood flow during cardiopulmonary resuscitation
  A. Cardiac pump mechanism
    1. CPR has traditionally been thought to produce systemic blood flow by selective compression of the heart (ventricles). If the heart does serve as a functional pump during CPR, the following hemodynamic findings and flow events would be expected:
      a) A significant central arteriovenous (aortic or left ventricular) (LV) to right atrial (RA) pressure gradient during thoracic compression
      b) A ventricular pressure gradient to assure atrioventricular valve closure during chest compression
      c) Left heart to systemic arterial flow and peripheral venous to right heart flow during thoracic compression.
    2. Presumably, artificial systole results when a higher pressure is generated in the ventricles than elsewhere in the thorax. The mitral and tricuspid valves close and the semilunar valves open. Blood is ejected into the great arteries, and a positive arteriovenous pressure difference is generated in the thorax.
    3. In artificial diastole, intracardiac pressure falls, the mitral and tricuspid valves open, and the heart fills from the systemic venous reservoir.
    4. Flow-limiting factors for the cardiac pump mechanism include those that limit filling and those that limit emptying of the pump.
      a) Filling of the pump depends on the pressure difference between the systemic veins and the right ventricle. Increasing this pressure gradient during CPR provides a rationale for

such measures as fluid loading to increase venous pressure, application of negative airway pressure during artificial diastole, and physical attempts, to *decrease* venous capacitance, such as use of abdominal compression bandaging.

b) Emptying of the ventricles depends on generating a left ventricular pressure higher than peripheral arterial pressure. Increasing this pressure difference is best accomplished by compression of the heart against the vertebrae and ribs by simultaneous ventilation and compression. Selective arteriolar dilating agents may also be used to decrease outflow resistance.

B. Thoracic pump mechanism

1. Recent studies in dogs have suggested that blood flow during CPR is a result of phasic alterations in intrapleural pressure (IPP) and that high IPP produced by simultaneous chest compression and lung inflation may be accompanied by an increase in systemic perfusion.
   a) The thoracic pump mechanism of blood flow during CPR notes that all blood-containing structures within the thorax are elastic tubes or chambers, which are susceptible to collapse by external pressure.
   b) The venae cavae that carry blood to the thoracic pump are easily collapsed by a small transmural pressure difference, whereas the aorta and its major branches tend to resist collapse.
2. The compression chamber of the thoracic pump includes the right ventricle, the pulmonary vasculature, the left atrium, and the left ventricle, all connected in series. The aortic valve and the tricuspid valve are critical to the operation of the thoracic pump; other cardiac valves are irrelevant.
3. Operation of the thoracic pump depends on the intermittent generation of global intrathoracic pressure greater than the prevailing extrathoracic arterial or venous pressures.
   a) Such pressure can be generated by thoracic compression as well as positive-pressure ventilation.
   b) As intrathoracic pressure rises, both forward and backward flow are possible, until the tricuspid valve closes. The action of the tricuspid valve is complemented by peripheral venous valves and collapse of the large central veins.

c) Forward flow occurs through the pulmonary vasculature and the left heart acts as a passive conduit. Generation of sufficient global intrathoracic pressures to move blood requires that venting of thoracic pressure via the airways be minimal as is certainly the case with simultaneous ventilation and chest compression.

C. Tissue perfusion
   1. Adequate blood flow to vital organs is essential for effective CPR.
   2. In dogs, the cardiac output during CPR is about one-fourth of normal. Flow to all organs is thus decreased during CPR and the relative decrease varies widely.
   3. The ratios of regional blood flow during CPR to regional blood flow during sinus rhythm are 90 percent for brain, 35 percent for heart, 15 percent for kidneys, 17 percent for adrenal glands, 14 percent for pancreas, 3 percent for spleen, and 33 percent for small intestine.

III. Rate of cardiac compression
   A. It is recommended that 60 thoracic compressions per minute be employed. Time must be allowed between compressions for diastolic filling of the ventricles.
   B. Maintaining an equal ratio between compression and relaxation of the thorax is more important in maintaining cardiac output than is the rate of compression. A general rule is to compress the thorax about 40 percent of the cycle and release 60 percent of the cycle.
   C. Thoracic compression with simultaneous ventilation should result in an improvement of mucous membrane color, a reduction of pupil size, and a palpable pulse with each compression. If the initial technique is not producing desired effects:
      1. Apply more or less pressure.
      2. Use a different position for the animal.
      3. Use a slower rate of compression.
      4. Increase fluid volume administration.

IV. Internal cardiac compression
   A. The decision to employ internal cardiac compression should be an individualized professional judgment.
   B. Ineffective CPR techniques can be a rationale for opening the thorax to apply direct cardiac compression but is infrequently employed.

C. In comparing conventional CPR techniques of augmented venous return (abdominal compression) and open-chest cardiac compression, the mean arterial pressure, systemic arterial pressure, systemic perfusion pressures (mean arterial pressure minus mean central venous pressure), carotid artery blood flow, and cerebral perfusion pressure (mean arterial pressure minus intracranial pressure) are superior in open thorax cardiac compression. If one is to employ internal cardiac compression, its use should neither be procrastinated nor a last-resort measure.

D. Technique
   1. In using internal cardiac compression, an incision is made in the fifth intercostal space with little or no aseptic preparation.
   2. Direct cardiac compression should be applied with force adequate to empty the ventricles and is repeated as soon as the ventricles refill with blood.
   3. With return of effective mechanical heart function, the incision site should be clipped and aseptically cleaned and the thorax should be thoroughly flushed and then closed in a routine fashion after insertion of a thoracic drain.
   4. A systemic antibiotic should be given.

Advanced Life Support

The primary responsibilities following cardiac arrest are concerned with CPR (basic life support) and reestablishing a normal sinus electrical rhythm. In order to establish this normal rhythm, it is necessary to have an intravenous infusion route, equipment for defibrillation, specific drugs and cardiac monitoring (Fig. 14-2).

Intravenous Fluids

Expansion of circulating blood volume is a critical component of ALS in patients that have sustained trauma or acute blood loss.

I. Fluid selection

A. Volume expansion is usually achieved with crystalloid solutions

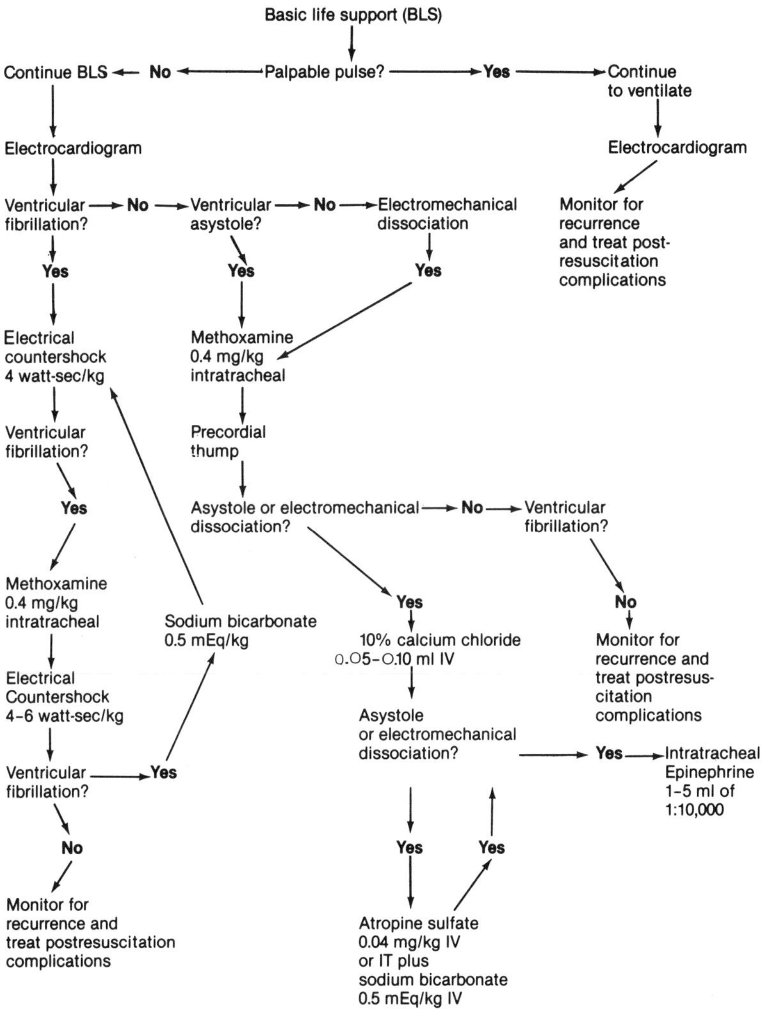

Fig. 14-2. Advanced life support in cardiopulmonary arrest.

such as Ringer's lactate solution or 0.9 percent sodium chloride, whole blood, or plasma. Whether to use a crystalloid or colloid solution remains controversial.

B. During resuscitation, it is accepted that replacement of oxygen carrying capacity is important.

C. It is accepted that some amount of a balanced salt solution is needed in addition to blood replacement. The availability of whole blood remains difficult for the practitioner and the expense of most synthetic colloids is usually prohibitive.

II. Route of administration

A. In most patients, the saphenous vein in the dog and the femoral vein in cats is the preferred site of intravenous infusion of fluid. This vein places the professional or paraprofessional out of the way of persons applying basic life support and is an easy vein to cannulate with a large-bore catheter (14 to 18 gauge).

B. If the intravenous line is to also be used for infusion of cardiac drugs, a more central catheter (e.g., jugular vein) should be employed to avoid hemodilution of the drugs being administered.

III. Rate of administration

A. Caution should be employed in the administration of intravenous volume. Although volume expansion is necessary, it may become excessive and hemodilution may complicate postresuscitation recovery.

B. As guidelines, calculate the initial volume to be administered at 90 ml/kg-hr (40 ml/lb-hr) in dogs and 50 ml/kg-hr (25 ml/lb-hr) in cats.

Defibrillation

Direct current countershock should be delivered as rapidly as possible to the arrest victim with ventricular fibrillation. This method of defibrillation will result in the most consistent success in resuscitation.

I. Energy

A. The energy necessary for external defibrillation is 0.5 to 10 watt-sec/kg body weight and 0.2-0.4 watt-sec/kg body weight for internally applied electrodes (Table 14-3).

B. Factors, including body weight, that influence success of counter-

TABLE 14-3. SUGGESTED PROTOCOL IN TREATING VENTRICULAR FIBRILLATION

1. Initiate basic life support (cardiopulmonary resuscitation).
2. Attach an electrocardiographic monitor to ensure the diagnosis of ventricular fibrillation.
3. Apply a liberal amount of conductive paste to the electrode paddles and chest wall. Do NOT use alcohol, as it is inflammable. For internal defibrillation, use saline-soaked sponges.
4. Place the paddles on the chest to maximize current flow through the myocardium.
5. Select an appropriate energy (approximately 4 watt-sec/kg body weight for external defibrillation and 0.03 watt-sec/kg for internal defibrillation).
6. Clear all personnel from the table and patient and discharge the machine.
7. Monitor the electrocardiogram and pulse to determine the effectiveness of the defibrillation attempt.
8. If additional attempts are required, use of adrenergic drugs (methoxamine), and possibly sodium bicarbonate, should supplement basic life support prior to electrical discharge.

shock therapy include the duration of fibrillation, degree of hypoxemia, concomitant drug therapy, acid–base, and electrolyte status.

II. Success versus failure of defibrillation
   A. In general, the incidence of defibrillation is inversely proportional to the duration of fibrillation. With increasing fibrillation duration, energy requirements for defibrillation proportionately increase.
      1. If electrical countershock is employed before 2 minutes of defibrillation, adrenergic drugs will usually not improve success of defibrillation. In most of these patients one should expect 90 to 100 percent success in defibrillation.
      2. Beyond 2 minutes of ventricular fibrillation, adrenergic drugs (i.e., epinephrine or methoxamine) will improve success in defibrillation but successful conversion may only result in 30 to 80 percent of the patients.
   B. Hypoxia is known to perpetuate arrhythmias. This is likely due to a sensitization of the myocardium to endogenous catecholamines and metabolic acidosis. Use of appropriate BLS and 100 percent oxygen will lessen problems of hypoxemia. By providing adequate ventilation and cardiac compression, in the absence of preexisting severe metabolic acidosis, the arterial pH can be maintained within reasonable limits for a considerable period during resuscitation without the addition of buffers. Immediately follow-

ing cardiac arrest, the arterial pH does rapidly decrease and a metabolic and respiratory acidosis ensues.

a) Only when the arrest is of prolonged duration or when the patient has preexisting severe illness with metabolic acidosis should sodium bicarbonate be given on a routine basis.

b) Metabolic acidosis will lower the threshold of the heart to ventricular fibrillation. Of itself, bicarbonate will not promote early restoration of spontaneous cardiac activity.

C. Administration of drugs will affect ventricular fibrillation occurrence. This is especially important if the animal is on these drugs prior to ventricular fibrillation.

1. Antiarrhythmic drugs such as lidocaine and quinidine increase the fibrillation threshold (i.e. decrease the susceptibility to defibrillation).
2. Animals on digitalis may be more easily defibrillated but have a higher frequency of occurrence of postresuscitation arrhythmias.
3. Potassium makes the heart more susceptible to defibrillation but also produces an unwanted negative inotropic effect.

D. In the absence of preexisting cardiac disease, cats may spontaneously revert their ventricular fibrillation to a sinus origin beat. Thus good BLS and monitoring are likely all that may be required in some cats.

III. Chemical defibrillation

A. Drugs that could induce prompt chemical defibrillation and return of cardiac function would be invaluable in the absence of an electrical defibrillator. Potassium and bretylium tosylate are the best known chemical defibrillators. Although successful in human patients, bretylium is reported to be uniformly unsuccessful in the dog.

B. The most consistent results in achieving chemical defibrillation have been in combining potassium chloride (1.0 mEq/kg) and acetylcholine chloride (6.0 mg/kg). Unfortunately when dogs have been premedicated with atropine sulfate, this combination has not been effective in converting the ventricular fibrillation.

Definitive Drug Therapy

All drugs administered to the cardiac arrest animal should follow initial BLS attempts.

I. Sodium bicarbonate
  A. Acidosis will rapidly develop following cardiac arrest. This acidosis has both a metabolic and a respiratory component and comes from lactic acid produced by anaerobic metabolism (metabolic) and hypercapnia due to ventilatory failure (respiratory).
  B. In the absence of preexisting severe acidosis, adequate ventilation alone can prevent acidosis.
  C. Administration of sodium bicarbonate in the absence of adequate ventilation will not result in a rise in the arterial pH but rather only substantial elevations in the arterial P_{CO_2} and serum osmolality. A rise in pH will only occur if the CO_2 produced in the process of buffering hydrogen ion is excreted via the lungs.
  D. Since CO_2 is known to permeate the cell membrane rapidly, it is likely that exogenous sodium bicarbonate initially aggravates intracellular acidosis as a result of the rise in arterial P_{CO_2}.
    1. The paradoxical fall in cerebrospinal fluid pH that occurs with the administration of bicarbonate appears to be an example of this phenomenon.
    2. Myocardial depression will also result when arterial P_{CO_2} increases and the pH remains constant.
    3. Thus, during the first few minutes after rapid administration of sodium bicarbonate, depression of myocardial function would occur if defibrillation and restoration of effective electrical activity occurred during this period.
  E. The principal value of sodium bicarbonate is to prevent metabolic acidosis from lowering the threshold of the heart to ventricular fibrillation.
    1. Ideally, bicarbonate administration should be based on measured values of arterial pH, P_{CO_2} and bicarbonate.
    2. In the absence of these values, administration of a dosage of 0.5 mEq/kg, of which only one-half is given over any 10-minute period, will be adequate.
    3. If the cardiac arrest is known to be less than 5 minutes in duration and if preexisting severe acidosis is unlikely, sodium bicarbonate is probably unnecessary.

II. Adrenergic drugs

Several adrenergic drugs have been used in cardiac arrest. Most frequently epinephrine and/or methoxamine are currently recommended.

A. Epinephrine will produce beneficial effects in the treatment of cardiac arrest, probably through both its α- and β-adrenergic receptor stimulating properties.
   1. Clinically, the drug elevates perfusion pressure generated during cardiac compression, enhances the contractile state of the heart, stimulates spontaneous contractions, and increases the vigor and intensity of ventricular fibrillation that may be more amenable to electrical countershock.
   2. Unfortunately, this increased vigor of fibrillation has the adverse effect of significant depressions in subendocardial blood flow and thereby worsens myocardial ischemia and hypoxia.
   3. The primary beneficial effect of epinephrine in cardiac arrest may in fact be secondary to its vasoconstrictor action leading to elevated diastolic pressures and improved coronary blood flow.
      a) Epinephrine's β-adrenergic effect in ventricular fibrillation leads to increased myocardial tone, a "coarse fibrillatory pattern" (an attribute previously thought desirable), increased oxygen consumption, and subendocardial vasoconstriction. These are disadvantageous, increasing myocardial ischemia.
   4. The recommended dosage of epinephrine is 0.05 to .5 mg (.5 to 5 ml of a 1 : 10,000 solution). It is necessary to repeat this dosage at approximately 5-minute intervals because of its short duration of action.
      a) There is convincing evidence that epinephrine is absorbed promptly after instillation into the tracheobronchial tree via an endotracheal tube.
         (1) The technique of administration involves the passage of a smaller tube through the endotracheal tube to the level of the bronchi.
         (2) The adrenergic drug is then ejected into the tube and residual fluid within the tube being blown out.
         (3) Cardiopulmonary resuscitation (BLS) is continued and the electrocardiograms monitored.
         (4) With direct access to the left heart and then to the systemic and coronary circulation, the epinephrine arrives rapidly at the site of effectiveness.
      b) Intravenous administration of epinephrine can be utilized with good CPR technique; it is considered the second preferred route.

c) The intracardiac route of injection should only be used if the endotracheal or intravenous sites are inaccessible. The intracardiac (IC) dose is 0.5 to 5 μg/kg. The hazards of intracardiac injection include coronary artery laceration, cardiac tamponade, pneumothorax, interruption of CPR, and intramyocardial injection.

5. The catecholamines are extremely pH sensitive with epinephrine showing decreased activity if the patient is acidotic. Epinephrine should not be infused with sodium bicarbonate as this too will inactivate the catecholamine.

B. Methoxamine is known to be as effective as epinephrine in resuscitation from ventricular asystole and is shown to be twice as effective as epinephrine in resuscitation from ventricular fibrillation.

1. Methoxamine is a pure α-agonist and this property likely explains methoxamine's superiority.

a) With its α-agonist effect, vasoconstriction of arterioles to nonessential vascular beds, including the skin, skeletal muscle, kidneys and gut, will provide vital organ perfusion following methoxamine.

2. The intratracheal dosage recommended for methoxamine is 0.4 mg/kg.

C. In contrast to epinephrine and methoxamine, drugs with pure beta adrenergic activity, such as isoproterenol, or alpha receptor blockade (phenothiazine tranquilizers), prevent resuscitation. With isoproterenol, blood flow is in fact shunted away from vital organs. Thus, use of these drugs should be reserved until cardiac function is restored. There should be no delay in using an appropriate vasoconstrictor during resuscitation from either aystole, electromechanical dissociation, or ventricular fibrillation.

III. Atropine sulfate is a parasympatholytic drug that reduces cardiac vagal tone and improves atrioventricular (AV) nodal conduction. It is useful in treating sinus bradycardia or in some patients with AV nodal block.

A. The recommended dosage of atropine sulfate is .01 to .02 mg/kg given intravenously and may be repeated at 5-minute intervals.

B. Because heart rate is a major determinant of myocardial oxygen requirements, atropine should be used cautiously in severe hypoxia.

C. The combined use of parasympatholytics and sympathomimetics may predispose to severe ventricular tachyarrhythmias and fibrillation.

D. Use of atropine sulfate should be limited to symptomatic bradyarrhythmias and close monitoring of the effect of atropine should be practiced.

IV. Calcium chloride

The calcium ion plays a critical role in excitation–contraction coupling. It will enhance the contractile state of the heart and is primarily indicated in the flabby or weakly beating heart. It may also be useful in the treatment of the severe hypotension and orderly electrical rhythm seen with electromechanical dissociation.

A. Dangerous levels of serum calcium have been documented following empirical administration of $CaCl_2$.

1. Calcium will enhance the excitability of the ventricles and will suppress sinus impulse formation.
2. Therefore, ventricular ectopy and ventricular tachyarrhythmias are frequently noted.

B. Another finding in use of $CaCl_2$ for dogs with cardiac arrest is the rapid increase in cerebrovascular resistance after restoration of circulation. In these dogs, the cerebrocortical blood flow approached zero 90 minutes after circulation was restored. Following administration of a calcium channel blocking agent, cerebrocortical blood flow returned to or was greater than the prearrest flow.

C. It seems likely that the administration of $CaCl_2$ is of no value in cardiac arrest and likely will reduce the likelihood of ultimate survival or increase the chances of survival with serious neurologic sequelae.

D. Previously digitalized patients are particularly susceptible to calcium due to the synergism between digitalis and calcium.

E. If there are indications for calcium administration, minimal dosages administered slowly should be practiced. The recommended dosage of $CaCl_2$ is 0.05 to 0.10 ml/kg of a 10 percent solution intravenous or by intracardial injection and this may be repeated at 10 minute intervals. Two other calcium salts are available: calcium gluceptate and calcium gluconate, however, calcium chloride is the preferable dosage form.

V. Calcium blocking drugs

Calcium blocking agents (e.g., verapamil) used during ALS are contrary to traditional teaching that recommends the use of calcium chloride to enhance myocardial contractility.

A. Although not widely accepted, at present, the calcium channel blocking drugs have several important effects

1. The postischemic myocardial lack of compliance is lessened as is the accumulation of calcium ion in the mitochondria. Following administration of calcium antagonists, there is an increase in blood flow to the ischemic area and a lessening of the area of myocardial damage.
2. Calcium antagonist drugs raise the threshold of the ischemic ventricle to ventricular fibrillation.
3. As vasodilators, the calcium antagonists will lower blood pressure but are shown to improve cerebral perfusion as noted above.
4. Calcium antagonists display slow conduction through the AV node and will be useful in management of supraventricular dysrhythmias.

B. The dosage of verapamil in the dog is currently 0.05 to 0.15 mg/kg over 2 minutes (5 mg total dose) given intravenously.

POSTRESUSCITATION CARE

The treatment of an animal during the period following resuscitation will depend on the initial postresuscitation status. It will vary from simple monitoring and observation to the management of single- or multiple-organ system failure. The first step then is the careful evaluation of the patient's postresuscitation status, particularly of neurologic and other deficits that were not present before cardiopulmonary arrest.

I. Maximal response to resuscitation

The animal is awake, responsive, and breathing spontaneously after resuscitation.

A. The electrocardiogram should be monitored continuously and an oxygen-rich environment provided.

B. An intravenous line should be available and an isotonic fluid administered.

C. If the arrest rhythm was ventricular fibrillation or ventricular tachycardia, a lidocaine bolus and constant rate infusion (25–75 μg/kg-min) is indicated.

D. If a serious bradycardia is present, atropine sulfate (0.01 to 0.02 mg/kg) may be used.
E. A postresuscitation laboratory profile should be collected. Particularly note serum blood urea nitrogen, creatinine, electrolytes, glucose, liver enzymes, and urinalysis.
F. The prearrest drug profile should be carefully reviewed.
G. A thoracic radiograph is useful to assess pulmonary status and evidence of resuscitative trauma.

II. Single- or multiple-organ system failure
A. An animal in this status will generally have an endotracheal tube in place.
B. Breathing may be present or absent.
C. The hemodynamic status may be unstable with respect to heart rate, rhythm, systemic blood pressure, and organ perfusion.
D. The animal may be in a coma or decreased responsiveness.
E. Monitoring should include a laboratory chemical profile, urinalysis, electrocardiogram, thoracic radiograph, and likely a central venous pressure.

III. Respiratory system
A. Postresuscitation thoracic radiographs should be performed to assess the presence of fractured ribs or sternebrae, pneumothorax, pulmonary contusions, and pulmonary edema.
B. If spontaneous ventilation is absent or appears inadequate, mechanical ventilation is initiated. If possible, arterial blood should be sampled for Po_2, Pco_2, and pH. Ventilatory adjustments can be made from these results.

IV. Cardiovascular system
A. A standard 10-lead electrocardiogram should be compared with previous tracings if available.
B. Thoracic radiographs, biochemical profile results, and previous drug therapy are assessed.
C. Measure the central venous pressure.
1. With the onset of pulmonary edema, the central venous pressure will rise and may reach 6 to 12 cm H_2O. With pulmonary edema, diuretics, morphine, or other drug therapy are indicated.
2. With a low central venous pressure (<5 cm H_2O) increased

volume replacement is indicated while continuing to monitor the central venous pressure.

V. Renal system
   A. The urinary bladder should be catheterized and urine output determined.
      1. Urine volume quantification is done on an hourly basis.
      2. Urine production should exceed 2 ml/kg-hr to ensure diuresis.
   B. The central venous pressure should be closely watched in order to avoid pulmonary edema.
   C. Drug therapy to promote urine production will include furosemide (2 mg/kg IV), mannitol, or 10 percent dextrose.
   D. Dopamine may also be used to promote diuresis. An evaluation of drug therapy should exclude nephrotoxic drugs and drugs eliminated predominantly via the kidneys.

VI. Central nervous system
   A. Cessation of circulation for 10 seconds results in a deficiency of oxygen supply to the brain that results in unconsciousness.
   B. Inadequate cardiopulmonary resuscitation techniques, vasoactive drugs, and excessive calcium administration are known to affect cerebral perfusion.
   C. Therapy for the unresponsive patient includes endotracheal intubation as well as hyperventilation to assist in reducing intracranial pressure.
      1. Osmotic and loop diuretics may also help reduce elevated intracranial pressures.
      2. Slight hypothermia and use of barbiturate anesthetics are shown to have sparing effects on the brain.
      3. Use of calcium channel blocking drugs will promote cerebral perfusion.
      4. Corticosteroids are useful in the management of cerebral edema.

COMPLICATIONS OF CARDIOPULMONARY ARREST

I. Complications of cardiopulmonary arrest will include vomiting, aspiration pneumonitis, fractured ribs or sternebrae, liver lacerations, gastric dilatation, pericardial tamponade, pulmonary edema, pulmonary contusions, pneumothorax, myocardial contusions, and postresuscitation arrhythmias.

II. The decision to terminate resuscitative efforts is a medical one and depends on the assessment by a veterinarian of the cerebral and cardiovascular status of the patient.
   A. Clinical criteria of the adequacy of cerebral circulation include the reactivity of the pupils, level of consciousness, presence of purposeful movement, and spontaneous respiration.
   B. Deep unconsciousness, absence of spontaneous respirations, and brain stem reflexes, and pupils that remain fixed and dilated for 15 to 30 minutes are usually ominous prognostic signs.

SUGGESTED READINGS

American Heart Association: Standards and guidelines for cardiopulmonary resuscitation (CPR) and emergency cardiac care (ECC). JAMA 244:453, 1980

Babbs CF: New versus old theories of blood flow during CPR. Crit Care Med 8:191, 1980

Bedell SE, Delbanco TL, Cook EF, Epstein, FH: Survival after cardiopulmonary resuscitation in the hospital. N Engl J Med 309:569, 1983

Bishop RL, Weisfeldt ML: Sodium bicarbonate administration during cardiac arrest. Effect on arterial pH, P_{CO_2} and osmolality. JAMA 235:506, 1976

Breznock EM, Kagan KG, Attix ES: Chemical cardioversion of electrically induced ventricular fibrillation in dogs. Am J Vet Res 39:971, 1978

Geddes LA, Tacker WA, Rosborough JP, et al: Electrical dose for ventricular defibrillation of large and small animals using precordial electrodes. J Clin Invest 53:310, 1974

Haskins, SC: Cardiopulmonary resuscitation. p. 377. In Kirk RW (ed): Current Veterinary Therapy—Small Animal Practice. Vol. 8. WB Saunders, Philadelphia, 1983

Holmes HR, Babbs CF, Voorhees WD, et al: Influence of adrenergic drugs upon vital organ perfusion during CPR. Crit Care Med 8:137, 1980

Livesay JJ, Follette DM, Fey KH, et al: Optimizing myocardial supply/demand balance with alpha-adrenergic drugs during cardiopulmonary resuscitation. J Thorac Cardiovasc Surg 76:244, 1978

Redding JS: Drug therapy in resuscitation from electromechanical dissociation. Crit Care Med 11:681, 1983

Redding JS: Cardiopulmonary resuscitation: an algorithm and some common pitfalls. Am Heart J 98:788, 1979

Safer P, Bleyaert A, Memoto EM, et al: Resuscitation after global brain ischemia–anoxia. Crit Care Med 6:215, 1978

Tilley LP: Essentials of Canine and Feline Electrocardiography. Interpretation and Treatment. ed. Lea & Febiger, Philadelphia, 1985

Voorhees WD, Babbs CF, Tacker WA: Regional blood flow during cardiopulmonary resuscitation in dogs. Crit Care Med 8:134, 1980

Yakaitis RW, Ewy GA, Otto CW, et al: Influence of time and therapy on ventricular defibrillation in dogs. Crit Care Med 8:157, 1980

Appendix
Common Cardiovascular Drugs*

Generic Name	Commonly Used Preparations	Approximate Dosage (for the dog unless otherwise noted)
Aminophylline	Aminophyllin (Searle Lab) 250 mg/10 ml injectable 100-, 200-mg tablets	4–6 mg/kg BID–QID IV, PO *For the cat* 4–6 mg/kg BID IV, PO
Atropine	Atropine sulfate (Eli Lilly) 0.4 mg/ml USP 0.4 mg tablets	0.01–0.02 mg/kg IV, IM 0.02–0.04 mg/kg SC, PO TID–QID *For the cat* 0.02–0.04 mg/kg IV, IM SQ QID
Calcium Chloride	Calcium chloride (Bristol) 10% solution (100 mg/ml) 10-ml vials	0.05–0.10 ml/kg IV or IC (dog, cat)
Captopril	Capoten (Squibb) 25-mg tablets	0.5–2 mg/kg TID (do not exceed 2 mg/kg TID) *For the cat* 6.25 mg BID–TID

*The authors and the publisher of this textbook have made every effort to ensure that the drug dosage schedules are accurate. The drug dosages are based on the standards accepted at the time of publication. The product information sheet included in the package of each drug should be checked before the drug is administered to be certain that changes have not been made in the recommended dose or in the contraindications for administration. Respective chapters should be reviewed for further details regarding dosages and side-effects. This advice is especially appropriate for new or infrequently used drugs.

Generic Name	Commonly Used Preparations	Approximate Dosage (for the dog unless otherwise noted)
Diethylcarbamazine citrate	Caricide (American Cyanamid) 60 mg/ml 50-, 200-, 400-mg tablets Diethylcarbamazine citrate (Beecham) 30-, 90-, 300-mg tablets Difil (Evsco), 60 mg/ml 50-, 200-, 400-mg tablets Filaribits (Norden) 60-, 180-mg tablets	5.5–6.5 mg/kg/day PO
Digitoxin	Foxalin (Halsom) 0.1-, 0.25-, 0.5-mg capsules Crystodigin (Eli Lilly) 0.2 mg/ml injectable 0.1-, 0.2-mg tablets	Oral maintenance (Foxalin): 0.04–0.1 mg/kg divided TID Rapid parenteral: 0.01–0.03 mg/kg, ½ of dose IV, wait 30–60 minutes and give ¼ of dose; wait 30–60 minutes and give remaining dose, if necessary
Digoxin	Lanoxin (Burroughs Welcome) 0.25 mg/ml injectable; elixir 0.05 mg/ml 0.125-, 0.25-, 0.5-mg tablets Cardoxin (Evsco) Elixirs 0.05, 0.15 mg/ml	Oral maintenance: 0.01–0.02 mg/kg divided BID, or 0.22 mg/m^2 of body surface area bid Rapid oral: 0.02–0.06 mg/kg divided BID for the first day and then go to maintenance Rapid IV: 0.01–0.02 mg/kg; administer ½ of calculated dose IV; wait 30 to 60 minutes and give ¼ of dose; wait 30 to 60 minutes and administer remaining dose, if necessary *For the cat* Oral maintenance: 0.007 to 0.015 mg/kg SID to every other day (average cat, ¼ of a 0.125-mg tablet every other day; liquid not well tolerated)

Generic Name	Commonly Used Preparations	Approximate Dosage (for the dog unless otherwise noted)
		Rapid IV: 0.005 mg/kg lean body weight divided between four doses or to effect; ½ the calculated dose IV; 60 minutes later ¼ of the calculated dose; and 60 minutes later the final ¼ dose, if necessary
Dithiazanine iodide	Dizan (Pitman Moore) 10-, 50-, 100-, 200-mg tablets	6–8 mg/kg/day PO for 7 days; if microfilaremia persists, the dose may be increased to 12–14 mg/kg for 7–10 additional days
Dobutamine hydrochloride	Dobutrex (Eli Lilly) 250 mg/20 ml	5–20 μg/kg/min IV
Dopamine	Inotropin (American Critical Care) 40 mg/ml	1–10 μg/kg/min IV
Epinephrine hydrochloride	Adrenalin (Parke-Davis) injection 1:1000 solution, 1 mg/ml	15–20 μg/kg IV, 0.5–5 μg/kg IC (dog and cat) dilute 1:10,000
Furosemide	Lasix (Hoechst-Roussel) 50 mg/ml injection, 10 mg/ml syrup 12.5-, 20-, 40-, 50-mg tablets	2–4 mg/kg (IV, IM, SQ, PO); BID–TID if needed *For the cat* 1–2 mg/kg BID–TID Maintenance dose: 0.5–2 mg/kg/day divided BID
Glycopyrrolate	Robinul (Robbins) injection 0.2 mg/ml	0.005–0.01 mg/kg IV, IM 0.01–0.02 mg/kg SC BID–TID
Hydralazine	Apresoline HCl (CIBA) 10-, 25-, 50-mg tablets	1–3 mg/kg PO BID *For the cat* 2.5 mg PO BID
Isopropamide	Darbid (Smith, Kine and French) 5-mg tablets	2.5–5.0 mg TID–QID

Generic Name	Commonly Used Preparations	Approximate Dosage (for the dog unless otherwise noted)
Isoproterenol hydrochloride	Isuprel (Breon) injection 0.2 mg/ml 1-, 5-ml ampule, 10-mg glossets Proterenol (Key) 20-, 40-mg tablets	0.4 mg in 250 ml 5% dextrose/water, drip slowly to effect Proternol: 10–20 mg q 4–6 hours Isuprel glossets: 5–10 mg per rectum q 4–6 hours *For the cat* 0.4 mg in 250 ml 5% dextrose/water, drip slowly to effect
Ivermectin	Ivomec (Merck Sharp & Dohme) (1 ml Ivomec to 9 ml propylene glycol)	0.05 mg/kg single PO dose as a microfilaricide (0.5 ml/20 kg of diluted solution)
Levamisole	Ripercol-L (Capri)	11 mg/kg PO once daily for 7 days; if microfilaremia persists, the same dosage is continued for 5 additional days
Lidocaine hydrochloride	Xylocaine (Astra) 2% (20 mg/ml) injectable	2–4 mg/kg slow IV, repeat every 10 minutes to a maximum of 8 mg/kg; constant rate infusion (CRI)$^{+}$: 25–75 μg/kg/min *For the cat* 0.5 mg/kg slow IV
Nitroprusside	Nipride (Roche)	1–5 μg/kg/min IV
Nitrates (ointment, isorbide dinitrate)	Nitro-BID ointment (Marion Labs) 2% ointment Isordil (Ives) 10-, 20-, 30-mg tablets	¼–2 in TID–QID ointment; ¼ – ½ in. topically (inside ear) for small dogs; 2 in. topically for giant dogs Isordil: 1–1.5 mg/kg TID–QID *For the cat* ⅛–¼ in. topically TID

$^{+}$Formula for CRI: Body weight (in kg) × dose (in μg/kg/min) × 0.36 = total dose in mg to administer intravenously over 6 hours; eg., 20-kg dog, 50 μg /kg/min infusion, etc., (20) (50) (0.36) = 360 mg over 6 hours.

Generic Name	Commonly Used Preparations	Approximate Dosage (for the dog unless otherwise noted)
Oxytriphylline	Choledyl (Parke-Davis) 50 mg/5 ml, 100 mg/5 ml 100-, 200-mg tablets	4–6 mg/kg BID–QID PO
Phenytoin	Dilantin (Parke-Davis) 50 mg/ml injectable, 125 mg/5 ml syrup 30-, 100-mg capsules	4 mg/kg slow IV, 4–8 mg/kg PO divided TID–QID
Prazosin	Minipress (Pfizer) 1-, 2-mg capsules	1 mg TID for dog weighing < 15 kg; 2 mg TID for dogs weighing > 15 kg
Probantheline	Pro-banthine (Searle) 7.5-, 15-mg tablets	7.5–15 mg BID–TID
Procainamide	Pronestyl (Squibb) injection 100, 500 mg/ml 200-, 500-mg tablet Procan-SR (Parke-Davis) 250-, 500-mg tablets	6–12 mg/kg IV slowly; CRI 25–40 μg/kg/min; 6–12 mg/kg IM q 6–8h (the initial dose may be doubled); 8–20 mg/kg q 6–8 h PO
Propranolol HCl	Inderal (Ayerst) 1 mg/ml injection, 10-, 20-, 40-, 80-mg tablets	0.04–0.06 mg/kg IV slowly 0.2–1.0 mg/kg orally TID (dog, cat)
Quinidine gluconate sulfate polygalacturonate	Quinidine gluconate (Eli Lilly) USP injection 80 mg/ml Quinidine sulfate (Parke-Davis) tablets USP 200 mg Quinidex (sustained release) tablets 300 mg Quinaglute Dura-tabs (Cooper) (quinidine gluconate) 324 mg Cardioquin (Purdue-Frederick) tablets (quinidine polygalacturonate), 275 mg	gluconate 6–20 mg/kg IM QID; sulfate 6–16 mg/kg PO QID, TID (Extentab); Quinaglute and Cardioquin 8–20 mg/kg PO TID–QID

Generic Name	Commonly Used Preparations	Approximate Dosage (for the dog unless otherwise noted)
Theophylline	Theophyl (Knoll) elixir 225 mg/30 ml 225 mg tablets	4–6 mg/kg BID–QID *For the cat* 4–6 mg/kg BID
Thiarcetamide sodium	Caparsolate Sodium (CEVA–Abbott) (Diamond) 10 mg/ml	2.2 mg/kg IV BID for 2 days
Verapamil	Verapamil HCl injectable 5 mg/2 ml Calan (Searle) 80-, 120-mg tablets Isoptin (Knoll) 2–5 mg/ml (2 ml ampule) 80-, 120-mg tablets	0.05 to 0.15 mg/kg over 2 min. IV, 5 mg total dose; oral dose not established

INDEX

Note: Numbers followed by f *denote figures; those followed by* t *denote tables.*